Biological Methylation and Drug Design

Experimental Biology and Medicine

Biological Methylation and Drug Design: *Experimental and Clinical Roles of S-Adenosylmethionine,* edited by **Ronald T. Borchardt, Cyrus R. Creveling, and Per Magne Ueland,** *1986*

Retroviruses and Human Pathology, edited by **Robert C. Gallo, Dominique Stehelin, and Oliviero E. Varnier,** *1985*

Directed Drug Delivery, edited by **Ronald T. Borchardt, Arnold Repta, and Valentino Stella,** *1985*

Immune Regulation, edited by **Marc Feldmann and N. A. Mitchison,** *1985*

Human T Cell Clones: *A New Approach to Immune Regulation,* edited by **Marc Feldmann, Jonathan R. Lamb, and James N. Woody,** *1985*

Inositol and Phosphoinositides: *Metabolism and Regulation,* edited by **John E. Bleasdale, Joseph Eichberg, and George Hauser,** *1985*

Growth, Cancer, and the Cell Cycle, edited by **Philip Skehan and Susan J. Friedman,** *1984*

Ir Genes: *Past, Present, and Future,* edited by **Carl W. Pierce, Susan E. Cullen, Judith A. Kapp, Benjamin D. Schwartz, and Donald C. Shreffler,** *1983*

Methods in Protein Sequence Analysis, edited by **Marshall Elzinga,** *1982*

Inflammatory Diseases and Copper, edited by **John R. J. Sorenson,** *1982*

Membrane Fluidity: *Biophysical Techniques and Cellular Regulation,* edited by **Morris Kates and Arnis Kuksis,** *1980*

Biological Methylation
and
Drug Design

Experimental and Clinical Role of S-Adenosylmethionine

Edited by

Ronald T. Borchardt, Cyrus R. Creveling,
and Per Magne Ueland

Humana Press · Clifton, New Jersey

Library of Congress Cataloging-in-Publication Data

Biological methylation and drug design.

(Experimental biology and medicine)
"This book has been developed from...the proceedings
of a symposium...held at the Solstrand Fjord Hotel in
Bergen, Norway on June 30-July 4, 1985"--Pref.
Includes index.
1. Adenosylmethionine--Metabolism--Congresses.
2. Methylation--Congresses. 3. Adenosylmethionine--
Therapeutic use--Congresses. 4. Nucleic acids--
Metabolism--Congresses. 5. Phospholipids--Metabolism--
Congresses. I. Borchardt, Ronald T. II. Creveling,
Cyrus R. III. Ueland, Per Magne. IV. Series:
Experimental biology and medicine (Clifton, N.J.)
QP563.A3B58 1986   574.19'283   86-7212

ISBN 0-89603-102-0

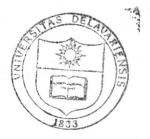

Copyright © 1986 by The Humana Press Inc.
Crescent Manor
PO Box 2148
Clifton, NJ 07015

Printed in the United States of America

Preface

This book has been developed from its earlier and far less formal presentment as the proceedings of a symposium entitled The Biochemistry of S-Adenosylmethionine as a Basis for Drug Design that was held at the Solstrand Fjord Hotel in Bergen, Norway on June 30–July 4, 1985. The purpose of the symposium was to bring together scientists from various disciplines (biochemistry, pharmacology, virology, immunology, chemistry, medicine, and so on) to discuss the recent advances that have been made in our understanding of the biological roles of S-adenosylmethionine (AdoMet) and to discuss the feasibility of utilizing AdoMet-dependent enzymes as targets for drug design. Thus the information provided herein will be of value not only to basic scientists involved in elucidating the role of AdoMet in biology, but also to medicinal chemists who are using this basic knowledge in the process of drug design. The volume should also be of interest to pharmacologists and clinicians involved in biological evaluation of potential therapeutic agents arising from the efforts of the biochemists and medicinal chemists.

Each plenary speaker at the symposium was requested to submit a chapter reviewing recent contributions of their discipline to our base of knowledge about the biological role of AdoMet. Topics covered in this volume include protein and phospholipid methylations (Section A), nucleic acid methylations (Section B), the regulation of AdoMet, S-adenosylhomocysteine, and methylthioadenosine metabolism (Section C), clinical aspects of AdoMet (Section D), and the design, synthesis, and biological evaluation of trans-methylation inhibitors (Section E).

The individual chapters in this volume represent comprehensive, up-to-date reviews of the subject material. However, to gain maximum appreciation for the pivotal role of AdoMet in biology, the editors suggest a thorough reading of the entire volume.

Ronald T. Borchardt
Cyrus R. Creveling
Per Magne Ueland

In Honor of Giulio Cantoni

The Executive Committee for the International Symposium entitled The Biochemistry of S-Adenosylmethionine as a Basis for Drug Design was privileged to select Dr. Giulio Cantoni as Honorary Chairman of the Symposium. The contributions of Dr. Cantoni to science began at the University of Milan, and continued at Oxford, The University of Michigan, New York University, Long Island College of Medicine, Western Reserve University, and the National Institute of Mental Health, where he has been the Chief of the Laboratory of General and Comparative Biochemistry since 1954. His initial studies on the methylation of nicotinamide were reported in 1951. In the same year he published a paper in the *Journal of the American Chemical Society* entitled The Nature of the Active Methyl Donor Formed Enzymatically from L-Methionine and Adenosine-Triphosphate. The crucial work appeared in the *Journal of Biological Chemistry* in 1953, S-Adenosyl-L-Methionine and ATP—and a new era in biochemistry began!

Dr. Cantoni has made many contributions since this seminal discovery, including the identification of S-adenosylhomocysteine, studies on S-adenosylhomocysteine hydrolase, studies on the enzymatic synthesis and decarboxylation of S-adenosylmethionine, the preparation of many unique and useful inhibitors of transmethylation, and studies on the role of methyltransferases in chemotaxis viral multiplication, cellular differentiation, and phospholipid methylation. Dr. Cantoni has materially contributed to many of the previous conferences on S-adenosylmethionine both as a speaker, a session chairman, and a valued member of organizing committees.

We have rightfully selected Dr. Cantoni as Honorary Chairman in recognition of the importance of his creative, persistent, and successful pursuit of the "active methyl donor." It is now clearly evident that S-adenosylmethionine ranks with ATP as one of the few truly pivotal molecules in biology.

The Editors

In Memory of Earl Usdin

We are all saddened by the recent death, on May 26, 1984, of Dr. Earl Usdin. The absence of his special leadership will be keenly felt in the many groups that he was instrumental in establishing, including our own "Conference on Transmethylation." Dr. Usdin began his career at the Johns Hopkins University. Then, upon receiving his doctorate in chemistry from the University of Ohio, he was a research fellow at the University of Pennsylvania; a research fellow at the Institute for Cancer Research, Philadelphia; Associate Professor at the University of New Mexico Highlands; Chief of Psychosomatic and Psychiatric Research at the Michael Reese Hospital; and worked for Melpar, Inc. Hazelton Laboratories, and Atlantic Research Corp. In 1968 he joined the National Institute of Mental Health, first as an Executive Secretary of the Preclinical Psychopharmacological Research Section and then Chief of the Pharmacology Section of Psychopharmacology Branch, NIMH. In 1981 Dr. Usdin was appointed Professor of Psychiatry at the California College of Medicine, University of California. In 1982 he became Chief of the Center for Education and International Research, International Institute on Brain and Behavior, University of California at Irvine.

Dr. Usdin's personal vision of his role in science was as a creator of "colleges." He saw the value and need for providing dynamic forums where scientists could meet, discuss, and subject their latest investigations to the critical eyes of knowledgeable colleagues. His own personal energy, humor, and sense of urgency was the moving force that made these groups function—finding the chairpersons, writing endless letters in his own piquant style to encourage their prompt action, forcefully maintaining discipline with authors to submit abstracts and manuscripts *on time*, and enforcing not only good but prompt editorial scholarship. The extent to which his efforts were successful is attested to by the number, more than sixty, of published proceedings of congresses, symposia, and conferences that bear his name.

Earl Usdin has left a legacy of friendships between scientists that extends across both disciplinary lines and national borders. His influence was truly international—he was at home in Scandianvia, in Europe, in Eastern Europe, the Orient, as well as throughout the United States. Many of those persons who had the privilege of working with Earl Usdin have not only acquired his techniques, but more important, his sense of mission and as such constitute a continuing memorial to this unique individual.

The Editors

Acknowledgments

The symposium entitled The Biochemistry of S-Adenosylmethionine as a Basis for Drug Design was organized and sponsored by the Department of Pharmaceutical Chemistry, S chool of Pharmacy, The University of Kansas, Lawrence, Kansas, USA and the Clinical Pharmacology Unit, University of Bergen, Bergen, Norway. We acknowledge with pleasure the assistance of Nancy Helm, Svein Helland, Asbjorn Svardal, Helga Refsum, and Halvard Bergesen in the organization of the symposium.

The symposium was made possible by the financial support provided by the following organizations:

AFI A/SFarmaceutisk Industri
AL A/S Apothekernes Laboratorium for Special Preparater
Astra Lakemedel AB
Beckman Instruments
BioResearch
Boehringer-Ingelheim, Ltd.
Burroughs Wellcome Company
CIBA-Geigy Pharma A/S
Glaxo A/S
Hewlett Packard
ICI-Pharma
Janssen Division ab Cikad
Lederle
NAF-Laboratoriene A/S
Norsk Pharmacia A/S
Norske Hoechst A/S
The Norwegian Cancer Society (LMK)
The Norwegian Society for Fighting Cancer (NftKB)
Norwegian Society for Science and the Humanities (NAVF)
Nyegaard & Co. A/S
Perkin-Elmer
Schering AG
G. D. Searle & Co.
Toyo Jozo Co.
The Upjohn Company

Contributors

V. Nambi Aiyar, *Duke University Medical Center, Durham, North Carolina*
Maqsudul Alam, *Biochemistry/Biophysics Program, Washington State University, Pullman, Washington*
R. D. Alarcon, *University of Alabama at Birmingham, Birmingham, Alabama*
R. Albers, *Department of Molecular Biology and Microbiology, Case Western Reserve University, Cleveland, Ohio*
*Jean-Herve Alix, *Institut de Biologie Physico-Chimique, Paris, France*
Vitauts Alks, *Grace Cancer Drug Center, Roswell Park Memorial Institute, Buffalo, New York*
D. Ayers, *Department of Molecular Biology and Microbiology, Case Western Reserve University, Cleveland, Ohio*
Carey D. Balaban, *Milton S. Hershey Medical Center, Pennsylvania State University, Hershey, Pennsylvania*
A. J. Bancroft, *University of Alabama at Birmingham, Birmingham, Alabama*
K. Benes, *Institute of Experimental Botany, Praha, Czechoslovakia*
Ralph J. Bernacki, *Grace Cancer Drug Center, Roswell Park Memorial Institute, Buffalo, New York*
*Melvin L. Billingsley, *Milton S. Hershey Medical Center, Pennsylvania State University, Hershey, Pennsylvania*
Pal Bjornstad, *Institute of Medical Biochemistry, University of Oslo, Oslo, Norway*
P. Blanchard, *Institut de Chimie des Substances Naturelles, CNRS, Gif-sur-Yvette, France*
Craig A. Bloch, *Howard Hughes Medical Institute Laboratories, Duke University Medical Center, Durham, North Carolina*
J. Blusztajn, *Massachusetts Institute of Technology, Cambridge, Massachusetts*
L. Boccassini, *Rheumatology Service, L. Sacco Hospital, Milan, Italy*
John Bollinger, *Biochemistry/Biophysics Program, Washington State University, Pullman , Washington*
*Ronald T. Borchardt, *Pharmaceutical Chemistry Department, The University of Kansas, Lawrence, Kansas*
*T. Bottiglieri, *King's College Hospital, London, UK*
*Jon Bremer, *Institute of Medical Biochemistry, University of Oslo, Oslo, Norway*
C. Cabrero, *Metabolismo, Nutricion Y Hormonas, Fundacion Jimenez Diaz, Madrid, Spain*
S. Camper, *Department of Molecular Biology and Microbiology, Case Western Reserve University, Cleveland, Ohio*
*Giulio L. Cantoni, *Laboratory of General and Comparative Biochemistry, National Institute of Mental Health, Bethesda, Maryland*

M. W. P. Carney, *King's College Hospital, London, UK*

Carlos J. Carrera, *Scripps Clinic and Research Foundation, La Jolla, California*

*Dennis A. Carson, *Scripps Clinic and Research Foundation, La Jolla, California*

Maria Carteni-Farina, *Department of Biochemistry of Macromolecules, University of Naples, Napoli, Italy*

*I. Caruso, *Rheumatology Service, L. Sacco Hospital, Milan, Italy*

Sara Chaffee, *Duke University Medical Center, Durham, North Carolina*

*Peter K. Chiang, *Division of Biochemistry, Walter Reed Army Institute of Research, Washington, DC*

*Steven Clarke, *Department of Chemistry and Biochemistry and the Molecular Biology Institute, University of California, Los Angeles, California*

*James K. Coward, *Department of Chemistry, Rensselaer Polytechnic Institute, Troy, New York*

Cyrus R. Creveling, *NIADDK, National Institutes of Health, Bethesda, Maryland*

Sylvia Curtis, *Duke University Medical Center, Durham, North Carolina*

E. DeClerq, *REGA Instituut, Leuven, Belgium*

N. Dodic, *Institut de Chimie des Substances Naturelles, CNRS, Gif-sur-Yvette, France*

Walter Doerfler, *Institute of Genetics, University of Cologne, Cologne, Germany*

J. Edeh, *King's College Hospital, London, UK*

J. Ferro, *Department of Microbiology, Oregon State University, Corvallis, Oregon*

*J. H. Fitchen, *Medical Research Service, Portland, Oregon*

J. L. Fourrey, *Institut de Chimie des Substances Naturelles, CNRS, Gif-sur-Yvette, France*

M. Fumagalli, *Rheumatology Service, L. Sacco Hospital, Milan, Italy*

Deborah Campano German, *Howard Hughes Medical Institute Laboratories, Duke University Medical Center, Durham, North Carolina*

M. Geze, *Institut de Chimie des Substances Naturelles, CNRS, Gif-sur-Yvette, France*

Robert N. Golden, *Laboratory of Clinical Science, National Institutes of Mental Health, Bethesda, Maryland*

R. Goodwin, *Department of Molecular Biology and Microbiology, Case Western Reserve University, Cleveland, Ohio*

Michael L. Greenberg, *Duke University Medical Center, Durham, North Carolina*

Masakazu Hatanaka, *Institute of Virus Research, Kyoto University, Kyoto, Japan*

*Gerald L. Hazelbauer, *Biochemistry/Biophysics Program and Program in Genetics and Cell Biology, Washington State University, Pullman, Washington*

S. Helland, *Department of Pharmacology, University of Bergen, Bergen, Norway*

*Michael S. Hershfield, *Duke University Medical Center, Durham, North Carolina*

*Fusao Hirata, *Laboratory of Cell Biology, National Institute of Mental Health, Bethesda, Maryland*

*Robert M. Hoffman, *Department of Pediatrics, University of California, San Diego, La Jolla, California*

P. Holbrook, *Massachusetts Institute of Technology, Cambridge, Massachusetts*

*A. Holy, *Institute of Biochemisty and Organic Chemistrty, Praha, Czechoslovakia*

S. Horowitz, *Department of Molecular Biology and Microbiology, Case Western Reserve University, Cleveland, Ohio*

Marie A. Iannone, *Wellcome Research Laboratories, Burroughs Wellcome Co., Research Triangle, North Carolina*

Taizo Iizasa, *Scripps Clinic and Research Foundation, La Jolla, California*

R. Jelinek, *Institute of Experimental Medicine, Praha, Czechoslovakia*

E. Olavi Kajander, *Scripps Clinic and Research Foundation, Ja Jolla, California*

Bradley T. Keller, *Pharmaceutical Chemistry Department, The University of Kansas, Lawrence, Kansas*

*H. Kersten, *Institut fur Physiologische Chemie, Universitat Erlangen-Nurnberg, Erlangen, West Germany*

Sangduk Kim, *Fels Research Institute, Temple University, Philadelphia, Pennsylvania*

Randall L. Kincaid, *NHLBI, National Institutes of Health, Bethesda, Maryland*

*Dagmar Knebel, *Institute of Genetics, University of Cologne, Cologne, West Germany*

Malak Kotb, *Howard Hughes Medical Institute Laboratories, Duke University Medical Center, Durham, North Carolina*

Debora L. Kramer, *Grace Cancer Drug Center, Roswell Park Memorial Institute, Buffalo, New York*

*Nicholas M. Kredich, *Howard Hughes Medical Institute Laboratories, Duke University Medical Center, Durham, North Carolina*

Masaru Kubota, *Scripps Clinic and Research Foundation, La Jolla, California*

*M. Lakher, *Massachusetts Institute of Technology, Cambridge, Massachusetts*

Klaus-Dieter Langner, *Institute of Genetics, University of Cologne, Cologne, West Germany*

M. Laundy, *King's College Hospital, London, UK*

F. Lawrence, *Institut de Chimie des Substances Naturelles, CNRS, Gif-sur-Yvette, France*

E. Lederer, *Institut de Chimie des Substances Naturelles, CNRS, Gif-sur-Yvette, France*

Hyang Woo Lee, *Fels Research Institute, Temple University, Philadelphia, Pennsylvania*

J. R. Lillehaug, *Department of Pharmacology, University of Bergen, Bergen, Norway*

M. Locati, *Rheumatology Service, L. Sacco Hospital, Milan, Italy*

J. B. Lombardini, *Department of Pharmacology, Texas Tech University, Lubbock, Texas*

Walter Lovenberg, *NHLBI, National Institutes of Health, Bethesda, Maryland*

J-C. Maire, *Massachusetts Institute of Technology, Cambridge, Massachusetts*

H. Malina, *Institut de Chimie des Substances Naturelles, CNRS, Gif-sur-Yvette, France*

P. Maroney, *Department of Molecular Biology and Microbiology, Case Western Reserve University, Cleveland, Ohio*

R. Martin, *King's College Hospital, London, UK*

*J. M. Mato, *Metabolismo, Nutricion Y Hormonas, Fundacion Jimenez Diaz, Madrid, Spain*

Keiichi Matsuda, *Laboratory of Cell Biology, National Institute of Mental Health, Bethesda, Maryland*

C. Mauron, *Massachusetts Institute of Technology, Cambridge, Massachusetts*

O. Melichar, *Institute of Organic Chemistry and Biochemistry, Praha, Czechoslovakia*

I. Merida, *Metabolismo, Nutricion Y Hormonas, Fundacion Jimenez Diaz, Madrid, Spain*

A. Merta, *Institute of Organic Chemistry and Biochemistry, Praha, Czechoslovakia*

George A. Miura, *Division of Biochemistry, Walter Reed Army Institute of Research, Washington, DC*

*John A. Montgomery, *Southern Research Institute, Birmingham, Alabama*

J. A. Monti, *University of Alabama, Birmingham, Alabama*

F. Montrone, *Rheumatology Service, L. Sacco Hospital, Milan, Italy*

D. A. Morere, *University of Alabama, Birmingham, Alabama*

P. Narayan, *Department of Molecular Biology and Microbiology, Case Western Reserve University, Cleveland, Ohio*

T. Nilsen, *Department of Molecular Biology and Microbiology, Case Western Reserve University, Cleveland, Ohio*

Kaare Norum, *Institute of Medical Biochemistry, University of Oslo, Oslo, Norway*

Dawn Nowlin, *Biochemistry/Biophysics Program, Washington State University, Pullman, Washington*

P. Ortiz, *Metabolismo, Nutricion Y Hormonas, Fundacion Jimenez Diaz, Madrid, Spain*

*Woon Ki Paik, *Fels Research Institute, Temple University, Philadelphia, Pennsylvania*

M. Pajares, *Metabolismo, Nutricion Y Hormonas, Fundacion Jimenez Diaz, Madrid, Spain*

P. Paolantonacci, *Institut de Chimie des Substances Naturelles, CNRS, Gif-sur-Yvette, France*

Chankyu Park, *Program in Genetics and Cell Biology, Washington State University, Pullman, Washington*

*Lionel A. Poirier, *Laboratory of Comparative Carcinogenesis, National Cancer Institute, Frederick, Maryland*

Carl W. Porter, *Grace Cancer Drug Center, Roswell Park Memorial Institute, Buffalo, New York*

William Z. Potter, *Laboratory of Clinical Science, National Institutes of Mental Health, Bethesda, Maryland*

Karen L. Prus, *Wellcome Research Laboratories, Burroughs Wellcome Co., Research Triangle, North Carolina*

Fulvio Della Ragione, *Department of Biochemistry of Macromolecules, University of Naples, Napoli, Italy*

*Aharon Razin, *Department of Cellular Biochemistry, The Hebrew University Medical School, Jerusalem, Israel*

H. Refsum, *Department of Pharmacology, University of Bergen, Bergen, Norway*

E. H. Reynolds, *King's College Hospital, London, UK*

Neale Ridgway, *Department of Biochemistry, University of British Columbia, Vancouver, Canada*

M. K. Riscoe, *Medical Research Service, Portland, Oregon*

*M. Robert-Gero, *Institut de Chimie des Substances Naturelles, CNRS, Gif-sur-Yvette, France*

Robert H. Roth, *Yale University School of Medicine, New Haven, Connecticut*

*F. Rottman, *Department of Molecular Biology and Microbiology, Case Western Reserve University, Cleveland, Ohio*

Contributors

*Matthew V. Rudorfer, *Laboratory of Clinical Science, National Institutes of Mental Health, Bethesda, Maryland*

S. Santandrea, *Rheumatology Service, L. Sacco Hospital, Milan, Italy*

P. Sarzi, *Rheumatology Service, L. Sacco Hospital, Milan, Italy*

J-S. Schanche, *Department of Pharmacology, University of Bergen, Bergen, Norway*

John A. Secrist, III, *Southern Research Institute, Birmingham, Alabama*

Michael A. Sherer, *Laboratory of Clinical Science, National Institutes of Mental Health, Bethesda, Maryland*

Narayan Shivapurkar, *Laboratory of Comparative Carcinogenesis, National Cancer Institute, Frederick, Maryland*

K. Slama, *Institute of Entomology, Praha, Czechoslovakia*

*J. R. Smythies, *University of Alabama, Birmingham, Alabama*

*Thomas W. Sneider, *Department of Biochemistry, Colorado State University, Fort Collins, Colorado*

Peter H. Stern, *Department of Pediatrics, University of California, San Diego, La Jolla, California*

Carolyn R. Stopford, *Wellcome Research Laboratories, Burroughs Wellcome Co., Research Triangle, North Carolina*

*Giorgio Stramentinoli, *BioResearch S.p.A. Research Laboratories, Milano, Italy*

*Janice R. Sufrin, *Department of Surgical Oncology and Grace Cancer Drug Center, Roswell Park Memorial Institute, Buffalo, New York*

A. Svardal, *Department of Pharmacology, University of Bergen, Bergen, Norway*

M. Tacconi, *Massachusetts Institute of Technology, Cambridge, Massachusetts*

C. Tempete, *Institut de Chimie des Substances Naturelles, CNRS, Gif-sur-Yvette, France*

C. Thomas, *King's College Hospital, London, UK*

L. C. Tolbert, *University of Alabama, Birmingham, Alabama*

B. K. Toone, *King's College Hospital, London, UK*

J. Traver, *Metabolismo, Nutricion Y Hormonas, Fundacion Jimenez Diaz, Madrid, Spain*

*P. M. Ueland, *Department of Pharmacology, University of Bergen, Bergen, Norway*

*Dennis E. Vance, *Department of Biochemistry, University of British Columbia, Vancouver, Canada*

I. Varela, *Metabolismo, Nutricion Y Hormonas, Fundacion Jimenez Diaz, Madrid, Spain*

M. Vedel, *Institut de Chimie des Substanzces Naturelles, CNRS, Gif-sur-Yvette, France*

M. Villalba, *Metabolismo, Nutricion Y Hormonas, Fundacion Jimenez Diaz, Madrid, Spain*

R. Volpato, *Rheumatology Service, L. Sacco Hospital, Milan, Italy*

I. Votruba, *Institute of Organic Chemistry and Biochemistry, Praha, Czechoslovakia*

W. G. Walter-Ryan, *University of Alabama, Birmingham, Alabama*

Yuji Wano, *Laboratory of Cell Biology, National Institute of Mental Health, Bethesda, Maryland*

Ulrike Weyer, *Institute of Genetics, University of Cologne, Cologne, West Germany*

Erik H. Willis, *Scripps Clinic and Research Foundation, La Jolla, California*

Mary J. Wilson, *Laboratory of Comparative Carcinogenesis, National Cancer Institute, Frederick, Maryland*

Gerald Wolberg, *Wellcome Research Laboratories, Burroughs Wellcome Co., Research Triangle, North Carolina*

Marina E. Wolf, *Yale University School of Medicine, New Haven, Connecticut*

R. J. Wurtman, *Massachusetts Institute of Technology, Cambridge, Massachusetts*

Hisashi Yamanaka, *Scripps Clinic and Research Foundation, La Jolla, California*

Y. Yao, *Department of Molecular Biology and Microbiology, Case Western Reserve University, Cleveland, Ohio*

*Vincenzo Zappia, *Department of Biochemistry of Macromolecules, University of Naples, Napoli, Italy*

*Thomas P. Zimmerman, *Wellcome Research Laboratories, Burroughs Wellcome Co., Research Triangle, North Carolina*

*Presenters

Contents

v   Preface

vii   Tributes

ix   Acknowledgments

xi   Contributors

A. Protein and Phospholipid Methylations

3   Protein Methylation at Abnormal Aspartyl Residues, **Steven Clark**

15   Enzymology of Protein Methylation: Recent Developments, **Woon Ki Paik, Sangduk Kim, and Hyang Woo Lee**

25   Is There a Function for Protein Carboxymethylation in the Nervous System? **Melvin L. Billingsley, Randall L. Kincaid, Marina E. Wolf, Robert H. Roth, Walter Lovenberg, and Carey D. Balaban**

43   Methyl-Accepting Chemotaxis Proteins in Bacteria, **Gerald L. Hazelbauer, John Bollinger, Chankyu Park, Dawn Nowlin, and Maqsudul Alam**

55   Biochemistry of Methylated Phospholipids, **Jon Bremer, Kaare Norum, and Pal Bjornstad**

67   Phospholipid Methylation and Cellular Differentiation, **Fusao Hirata, Masakazu Hatanaka, Yuji Wano, and Keiichi Matsuda**

75   Methylation of Phosphatidylethanolamine: Enzyme Characterization,
     Regulation, and Physiological Function, **Dennis E. Vance and
     Neale Ridgway**

89   Regulation of Phospholipid Methylation by Reversible
     Phosphorylation, **I. Varela, M. Pajares, I. Merida,
     M. Vaillalba, C. Cabrero, P. Ortiz, J. Traver, and
     J. M. Mato**

101 Brain Phosphatidylcholine Pools as Possible Sources of Free Choline
     for Acetylcholine Synthesis, **M. Lakher,
     R. J. Wurtman, J. Blusztajn, P. Holbrook,
     J-C. Maire, C. Mauron, and M. Tacconi**

B. Nucleic Acid Methylations

113 DNA Methylation: Overview and Prospectives, **Thomas W.
     Sneider**

127 Tissue-Specific DNA Methylation Patterns: Biochemistry of
     Formation and Possible Role, **Aharon Razin**

139 Regulation of Gene Expression by Site-Specific Promoter
     Methylation, **Walter Doerfler, Klaus-Dieter Langner,
     Dagmar Knebel, and Ulrike Weyer**

151 Carcinogenesis and DNA Hypomethylation in Methyl-Deficient
     Animals, **Lionel A. Poirier, Mary J. Wilson, and Narayan
     Shivapurkar**

163 The Role of Coenzymes and tRNA Modifications in Metabolic
     Control of Gene Expression, **H. Kersten**

175 Relationship Between Methylation and Maturation of Ribosomal
     RNA in Prokaryotic and Eukaryotic Cells, **Jean-Herve Alix**

189 Distribution of m^6A in RNA and Its Possible Biological Role,
     **F. Rottman, P. Narayan, R. Goodwin, S. Camper,
     Y. Yao, S. Horowitz, R. Albers, D. Ayers,
     P. Maroney, and T. Nilsen**

C. Regulation of S-Adenosylmethionine, S-Adenosylhomocysteine, and Methylthioadenosine Metabolism

203 Regulation of S-Adenosylmethionine Synthesis in Human Lymphocytes, **Nicholas M. Kredich, Malak Kotb, Deborah Campano German, and Craig A. Bloch**

215 Cancer, Methionine, and Transmethylation, **Robert M. Hoffman and Peter H. Stern**

227 The Centrality of S-Adenosylhomocysteinase in the Regulation of the Biological Utilization of S-Adenosylmethionine, **Giulio L. Cantoni**

239 S-Adenosylhomocysteine Hydrolase, **Peter K. Chiang and George A. Miura**

253 Probes for Examining the Structure and Function of Human S-Adenosylhomocysteine Hydrolase, and for Isolation of cDNA, **Michael S. Hershfield, V. Nambi Aiyar, Sara Chaffee, Sylvia Curtis, and Michael L. Greenberg**

263 Disposition of Endogenous S-Adenosylhomocysteine and Homocysteine Following Exposure to Nucleoside Analogs and Methotrexate, **P. M. Ueland, A. Svardal, H. Refsum, J. R. Lillehaug, J-S. Schanche, and S. Helland**

275 Regulation of S-Adenosylmethionine and Methylthioadenosine Metabolism in Methylthioadenosine Phosphorylase-Deficient Malignant Cells, **Dennis A. Carson, E. Olavi Kajander, Carlos J. Carrera, Hisashi Yamanaka, Taizo Iizasa, Masaru Kubota, Erik H. Willis, and John A. Montgomery**

287 Purification and Properties of Mammalian 5'-Methylthioadenosine Phosphorylase and Bacterial 5'-Methylthioadenosine Nucleosidase: Pharmacological Implications and Perspectives, **Vincenzo Zappia, Fulvio Della Ragione, and Maria Carteni-Farina**

301 Uncoupling of Granulopoietic Cell Proliferation and Differentiation by Methylthioadenosine, **J. H. Fitchen, M. K. Riscoe, and A. J. Ferro**

D. Clinical Aspects of S-Adenosylmethionine

315   AdoMet as a Drug: Pharmacokinetic and Pharmacological Aspects,
      Giorgio Stramentinoli

327   A Biochemical Study of Depressed Patients Receiving S-Adenosyl- L-
      methionine (SAM), **T. Bottiglieri,
      M.W. P. Carney, J. Edeh, M. Laundy, R. Martin,
      E. H. Reynolds, C. Thomas, and B. K. Toone**

339   Noradrenergic and Cardiovascular Effects of Chronic S-Adenosyl-
      methionine in Healthy Volunteers, **Michael A. Sherer, Matthew
      V. Rudorfer, Giulio L. Cantoni, Robert N. Golden, and
      William Z. Potter**

351   Role of the One-Carbon Cycle in Neuropsychiatry,
      **J. R. Smythies, R. D. Alarcon, A. J. Bancroft,
      J. A. Monti, D. A. Morere, L. C. Tolbert, and
      W. G. Walter-Ryan**

363   Double-Blind Study of S-Adenosylmethionine Versus Placebo in Hip
      and Knee Arthrosis, **I. Caruso, F. Montrone,
      F. Fumagalli, P. Sarzi, L. Boccassini, S. Santandrea, M.
      Locati, and R. Volpato**

E. Design, Synthesis, and Biological Evaluation of Transmethylation Inhibitors

373   Methionine Analog Inhibitors of S-Adenosylmethionine Biosynthesis
      as Potential Antitumor Agents, **Janice R. Sufrin,
      J. B. Lombardini, Debora L. Kramer, Vitauts Alks,
      Ralph J. Bernacki, and Carl W. Porter**

385   Metabolism and Mechanism of Action of Neplanocin A—A Potent
      Inhibitor of S-Adenosylhomocysteine Hydrolase, **Bradley T.
      Keller and Ronald T. Borchardt**

397   Biological Consequences of S-Adenosyl-L-homocysteinase Inhibition
      by Acyclic Adenosine Analogs, **A. Holy,
      I. Votruba, A. Merta, E. DeClercq, R. Jelinek,
      K. Slama, K. Benes, and O. Melichar**

Contents

409 Nucleoside Analogs as Antiviral Agents, **John A. Montgomery and John A. Secrist, III**

417 Studies Concerning the Mechanism of Action of 3-Deazaadenosine in Leukocytes, **Thomas P. Zimmerman, Gerald Wolberg, Carolyn R. Stopford, Karen L. Prus, and Marie A. Iannone**

427 Mechanism-Based Inhibitors of Alkyltransferase, **James K. Coward**

435 Sinefungin and Derivatives: Synthesis, Biosynthesis, and Molecular Target Studies in Leishmania, **P. Blanchard, N. Dodic, J. L. Fourrey, M. Geze, F. Lawrence, H. Malina, P. Paolantonacci, M. Vedel, C. Tempete, M. Robert-Gero, and E. Lederer**

447 **Index**

A. Protein and Phospholipid Methylations

PROTEIN METHYLATION AT ABNORMAL ASPARTYL RESIDUES

Steven Clarke

Department of Chemistry and Biochemistry
and the Molecular Biology Institute
University of California
Los Angeles, California   90024

Enzymes that catalyze the formation of protein methyl esters have been found in all tissues examined to date. It had been reasonably assumed that all of these enzymes would function as components of reversible covalent modification systems to regulate the activity of various methyl-accepting proteins (Gagnon and Heisler, 1979; Paik and Kim, 1980; O'Dea et al., 1981). Although this does appear to be the case for a class of bacterial methyltransferases which catalyze the formation of L-glutamyl γ-methyl esters on membrane chemoreceptors (Clarke et al., 1980; Terwilliger & Koshland, 1984; Kehry et al., 1983), this assumption does not seem to hold for a second potentially widespread class of enzymes, found both in bacteria and higher cells (Clarke, 1985a). These enzymes appear to catalyze the formation of D-aspartyl β-methyl esters and L-isoaspartyl α-methyl esters on proteins containing these abnormal amino acids (McFadden and Clarke, 1982; Aswad, 1984; Murray & Clarke, 1984; O'Connor et al., 1984).

Both classes of protein carboxyl methyltransferases were previously listed under E.C. 2.1.1.24. This designation has now been reserved for enzymes specific for L-glutamate residues. The only examples so far of enzymes in this class are the bacterial methyltransferases involved in chemotaxis. A new number (E.C. 2.1.1.77) has been established for enzymes capable of forming D-aspartyl/ L-isoaspartyl methyl esters (Enzyme Nomenclature, 1984). Although it is clear that the enzymes from human red blood

3

cells and bovine brain represent methyltransferases of this latter type, sufficient information has not been obtained to allow a distinction to be made for many of the other protein carboxyl methyltransferases characterized from various sources to date (Clarke, 1985a). Table I summarizes the differences in these two types of enzymes.

Research in our laboratory has focused on the role of the D-aspartyl/L-isoaspartyl protein carboxyl methyltransferase in human erythrocytes. We detect little or no enzyme activity in the membrane fraction, but do detect two isozymes in the cytosol that can be separated by isoelectric focusing gels (pI 5.5, 6.6) or DEAE-cellulose chromatography (I. Ota and S. Clarke, unpublished). These isozymes have similar properties to the purified enzyme preparation of Kim et al. (1983) which may represent a mixture of both isozymes. The substrate specificity of these enzymes has been studied both in intact cells, labelled with [methyl-^{3}H]methionine, and in broken cell and purified systems where S-adenosyl[methyl-^{3}H]methionine is used as a methyl donor. In all cases, D-aspartic acid [^{3}H] β-methyl ester can be isolated in 0.1% to 15% yield by proteolytic digestion (McFadden & Clarke, 1982; O'Connor & Clarke, 1983; O'Connor and Clarke, 1984; Clarke et al., 1984). A second type of activity of these enzymes has recently been discovered using synthetic hexapeptides and deamidated ACTH derivatives (Aswad, 1984; Murray and Clarke, 1984). Here, methylation of L-isoaspartyl residues, but not at normal L-aspartyl or L-asparaginyl residues, is detected. Although L-isoaspartyl α-methyl esters have not been detected so far in cellular proteins, a fraction of the methyl esters seen in intact erythrocytes labelled with [methyl-^{3}H]methionine may occur in this form.

It seems unlikely at first that a single enzyme could catalyze the methylation of both D-aspartyl and L-isoaspartyl residues. However, these sites do share some stereochemical features, as shown in Fig. 1. In the indicated configuration, the only difference is in the placement of the α-amino group, which is attached to either the α- or β-carbon but which in both cases is behind the plane of the paper. There is, however, one result which does not appear to fit in with this picture. Although the hexapeptide L-Val-L-Tyr-L-Pro-L-isoAsp-Gly-L-Ala is an excellent substrate for the red cell protein carboxyl methyltransferase (Km = 6.2 μM, Murray & Clarke, 1984), the corresponding

TABLE I[a]

TWO DISTINCT CLASSES OF PROTEIN CARBOXYL METHYLTRANSFERASES

	Class I (E.C. 2.1.1.24)	Class II (E.C. 2.1.1.77)
Residue methylated	L-Glutamyl	D-Aspartyl[b] L-Isoaspartyl Others?
Methyl accepting protein Substrates	Specific for 60,000 dalton membrane chemo-receptors	Relatively non-specific--ovalbumin, calmodulin, gelatin, ACTH, ribonuclease, glucagon can serve as substrates
Stoichiometry of methylation	Stoichiometric--up to 4 methyl groups per polypeptide	Substoichiometric--generally 1 methyl group per 100 to 1,000,000 polypeptides
Function	Modulates activity of methyl accepting protein	Metabolism of altered proteins, possible repair
Examples and distribution	Only found so far in bacteria--che R methyltransferase of Escherichia coli, Salmonella typhimurium, Bacillus subtilus	Widespread (?) Human red blood cells, bovine brain, Salmonella typhimurium, etc.

[a] For references and fuller descriptions, see Table III of Clarke (1985a).

[b] Based on the isolation of D-aspartic acid β-methyl ester from proteolytic digests of erythrocyte proteins.

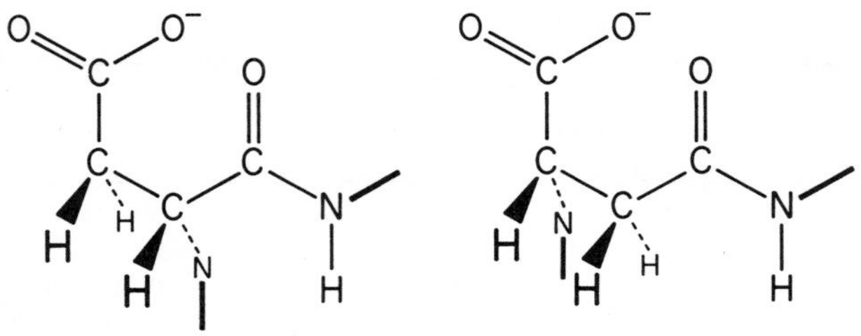

D-Asp   L-isoAsp

Figure 1. Relative Conformation of D-Aspartyl and L-isoAspartyl Residues.

D-Asp derivative does not appear to be a substrate. It is possible that specific sequences or three-dimensional structures are needed for the D-aspartyl methylation reaction. We have also considered the possibility that the D-aspartic acid β-[^{3}H]methyl ester isolated from enzymatic digests of red cell proteins may be artifactually formed from L-isoaspartyl α-[^{3}H]methyl esters during the sample work up. (We do not detect any L- or D-aspartic acid β-methyl ester formation from proteolytic digests of the synthetic L-isoaspartyl hexapeptide α-methyl ester, however). Alternatively, the actual substrate of the methylation reaction in cells may be a D-asparagine or otherwise modified D-aspartic acid residue. For example, the enzyme could catalyze both a deamidation and a methyl transfer reaction with D-asparagine residues to produce D-aspartic acid β-methyl ester residues.

The two isoenzymes of bovine brain carboxyl methyltransferase purified by Aswad and Deight (1983) appear to be very similar to the erythrocyte enzyme. For instance both isozymes catalyze the methylation of L-Val-L-Tyr-L-Pro-LisoAsp-Gly-L-Ala (Aswad, 1984; Murray & Clarke, 1984) and result in the formation of D-aspartic acid β-methyl esters on red cell membrane proteins (O'Connor et al., 1984). Many other protein carboxyl methyltransferases have been isolated which share at least some of the properties of the red cell and brain enzymes, especially with regard to the substoichiometric methylation of a variety of methyl accepting proteins (Clarke, 1985a). We have recently shown that extracts of an adrenal medulla-derived cell line

(PC-12), as well as extracts of <u>Xenopus</u> oocytes and
<u>Salmonella typhimurium</u> catalyze the specific methylation of
L-Val-L-Tyr-L-Pro-L-isoAsp-Gly-L-Ala (C. M. O'Connor and
S. Clarke, to be published). Thus, Class II methyltrans-
ases appear to have a wide distribution in nature.

We have not detected L-glutamyl γ-[^{3}H]methyl esters or
L-aspartyl β-methyl esters in proteolytic digests of erythrocyte proteins (Clarke et al., 1984). With the exception
of the bacterial chemotaxis proteins, there are no other
reports of the isolation of methyl ester derivatives in
these "natural" L-configurations. The isolation of such
derivatives in a given cell type would be good evidence for
the presence of a "regulatory" Class I methyltransferase
(Table I). Other criteria for establishing new regulatory
methyltransferases have been discussed previously (Clarke,
1985a). Although it would be very surprising if L-specific
methyltransferases are limited to the bacterial <u>che R</u>
enzymes, we do not have any clear evidence that these
enzymes exist in other cell types (Clarke, 1985a).

One of the areas in which we are presently focusing
our interest concerns the origin of D-aspartyl and L-isoaspartyl residues (Clarke, 1985b). The former residue can
be formed by the slow racemization of an L-aspartyl residue
(Bada, 1984), and the latter residue can form from the slow
deamidation of asparagine residues (Aswad, 1984). One
would therefore expect that these residues would tend to
accumulate in long-lived proteins, especially in tissues
like red cell or eye lens where the capacity for protein
synthesis has been lost and protein turnover is minimal.
If this were the case, then these altered sites could be
recognized by the protein carboxyl methyltransferase and
provide a signal to the cell either to degrade the "damaged
protein" or to possibly repair the damage (McFadden and
Clarke, 1982). The finding that the D-aspartyl/L-isoaspar-
tyl methyltransferases are present in tissues where protein
synthesis and turnover do occur is then puzzling. It is
possible that the rate of aspartyl residue degradation in
certain proteins is rapid, and might necessitate the
recognition of damage by a methyltransferase. On the other
hand, L-isoaspartyl residues and D-aspartyl residues may
represent side-products of protein biosynthesis, and might
be expected to be present in "young" as well as "old"
proteins. For example, if an L-aspartyl residue is
attached to its cognate tRNA via the β-carboxyl group, an

L-isoaspartyl residue may be introduced into the protein.
Alternatively, the rate of racemization on the ribosome may
be significant. In either case, altered aspartyl residues
would be incorporated and may be detected by cytosolic
methyltransferases. Chen et al. (1978) have demonstrated,
in fact, that carboxyl methylation can occur on nascent
polypeptide chains still attached to ribosomes.

     Thus, it appears that protein carboxyl methyltransfer-
ases can recognize proteins with altered aspartyl residues. The question concerning the fate of the methylated
protein remains. Specific roles have been proposed, including that the methylated protein is a substrate for a
repair reaction which partially or fully returns the modified aspartyl residue to the original L-aspartic and/or
L-asparagine configuration (McFadden and Clarke, 1982).
Such a role would be important in red blood cells or the
eye lens, where no capacity exists for protein renewal by
synthesis. The situation may be more complicated for nucleated cells. In these cells, the presence of L-isoaspartyl
or D-aspartyl residue may simply mark the oldest cellular
proteins.   These proteins may also contain significant
amounts of racemized Ser, Thr, Glu, and Phe residues
(Whitaker, 1980) as well as other covalent alterations
(Clarke, 1985b).   A logical scenario would be that the
methylation reaction provides a signal to the cell to
proteolyze these modified polypeptides.

     To test whether methylation is part of a repair path-
way or signals protein degradation, the metabolism of protein methyl esters in cells and cellular extracts must be
examined. The first step of this process appears to be the
loss of the methyl group. Although most methyl esters,
including the methylated L-glutamyl chemoreceptors (Kleene
et al., 1977), are stable under physiological conditions
(pH 7.4, 37°C), the methylated protein products of the
erythrocyte, brain, and other eukaryotic protein carboxyl
methyltransferases appear to be quite unstable. The data
in Table II show that model compounds such as methyl pro-
pionate and N-benzoyl L-aspartic acid β-methyl ester hydrolyze under physiological conditions with half times of
5,600 and 50,000 minutes, respectively. In contrast, the
half-times for a number of methyl accepting proteins of red
blood cell membranes, calmodulin, glucagon, and peptide
substrates range from 4 to 120 minutes. Although it is
possible that these rate enhancements are a product of

TABLE II
DEMETHYLATION RATES OF PROTEIN METHYL ESTERS AND MODEL
COMPOUNDS

Compound	t1/2 (pH 7.4, 37°C) min
Methyl propionate[a]	5,600
L-Aspartic acid β-methyl ester[a]	1,500
N-Benzoyl L-aspartic acid β-methyl ester[a]	50,000
N-Benzoyl L-aspartic acid β-methyl ester glycylamide[a]	95[b]
Calmodulin methyl ester[c]	120
Glucagon methyl ester[d]	55
Deamidated ACTH methyl ester[e]	7.2
L-Val-L-Tyr-L-Pro-L-isoAsp α-methyl ester-Gly-L-Ala[f]	4
Red blood cell membranes[g]	About 45

[a] Data of Terwilliger and Clarke (1981).
[b] This value represents the rate of hydrolysis. As the reaction is likely to go through a succinimide intermediate, the rate of demethylation is probably on the order
of 10 times faster (Bernhard, 1983).
[c] Methylated with the erythrocyte protein carboxyl methyltransferase (L.S. Brunauer and S. Clarke, unpublished).
[d] Methylated with the erythrocyte protein carboxyl methyltransferase (K.L. Oden and S. Clarke, unpublished).
[e] Data of Johnson and Aswad (1985).
[f] E.D. Murray, Jr. and S. Clarke, to be published.
[g] Data of Barber and Clarke (1985) for [^{3}H]-methylated membranes purified from intact cells incubated with [methyl-
^{3}H]methionine.

steric and electronic effects of neighboring groups,
aspartyl esters in peptides can undergo demethylation by
intramolecular ring forming reactions that are much more
rapid than demethylation mechanisms based on water or
hydroxide ion attack on the ester group (Bernhard, 1983).

These intramolecular mechanisms are discussed more fully below and in Table III.

The rapid spontaneous demethylation rate observed for protein methyl esters suggests that the cellular removal of methyl groups may be a non-enzymatic process. We have recently tested this hypothesis by comparing the rate of turnover of methyl groups in the membrane proteins of intact erythrocytes with the rate of demethylation of the isolated membrane fraction. We found that the presumably spontaneous demethylation of the isolated membrane proteins could account for the methyl group turnover in intact cells and that the addition of cell lysate to the membrane fraction did not increase the rate of demethylation (Barber and Clarke, 1985). Similarly, we have not found evidence for methyl esterase activity in red cell lysates using L-Val-L-Tyr-L-Pro-L-isoAsp-α-methyl ester-Gly-L-Ala as a substrate (E.D. Murray, Jr. and S. Clarke, to be published). In contrast to these results from a homologous erythrocyte system, Gagnon et al. (1984) have purified an enzyme from rat kidney which catalyzes the demethylation of gelatin methyl esters formed by the red cell protein methyltransferase. This enzyme is most active at acidic pH values.

If one considers both the rapid rates of hydrolysis of protein methyl esters and the likely formation of intermediates such as succinimides during the demethylation reactions (Bernhard, 1983), one can hypothesize that these intermediates themselves may have physiological importance. Johnson and Aswad (1985) have provided evidence to support a succinimide intermediate in the spontaneous hydrolysis of the methylated deamidated form of ACTH in buffer, and we have also obtained evidence for a succinimide intermediate in the demethylation of the synthetic peptide L-Val-L-Tyr-L-Pro-L-isoAsp-α-methylester-Gly-L-Ala in erythrocyte cytosolic extracts (E.D. Murray, Jr. and S. Clarke, to be published). It is presently unknown whether such succinimides are formed from cellular protein methyl esters. Additionally, there are other possible intramolecular reactions that can account for the rapid hydrolysis rates. These reactions would form the other three intermediates shown in Table III. Some of these intermediates have chemical properties that may be highly relevant to the function of protein carboxyl methylation. In the first place, the succinimide can hydrolyze to give both normal aspartyl residues as well as isoaspartyl residues. It is

TABLE III

POSSIBLE INTRAMOLECULAR DEMETHYLATION PRODUCTS OF
ASPARTYL AND ISOASPARTYL METHYL ESTERS IN PROTEINS

Product	Formed from	Racemization Prone?	Products of Hydrolysis
SUCCINIMIDE	Asp β-methyl ester or isoAsp α-methyl ester	?	DL(?)-Asp (30%) and DL(?)-isoAsp (70%)
"ANHYDRIDE" (4,5-diamino-2-oxolanone)	Asp β-methyl ester	?	(DL)?-Asp
"ISOANHYDRIDE" (3,5-diamino-2-oxolanone)	IsoAsp α-methyl ester	?	DL(?)-isoAsp
5-(4H)OXAZOLONE	IsoAsp α-methyl ester	YES	DL-isoAsp

simple to envision how the methylation system may then function to generate L-aspartyl residues from L-isoaspartyl residues in a "repair" reaction. However, a second property of some or all of these intermediates may complicate this role. For example, if an L-isoaspartyl α-methylester is hydrolyzed via a 5(4H)oxazolone intermediate (Benoiton, 1983), this intermediate can racemize extremely rapidly and the reaction product would be a DL-mixture of isoaspartic acid. The degree of racemization of the succinimide and "anhydride" derivatives is not established but may result in the formation of D and L products here as well. The end result of such reactions would then be to form proteins containing all four aspartyl derivatives—L-Asp, D-Asp, L-isoAsp, D-isoAsp. Since the D-Asp and L-isoAsp derivatives would be recycled by the methyltransferase, the net result of these reactions would then be the conversion of D-aspartyl and L-isoaspartyl residues to L-aspartyl and D-isoaspartyl residues (Fig. 2).

It should be noted that the demethylation of L-glutamyl γ-methyl esters in bacterial chemoreceptors is a much more straightforward process. Here, the esters are relatively stable under physiological conditions (Kleene et al. 1977) and a specific enzyme exists which catalyzes the hydrolysis and reformation of L-glutamyl residues (Snyder et al., 1984). There is no indication that intramolecular reactions analogous to those in Table III occur.

One very intriguing aspect of the hypothesized reaction in Fig. 2 is that the configuration of a D-isoAsp

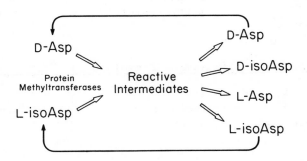

Figure 2. Possible Cellular Fates of Protein D-Aspartyl and L-isoAspartyl Residues.

residue is similar to that of an L-Asp residue in the same
way that the configuration of a D-Asp residue is similar to
an L-isoAsp residue (Fig. 3, cf. Fig. 1). It is thus
possible that a D-isoaspartyl residue fits into the protein
structures better than a D-aspartyl or an L-isoaspartyl
residue and would not have to be further "repaired".

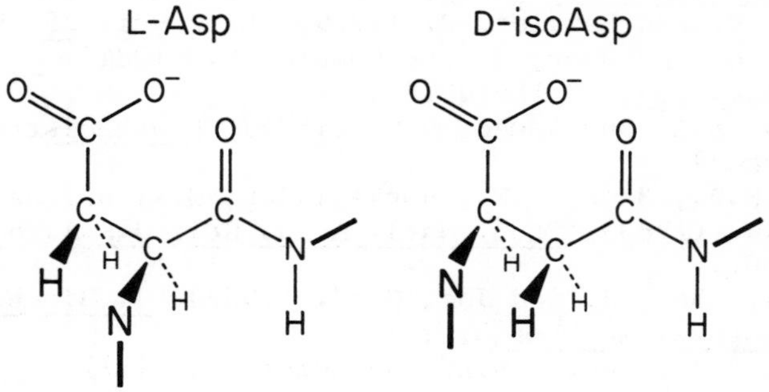

Figure 3. Relative Conformation of L-Aspartyl and
D-isoAspartyl Residues.

        Additional work is clearly needed to determine which,
if any, of the intermediates shown in Table III actually
occur as demethylation products of protein methylesters,
and whether these intermediates are recognized by specific
cellular enzymes which may direct their hydrolysis.

REFERENCES

Aswad, D.W. (1984) J. Biol. Chem. 259, 10714-10721.
Aswad, D.W. and Deight, E.A. (1983) J. Neurochem. 40, 1718-
     1726.
Bada, J.L. (1984) Methods Enzymol. 106, 98-115.
Barber, J.R. and Clarke, S. (1985) Biochemistry 24 (in
press).
Benoiton, N.L. (1983) The Peptides 5, 217-284.
Bernhard, S.A. (1983) Anal. N.Y. Acad. Sci. 421, 28-40.
Chen, J.-K. and Liss, M. (1978) Biochem. Biophys. Res.
     Commun. 84, 261-268.
Clarke, S. (1985a) Ann. Rev. Biochem. 54, 479-506.

Clarke, S. (1985b) in Cellular and Molecular Aspects of
    Aging: The Red Cell as a Model (Eaton, J., Ed.), Alan
    R. Liss, New York (in press).
Clarke, S., McFadden, P.N., O'Connor, C.M. and Lou, L.L.
    (1984) Methods Enzymol. 106, 330-344.
Clarke, S., Sparrow, K., Panasenko, S. and Koshland, D.E.,
    Jr. (1980) J. Supramol. Struct. 13, 315-328.
Enzyme Nomenclature (1984) Academic Press, New York.
Gagnon, C. and Heisler, S. (1979) Life Sci. 25, 993-1000.
Gagnon, C., Harbour, D. and Camato, R. (1984) J. Biol.
    Chem. 259, 10212-10215.
Johnson, B.A. and Aswad, D.W. (1985) Biochemistry 24 (in
    press).
Kehry, M.R., Bond, M.W., Hunkapiller, M.W. and Dahlquist,
    F.W. (1983) Proc. Natl. Acad. Sci. U.S.A. 80, 3599-
    3602.
Kim, S., Choi, J. and Jun, G.-J. (1983) J. Biochem.
    Biophys. Methods 8, 9-14.
Kleene, S.J., Toews, M.L. and Adler, J. (1977) J. Biol.
    Chem. 252, 3214-3218.
McFadden, P.N. and Clarke, S. (1982) Proc. Natl. Acad.
    Sci. U.S.A. 79, 2460-2464.
Murray, E.D., Jr. and Clarke, S. (1984) J. Biol. Chem.
    259, 10722-10731.
O'Connor, C.M. and Clarke, S. (1983) J. Biol. Chem. 258,
    8485-8492.
O'Connor, C.M. and Clarke, S. (1984) J. Biol. Chem. 259,
    2570-2578.
O'Connor, C.M., Aswad, D.W. and Clarke, S. (1984) Proc.
    Natl. Acad. Sci. U.S.A. 82, 7557-7564.
O'Dea, R.F., Viveros, O.H., and Diliberto, E.J., Jr. (1981)
    Biochem. Pharmacol. 30, 1163-1168.
Paik, W.K. and Kim, S. (1980) Protein Methylation, pp.
    202-231, John Wiley and Sons, New York.
Snyder, M.A., Stock, J.B. and Koshland, D.E., Jr. (1984)
    Methods Enzymol. 106, 321-330.
Terwilliger, T.C. and Clarke, S. (1981) J. Biol. Chem.
    256, 3067-3076.
Terwilliger, T.C. and Koshland, D.E., Jr. (1984) J.
    Biol.Chem. 259, 7719-7725.
Whitaker, J.R. (1980) in Chemical Deterioration of Pro-
    teins (Whitaker, J.R. and Fujimike, M., Eds.), pp.
    165-194, American Chemical Society, Washington, D.C.

ENZYMOLOGY OF PROTEIN METHYLATION: RECENT DEVELOPMENT

Woon Ki Paik, Sangduk Kim, and Hyang Woo Lee

Fels Research Institute, Temple University
School of Medicine
3420 North Broad Street, Philadelphia, PA

The presence of ε-N-methyllysine was first observed in
Salmonella typhimurium in 1959. Since this discovery the
ubiquitous occurrence of protein methylation in nature has
been well established (Paik & Kim, 1980). It involves N-
methylation of lysine, arginine, histidine, alanine, proli-
ne, and glutamine, O-methylation of glutamic and aspartic
acid, and S-methylation of methionine and cysteine (Paik &
Kim, 1985). As shown in Table I, methylated amino acids
occur in highly specialized proteins such as histones, flagella protein, myosin, actin, ribosomal proteins, opsin,
EF1α(Tu), HnRNP protein, HMG-1 and HMG-2 protein, fungal
and plant cytochrome c, myelin basic protein, porcine heart
citrate synthase, heat-shock proteins, nucleolar protein,
ferredoxin, wheat α-amylase, and calmodulin.

It has been realized during the past 15 years that
these methylations are carried out by several classes of
highly specific methyltransferases. For example, protein
methylase I (S-Adenosyl-L-methionine:protein-arginine N-
methyltransferase; EC 2.1.1.23), representing one such class,
methylates the guanidino group of arginine residues; protein
methylase II (S-Adenosyl-L-methionine:protein-carboxyl O-
methyltransferase; EC 2.1.1.24) methylates the carboxyl
group of glutamyl or aspartyl residues; and protein methylase III (S-Adenosyl-L-methionine:protein-lysine N-methyltransferase; EC 2.1.1.43) methylates the ε-amino group of
lysine residues (Paik & Kim, 1980 and 1985).

The most remarkable characteristics of these methyltransferases are undoubtedly the high degree of specificity

15

Table I

Natural Occurrence of Various Methylated Amino Acids

Methylated amino acids	Proteins
ε-N-Monomethyl-L-lysine	Flagella protein, histones, myosin, actin, ribosomal proteins, opsin, tooth matrix protein, EF 1α (fungus Mucor), ferredoxin (Sulfolobus acidocaldarius)
ε-N-Dimethyl-L-lysine	Flagella protein, histones, myosin, actin, opsin, ribosomal proteins, EF 1α (fungus Mucor)
ε-N-Trimethyl-L-lysine	Histones, cytochrome c (Ascomycetes), myosin, actin, ribosomal proteins, calmodulin, EF-Tu, citrate synthase (porcine heart), heat-shock proteins, EF 1α (fungus Mucor), α-amylase (wheat)
N^G-Monomethyl-L-arginine	Histones, acidic nuclear protein, myelin basic protein, heat-shock protein
N^G,N^G-Dimethyl-L-arginine	Histones, myelin basic protein, myosin, HnRNP protein, ribosomal proteins, tooth matrix protein, HMG-1 and HMG-2 protein, nucleolar protein C23
N^G,N'^G-Dimethyl-L-arginine	Histones, myelin basic protein, tooth matrix protein, myosin, actin, opsin
3-N-Methyl-L-histidine	Myosin, actin, histone, opsin
δ-N-Methylglutamine	Ribosomal protein
Glutamyl or aspartyl ester	Membrane proteins of bacteria, and erythrocytes

toward a particular amino acid residue in the substrate protein. However, evidence is fast accumulating to demonstrate that an additional level of specificity is endowed in the identity of the methyl-acceptor protein species. At least several examples within each of these methyltransferase classes have been well characterized. A brief account

of the specificity of the enzyme concerned will be the
major topic of this article.

Methyltransferases are not only specific for the amino acid residues, but also for the protein species

It has long been thought that a single protein methylase I is responsible for in vivo methylation of arginine
residues of all the proteins which contain N^G-methylargini-
ne residues (Table I). However, it is increasingly evident
that the enzyme responsible for methylating histones is
distinctly different from the myelin basic protein (MBP)-
methylating enzyme. During purification of protein methylase I from calf brain, the ratio of the enzyme activities
determined using histone and MBP as substrates varied significantly (Lee et al., 1977). Also, the protein methylase I
purified from wheat germ methylates histone, but not MBP
(Gupta et al., 1982). In addition, the protein methylase I
activity using these two protein substrates varied significantly during the normal development of mouse spinal cord
(Crang & Jacobson, 1982) and in jimpy mice brains (Kim et
al., 1984).

Recently, we have purified an enzyme from Euglena
gracilis which methylates a arginine residue of cytochrome
c only (Farooqui et al., 1985) (Table II).

Table III and IV lists the properties of protein methylase III (protein-lysine methylating) isolated from various
sources. These enzymes are highly protein-specific. Protein methylase III purified from Crithidia oncopelti is
completely inert toward horse heart cytochrome c, however,
strongly active with its own cytochrome c-557 (Valentine &
Pettigrew, 1982). Likewise, the enzyme from Euglena gracilis methylates only histone H1 (lysine-rich), but not
histone H4 (arginine-rich) (Tuck et al., 1985).

Although protein methylase II (protein-carboxyl methylating) in prokaryotes methylesterifies primarily the membrane proteins of Gram-negative and -positive bacteria as a
biochemical signal for chemotactic action (Kleene et al.,
1977; Van der Werf & Koshland, 1977; Ahlgren & Ordal, 1983),
the enzyme in eukaryotes methylates a wide variety of proteins (Paik & Kim, 1980), including membrane proteins
(Galletti et al., 1979). No evidence is presently available
to indicate that these substrate proteins are methylated by
separate enzymes in vivo or in vitro, although several molecular species with different pI values of protein methylase
II have been reported (Kim, 1973; Kim, et al., 1978; Aswad
& Deight, 1983).

Table II

Properties of Protein Methylase I from Different
Sources[a]

Properties	Source of enzyme		
	Calf brain	Wheat germ	E. gracilis
Subcellular location	Cytosol	Cell sap	Cytosol
In vitro protein substrate	Histone:MBP [b]	Histone	Cytochrome c[c]
Purification achieved (fold)	120	90	52
pH optimum	7.2	9.0	7.0
K_m for S-adenosyl-L-methionine	7.6×10^{-6} M	5.7×10^{-6} M	40×10^{-6} M
K_m for protein substrate	2.5×10^{-5} M (histone)	5×10^{-4} M	8.3×10^{-5} M
K_i for S-adenosyl-L-homocyst.	2.6×10^{-6} M	1×10^{-6} M	1.2×10^{-5} M
Ratio of N^G-mono:N^G,N^G-di: N^G,N'^G-methylarginine	55:5:40	73:27:0	100:0:0
Reference	Lee et al (1977)	Gupta et al (1982)	Farooqui et al. (1985)

a. For extensive information, see Paik & Kim (1985)
b. Relative rate; 1:0.3.

Table III

Properties of Protein Methylase III from Higher Organisms [a]

Properties	Sources of enzyme	
	Calf thymus	Rat brain
Subcellular location	Chromatin	Cytosol
In vitro protein substrate	Histone H4	Calmodulin
Residue modified	Lys-20	—
Molecular weight (Da)	—	—
pH optimum	7.5–9.0	8.1
K_m for S-adenosyl-L-methionine	3×10^{-6} M	—
K_m for protein substrate	—	1.1×10^{-5} M
K_i for S-adenosyl-L-homocysteine	—	—
Ratio of ε-N-mono:di:trimethyl-lysine in product	—	Mostly tri-
Reference	Paik & Kim (1970)	Sitaramayya et al (1980)

a. For more information, see Paik & Kim (1985)

Table IV

Properties of Protein Methylase III from Lower Organisms [a]

Properties	Source of enzymes		
	E. gracilis	N. crassa	C. oncopelti
Subcellular location	Cytosol	Cytosol	–
In vitro protein substrate	Histone H1	Cytochrome c	Cytochrome c-557
Residue modified	–	Lys-72	Lys-2
Molecular weight (Da)	34,000	120,000	–
pH optimum	9.0	9.0	9.0
K_m for S-adenosyl-L-methionine	3×10^{-5} M	2×10^{-5} M	–
K_m for protein substrate	4×10^{-7} M	2×10^{-3} M	–
K_i for S-adenosyl-L-homocysteine	2×10^{-6} M	2×10^{-6} M	–
Ratio of ε-N-mono:di:trimethyl-lysine in product	38:39:23	12:38:50	Mostly tri-
Reference	Tuck et al. (1985)	Durban et al. (1978)	Valentine & Pettigrew (1982)

a. For more information, see Paik & Kim (1985).

Multiple methylation of a protein

As described in Tables II, III and IV, histones can be methylated at arginine and lysine residues by protein methylase I and III, respectively. However, the most glaring example of such multiple methylation of a protein by several different enzymes has been witnessed in the enzymatic methylation of cytochrome c.

It has earlier been shown that protein methylase III isolated from Neurospora crassa, wheat germ or Saccharomyces cerevisiae methylates the lysine residue-72 of horse heart cytochrome c in vitro (Durban et al., 1978; DiMaria et al., 1979 & 1982). Recently, however, we have identified two additional enzymes from Euglena gracilis, one of which methylates specifically methionine-65 and the other the arginine-38 residue of cytochrome c (Farooqui et al., 1985). These enzymes are highly specific in that only cytochrome c serves as an in vitro substrate.

What biochemical influence these enzymes bring about on the function of cytochrome c is not clear at present. However, as shown in Table V, the most remarkable feature of enzymatic methylation is the tendency to lower the pI values of the hemoprotein.

Table V

Effect of Enzymatic Methylation on Isoelectric Point (pI value) of Cytochrome c

Cytochrome c methylated at:	pI	Decrease	Reference
Native	10.03		
Lysine-72	9.49	0.54	Kim et al. (1980)
Arginine-38	9.33	0.70	Farooqui et al.
Methionine-65	9.23	0.80	ibid. (1985)

Conclusion

Although the presence of ε-N-methyllysine in the flagella protein of Salmonella typhimurium was first described more than 25 years ago, the concept of Protein Methylation emerged only after our demonstration in 1966 that the ε-N-methyllysine in histones resulted from post-synthetic methylation of the protein by S-adenosyl-L-methionine.

During the intervening years, protein methylation has

been implicated in a number of biochemical phenomena. However, its precise function is known only in a few systems;
in carnitine biosynthesis by providing the metabolic precursor, ε-N-trimethyl-L-lysine, in chemotactic action by
signaling biochemical sensory input, and in the repair of
damaged DNA.

In the present article, space did not allow us to
indulge ourselves in a comprehensive review of the enzymology of protein methylation [for detailed discussion, the
readers are advised to consult our recent publication; Paik
& Kim, 1985]. However, we have attempted to draw attention
in this thesis that protein methyltransferases are not only
highly specific for the amino acid residues involved, but
also for the tertiary structure of the substrate proteins.
Naturally, we strongly envisage that most of the proteins,
if not all, listed in Table I should have their own specific methyltransferases.

Acknowledgements

This work was supported by Research Grants AM09602,
CA12226 and CA12227 from National Institute of Health.

References

Ahlgren, J. A. and Ordal, G. W. (1983) Biochem. J. 213,759.
Aswad, D. W. and Deight, W. A. (1983) J. Neurochem. 40,
    1718.
Crang, A. J. and Jacobson, W. (1982) J. Neurochem. 39, 244.
DiMaria, P., Kim, S. and Paik, W. K. (1982) Biochemistry
    21, 1036.
DiMaria, P., Polastro, E., DeLange, R. J., Kim, S. and Paik,
    W. K. (1979) J. Biol. Chem. 254, 4645.
Durban, E., Nochumson, S., Kim, S. and Paik, W. K. (1978)
    J. Biol. Chem. 253, 1427.
Farooqui, J., Tuck, M. and Paik, W. K. (1985) J. Biol. Chem
    260, 537.
Galletti, P., Paik, W. K. and Kim, S. (1979) Eur. J. Biochem
    97, 221.
Gupta, A., Jensen, D., Kim, S. and Paik, W. K. (1982) J.
    Biol. Chem. 257, 9677.
Kim, C.-S., Kueppers, F., DiMaria, P., Farooqui, J., Kim,
    S., and Paik, W. K. (1980) Biochim. Biophys. Acta 622,
    144.
Kim, S. (1974) Arch. Biochem. Biophys. 161, 652.
Kim, S., Nochumson, S., Chin, W. and Paik, W. K. (1978)
    Anal. Biochem. 84, 415.

Kim, S., Tuck, M., Kim, M., Campagnoni, A. T. and Paik, W.
    K. (1984) Biochem. Biophys. Res. Communs. 123, 468.
Kleene, S. J., Toews, M. L. and Adler, J. (1977) J. Biol.
    Chem. 252, 3214.
Lee, H. W., Kim, S. and Paik, W. K. (1977) Biochemistry
    16, 78.
Paik, W. K. and Kim, S. (1970) J. Biol. Chem. 245, 6010.
Paik, W. K. and Kim, S. (1980) Protein Methylation, John
    Wiley & Sons, New York.
Paik, W. K. and Kim, S. (1985) The Enzymology of Post-Trans-
    lational Modification of Proteins, Vol. 2 (Freedman,
    R. and Hawkins, H. C., Ed.), Academic Press (London),
    in press
Sitaramayya, A., Wright, L. S. and Siegel, F. L. (1980) J.
    Biol. Chem. 255, 8894.
Tuck, M., Farooqui, J. and Paik, W. K. (1985) J. Biol.
    Chem. 260, 7114.
Valentine, J. and Pettigrew, G. W. (1982) Biochem. J. 201,
    329.
Van der Werf, P. and Koshland, D. E. jr. (1977) J. Biol.
    Chem. 252, 2793.

IS THERE A FUNCTION FOR PROTEIN CARBOXYLMETHYLATION IN THE NERVOUS SYSTEM?

Melvin L. Billingsley,* Randall L. Kincaid,[†]
Marina E. Wolf,[§] Robert H. Roth,[§] Walter
Lovenberg[†] and Carey D. Balaban.* Milton S.
Hershey Medical Center, Penn State University,
Hershey,* PA 17033; NHLBI, NIH,[†] Bethesda, MD
20205; and Yale University School of Medicine,[§]
New Haven, CT 06510.

INTRODUCTION

The functional aspects of protein carboxylmethylation in eucaryotic cells have remained enigmatic. Some of the major issues which obscure the possible role of this enzyme are 1) the nature and specificity of relevant in vivo protein substrates; 2) the stoichiometry of protein carboxylmethylation and 3) the rapid hydrolysis of carboxylmethylesters under conditions of neutral and basic pH (Billingsley and Lovenberg, 1985). Thus, two major schools of thought have arisen which attempt to address these issues-the functionalists, who look for revelant substrates which may be regulated by rapid carboxyl-methylation, and the structuralists, who suggest that protein carboxylmethylation recognizes and/or repairs either reacemized aspartyl (Terwilliger and Clarke, 1981; McFadden and Clarke, 1982; Murray and Clarke, 1984) or beta isopeptide links (Aswad, 1984; O'Connor, et al., 1984) in a wide range of substrates. We will present evidence which suggests a possible functional role for protein-O-carboxylmethyltransferase (PCM; E.C.2.1.1.24) in nervous tissue based on the following findings.

We produced polyclonal antibodies against bovine brain PCM (PCM 1) and used the antisera to explore the distribution of PCM in nervous tissue, finding that PCM was localized primarily in neurons (Billingsley, et al., 1985a). Further, PCM immunoreactivity was markedly different between

25

several brain regions, suggesting selective gene expression
of PCM (Billingsley and Balaban, 1985).   Calcineurin, a
calmodulin-dependent protein phosphatase (Stewart et al.,
1982), has been reported to be a substrate for PCM (Gagnon,
1984).   We have found that calcineurin was able to
incorporate between 0.3 - 2.0 mol CH_3/mol protein using in
vitro assays with purified bovine brain PCM; all of the
methyl groups were located on the 61,000 dalton catalytic
subunit (Billingsley et al., 1985b).   Carboxylmethylesters
on calcineurin were rapidly hydrolysed at neutral pH (t 1/2
= 3.0 min at pH 7.4), and the carboxylmethylation was
inhibited   by   S-adenosylhomocysteine   (AdoHcy).   When
carboxylmethylated calcineurin was assayed for phosphatase
activity, a marked reduction was observed in calmodulin
stimulated, but not basal activity. We have used affinity-
purified antibodies against calcineurin to localize this
protein in brain, and have found that it is distributed in a
pattern similar to that of PCM (Kincaid, et al., 1985).
Finally, we have used drug probes for dopaminergic systems
to   stimulate   or   inhibit   PCM   activity   in   nigrostriatal
dopamine neurons in tissue slices (Wolf and Roth, 1985).
The   nigrostriatal   system   has   high   concentrations   of
immunoreactive PCM which are colocalized in neurons which
are positive for tyrosine hydroxylase.

MATERIALS AND METHODS

Materials

[^{3}H-methyl]-S-adenosylmethionine (62 and 15 Ci/mmol) was
purchased from Amersham.   S-adenosylmethionine (AdoMet),
AdoHcy, and diaminobenzidine were purchased from Sigma
Chemical Co., 2-(N-morpholino)-ethane sulfonic acid (MES)
from Calbiochem, AdoHcy-agarose from Bethesda Research labs,
and electrophoresis chemicals were purchased from BioRad
Labs.   Immunochemical kits (Vectastain-ABC peroxidase) were
purchased from Vector Labs.   Horseradish peroxidase goat
antirabbit IgG was purchased from BioRad, and nitrocellulose
sheets were purchased from Schleichter and Schuell.   All
other reagents were obtained from local suppliers.

Preparation of Enzymes

Calcineurin was prepared from bovine brain as described

by Kincaid, et al. (1984). The enzyme was homogeneous following sodium dodecyl sulfate-polyacrylamide gel electrophoresis (SDS-PAGE), consisting of a 61,000 and 18,000 dalton subunits (Kincaid, et. al., 1984). Calmodulin and calmodulin-Sepharose were prepared as described (Kincaid and Vaughan, 1979). Bovine brain, rat brain and human erythrocyte PCM was purified from cytosolic fractions of tissue, using anion exchange chromatography (DEAE-Trisacryl; LKB Instruments), AdoHcy-agarose inhibitor chromatography, and molecular sizing (Biogel P-30; BioRad; or Fractogel TSKHW-55; EM Reagents) using minor modifications of published methods (Kim, et al., 1978). In several studies, purified PCM was chromatographed over concanavallin-A, Wheat germ agglutin or lentil lectin-Sepharose (Pharmacia) in order to characterize potential glycoside moieties.

SDS-PAGE and Immunoblotting Procedures

Protein samples were solubilized in an SDS buffer containing mercaptoethanol, and electrophoresed at constant current. Unfixed gels were used for immunoblotting, which was performed as described by Towbin, et al. (1981). After the transfer was complete, the paper was incubated in blocking buffer (5% nonfat dry milk in 50 mM Tris-HCl, 150 mM NaCl, pH 7.4) to block excess protein binding sites, and the antibody solution (1:500 in blocking buffer) was incubated overnight with the transfer. Immune complexes were detected using either horseradish peroxidase coupled with the second antibody or by using biotinylated second antibodies followed by avidin-horseradish peroxidase. Either diaminobenzidine or p-chloronapthol was used as a chromogen for peroxidase, using 0.03% H_2O_2.

Antibody Preparations

Purified bovine brain PCM was electrophoresed in 12.5% SDS-PAGE, lightly stained with Coomassie Blue, the bands excised and homogenized in Complete Freund's adjuvant (Billingsley, et al., 1985a). Male rabbits were injected subcutaneously with 50-100 µg of enzyme, and were boosted with 25 µg in incomplete Freund's adjuvant at three week intervals. Antiserum was stored in 40% glycerol at -20°C. Some antisera preparations were purified into IgG fractions

using CM-Affigel-Blue (BioRad). Polyclonal antibodies to
purified calcineurin were raised in a goat as described, and
the antibody was purified using calcineurin-Sepharose
affinity chromatography followed by further purification
using protein-A-Sepharose (Kincaid, et al., 1985). This
antibody did not significantly cross-react with any other
protein.

Immunohistochemistry

Adult male Sprague-Dawley rats were perfused with
phosphate-buffered saline (PBS) followed by 10% buffered
formalin. Coronal sections (50-100 µm) were prepared using
a vibratome (Oxford), and the free-floating sections were
rinsed in PBS containing 0.5% triton-X-100 (TPBS), followed
by overnight incubation with antisera (1:500) in TPBS and 1%
normal rabbit (PCM) or goat (calcineurin) serum. Sections
were then washed in PBS, incubated with biotinylated second
antibody, followed by avidin-peroxidase, and color was
developed using diaminobenzidine as a chromogen. Sections
were mounted on slides, dehydrated through a graded series
of alcohol, and cleared in xylene. Photomicrographs were
taken using Kodak technical pan film at ASA 25.

Carboxylmethylation Assays

Purified calcineurin was incubated at $30^{\circ}C$ with
purified bovine brain PCM (2-14 µM) in a 100 µl reaction
volume containing: calcineurin (1.25 -62.5 pmol), [^{3}H-
methyl]-AdoMet (1-200 µM) in 50 mM MES, pH 6.25, for 10-15
min. 10% trichloroacetic acid was used to terminate the
reaction, and the pellet was washed twice with additional
trichloroacetic acid, once with acetone, and solubilized in
1.5 M Tris-HCl, pH 8.8, 0.4% SDS for radiometric assay. For
reactions where calcineurin activity was measured following
methylation, the reaction was terminated by addition of 200
µM AdoHcy (final concentration).

Calcineurin Phosphatase Activity

The ability of calcineurin to hydrolyse p-nitrophenyl
phosphate (PNPP) was determined spectrophotometrically
(Pallen and Wang 1983) at pH 6.5 (to minimize methylester

hydrolysis. Calcinerin (6.25 pmol) was first incubated at 30°C with 200 µM AdoMet, 50 mM MES, 0.1 mM EGTA, in a volume of 50 µl, with or without PCM ($9-14$ µM) for 15 min. AdoHcy was added (200 µM), and 1 mM Mn^{+2}, 2 µM calmodulin, and 100 mM PNPP were added and incubated at 30°C for 3 min. Reactions were terminated with 2 M Na_2CO_3, and the product released determined by absorbance at 410 nm. Stoichiometry was determined in parallel samples which contained [^{3}H-methyl]-AdoMet (1100 DPM/pmol). Protein was measured using the method of Bradford (1976).

Dopamine Release from Striatal Slices

Striata from male rats were removed, processed into slices (200 µm) using a Sorvall tissue chopper, and incubated in a modified, oxygenated Krebs-Ringer buffer as described by Wolf and Roth (1985). The slices were preloaded with [^{3}H]-dopamine and superfused with Krebs-Ringer buffer. Release was stimulated twice in each experiment via 30 sec superfusion with 30 mM K^+ (S1 and S2), and the radioactivity released was expressed as percent fractional release per fraction. Drugs were added prior to S2 (10-20 min), and results analysed using a ratio of peak area of radioactivity in S1/S2. Dopa accumulation was used as an index of tyrosine hydroxylation as described (Bannon, et al., 1981).

RESULTS

Characterization of PCM

PCM was purified from rat and bovine brain, and human erythrocyte using AdoHcy inhibitor chromatography. The protein patterns after 15% SDS-PAGE and immunoblotting with antiserum against bovine brain PCM are shown for the three types of the enzyme in Figure 1. Lane 2 is bovine brain cytosol protein which passed through a DEAE column, and lane 3 is the effluent of bovine brain cytosol protein from an AdoHcy column (post DEAE). Lane 4 shows rat brain PCM specifically eluted from an AdoHcy column before molecular sizing, while lane 6 is the same fraction following chromatography on BioGel P-30 to remove contaminants. Lanes 5 and 8 show purified bovine brain PCM, and lane 7 is human erythrocyte PCM. All forms exhibited slightly different molecular weights, suggesting subtle differences in

structure or posttranslational modification. All enzymes
were prepared from material which did not bind to DEAE (PCM
I; Aswad and Deight, 1983). Immunostaining of protein blots
revealed that antisera against bovine PCM crossreacted with
both rat brain and human erythrocyte forms of the enzyme;
this antiserum was used in subsequent immunochemical
studies. The antisera did not cross-react with bands in
crude fractionations of brain cytosol, as shown in Figure 2
(lanes 2 and 3); the antiserum did recognize bands which
comigrated with purified bovine PCM in these crude
preparations, however.

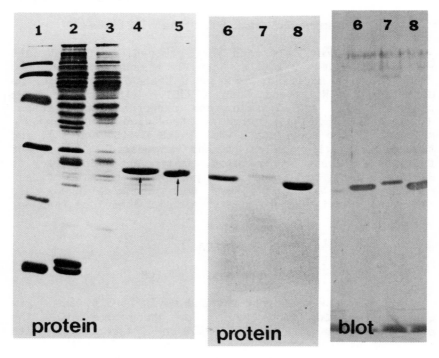

Figure 1: SDS-PAGE and Immunoblot of PCM: PCM was purified
from rat brain (lanes 4 and 6), bovine brain (lanes 5 and 8)
and human erythrocyte (lane 7) as described and following
electrophoresis, was electroblotted onto nitrocellulose and
reacted with antiserum against bovine brain PCM. lanes 2,
3-cytosolic protein effluent post DEAE chromatography and
post AdoHcy chromatography. Lane 1 = MW Stds (94,000;
67,000; 43,000; 30,000; 21,100; and 14,400 daltons).

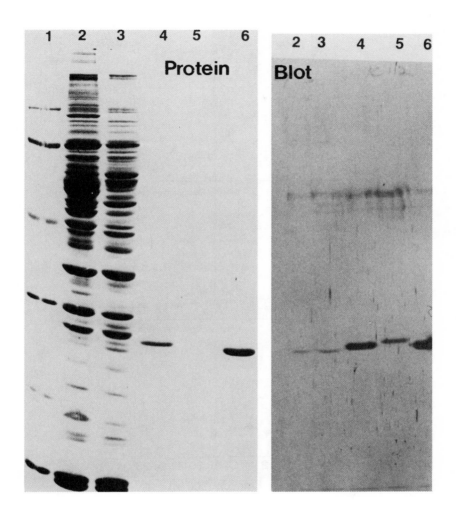

Figure 2: SDS-PAGE and Immunoblot of PCM: Following 12%
SDS-PAGE, crude bovine brain cytosol (lanes 2 and 3) was
electroblotted, and incubated with antiserum against bovine
brain PCM.   Lane 4 = rat brain PCM (4 μg), lane 5 =
humanerythrocyte PCM (0.5 μg), Lane 6 = bovine brain PCM (5
μg).   Lane 1 = MW Stds. as in Figure 1.

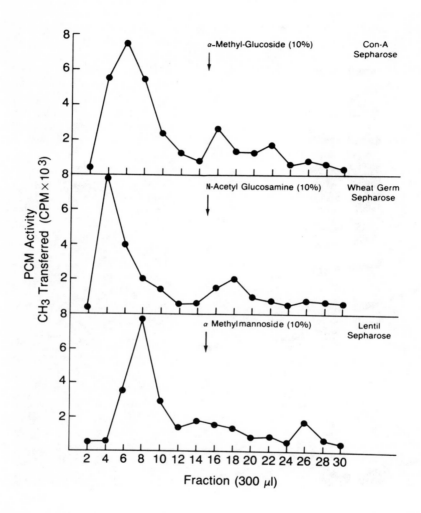

Figure 3: Lectin Chromatography of Bovine PCM: Purified bovine brain PCM (25 μg) in 20 mM Tris-acetate (pH 6.5) was applied lectin columns (2.0 ml bed volume), and washed with 6 ml of Tris-acetate buffer. Columns were eluted with 10% solutions of the listed sugar in Tris-acetate buffer. Fractions were collected and assayed for PCM activity using 5 μM ^{3}H-AdoMet and gelatin (25 mg/ml) as a substrate. Recovery of activity was constant for each column.

In order to determine if the differences in the apparent molecular weights of bovine, rat, and human PCM was the result of glycosylation, we chromatographed purified bovine PCM over various lectin columns which are specific for sugar residues. As can be seen in Figure 3, bovine brain PCM did not bind to concanavallin A- Wheat germ agglutin-, or lentil lectin-Sepharose, as determined by elution of the columns with either alpha-methylglucoside, N-acetyl glucosamine or alpha-methylmannoside. Other forms of the enzyme did not bind (data not presented), suggesting that differences in molecular weight may not be the result of differential glycosylation.

Carboxylmethylation of Calcineurin

We have previously observed that calmodulin binding proteins specifically eluted from calmodulin-Sepharose affinity resins were good substrates for protein methylation relative to calmodulin itself and cytosol (Billingsley, et al. 1984). Calcineurin is one of the more abundant calmodulin binding proteins in brain (Klee, et al., 1979). When purified calcineurin was carboxylmethylated, we found that at low concentrations of PCM, 30-40% of the calcineurin molecules were carboxylmethylated; this percentage of methylation could be increased by increasing the PCM concentrations, reaching a maximum of 2 mol CH_3/mol calcineurin (Billingsley, et al., 1985b). Acidic gel electrophoresis demonstrated that the majority of methylation occurred on the 61,000 dalton catalytic subunit, which binds calmodulin. We designed experiments to determine if the phosphatase activity of calcineurin was altered by prior carboxylmethylation. One such experiment is shown in Figure 4. Calcineurin phosphatase activity was stimulated 2.5 fold from basal (Mn^{+2}-supported) levels when 2.0 µM calmodulin was added in the absence of PCM; neither activity state was affected by either AdoHcy or Adomet alone. When calcineurin was carboxylmethylated by purified bovine brain PCM (6, 4, 2 and 1 µM), calmodulin stimulated, but not basal phosphatase activity was inhibited. The degree of inhibition was dependent on the concentration of PCM, which altered the stoichiometry of methylation (Figure 4). The stoichiometric determinations were made in parallel samples which were incubated with [^{3}H-methyl]-AdoMet and the standard components of the reaction. Since excess AdoHcy was present in the phosphatase assay, it is unlikely that calmodulin

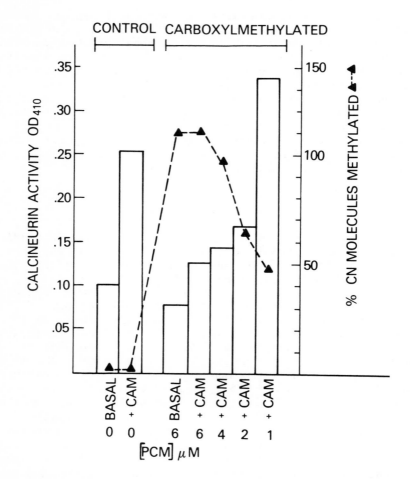

Figure 4:   Effects of Carboxylmethylation on Calcineurin:
Purified calcineurin was first incubated with or without
bovine brain PCM, and AdoMet.   All tubes received AdoHcy,
and phosphatase activity was determined using PNPP as a
substrate.   Open bars depict phosphatase activity, and the
triangles show the extent of carboxylmethylation in parallel
samples.

carboxylmethylation   significantly   contributed   to   the
observed inhibition of calmodulin-stimulated phosphatase
activity.

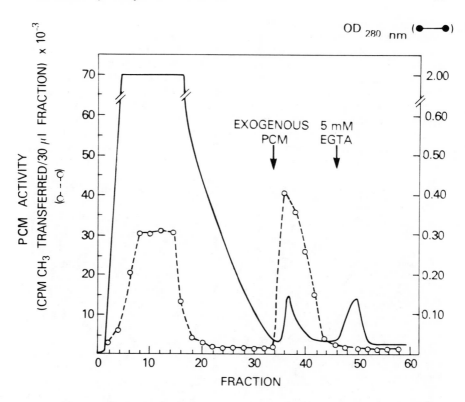

Figure 5: Lack of PCM binding to Calmodulin-Sepharose: Rat
brain cytosol was depleted of calmodulin and applied to a
calmodulin affinity column. Exogenous bovine brain PCM (50
μg) was loaded when most of the effluent (fractions 0-30)
was washed from the column. Calmodulin binding proteins
were eluted using 5 mM EGTA, and alternate fractions were
assayed for PCM activity.

     We investigated whether PCM activity would be retained
on either calmodulin-Sepharose or brain calmodulin binding
proteins immobilized on calmodulin-Sepharose. Rat brain
cytosol was depleted of calmodulin by phenothiazine affinity
chromatography.   The calmodulin-depleted cytosol was
chromatographed on calmodulin-Sepharose in the presence of
Ca^{+2}, and PCM activity and absorbance at 280 nm was
monitored (Figure 5).   After the majority of cytosolic
proteins passed through the calmodulin-Sepharose column,

exogenous bovine brain PCM was loaded onto the column which
contained calmodulin binding proteins.   The calmodulin
binding proteins were eluted with 5 mM EGTA. As can be seen
in Figure 6, endogenous rat brain PCM did not adsorb onto
either   calmodulin-Sepharose   (fractions   2-20)   or   onto
immobilized   calmodulin   binding   proteins.   Similarly,
exogenous   bovine   brain   PCM   did   not   adsorb   to   either
calmodulin-Sepharose   (fractions   34-42)   or   immobilized
calmodulin binding proteins (fractions 46-52), indicating
that, under these conditions, PCM does not bind to calmodulin or calmodulin binding proteins with high affinity.

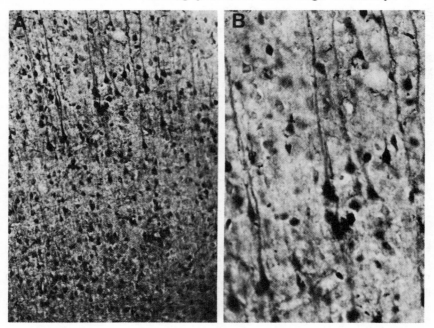

Figure 6: Immunoreactive PCM in Rat Cortex. Formalin-fixed
coronal brain slices were incubated with atiserum against
PCM, and stained as described.   Panel A - Cortical neurons
(200X); Panel B - cortical neurons and processess (400X).

Immunocytochemical Studies

    Antisera   against   bovine   brain   PCM   was   used   to
demonstrate that PCM is localized primarily in rat brain

neurons, and this is shown in Figure 6. Panels A and B show the patterns of PCM immunoreactivity in the cortex of the rat (layers 3-5), illustrating that PCM is found in neuronal cell bodies and processes.   Immunocytochemistry was also used to show that PCM and calcineurin (CN) are localized in similar populations of pyramidal neurons in the CA1 region of the hippocampus (Figure 7). Calcineurin immunoreactivity was   punctate   in   appearance,   and   appeared   to   be compartmentalized   in   the   cell   body;   some   staining   of dendrites was noted.   PCM immunoreactivity was concentrated over the cell body.   Thus, both PCM and calcineurin are localized in similar populations of neurons, but may be compartmentalized in different regions of the cell.

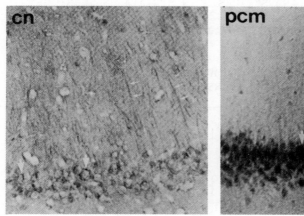
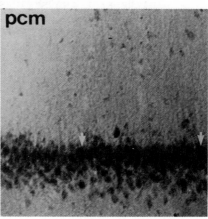

Figure   7:   Co-localization   of   PCM   and   Calcineurin: Immunocytochemical staining of hippocampal pyramidal cells for calcineurin (cn) and PCM.   large arrows depict pyramidal cell bodies in CA1 neurons, small arrows show dendritic staining with CN (400X).

Effects of PCM Inhibition on Dopamine Release and Synthesis

Superfusion of striatal slices with 30 mM K^+ released dopamine into the superfusate. When L-sulpiride, a dopamine antagonist, was added to the medium 10 min before a second stimulation, increases in both release of dopamine and accumulation of DOPA were observed (Table 1); addition of EMD 23 448, an autoreceptor agonist, decreased K^+-stimulated release of dopamine and DOPA accumulation. If PCM is involved in autoreceptor mediated inhibition of release and synthesis, then addition of PCM inhibitors should result in enhanced release of dopamine and accumulation of DOPA, similar to that seen with sulpiride. As is summarized in Table 1, 200 μM AdoHcy enhanced K^+-stimulated dopamine release, but did not enhance DOPA accumulation; this treatment results in 80% inhibition of methylester formation in striatal slices. Thus, PCM may be involved in the auto-receptor-mediated control of dopamine release in striatal slices.

TABLE 1

DA RELEASE AND SYNTHESIS IN STRIATAL SLICES:

MODULATION BY AGONISTS, ANTAGONISTS, AND PCM INHIBITORS

TREATMENT	K^+-STIMULATED ^{3}H-DA RELEASE	K^+-STIMULATED DOPA ACCUMULATION
1. SULPIRIDE (DA ANTAGONIST)	↑ ↑	↑ ↑
2. EMD 23 448 (AUTORECEPTOR-SPECIFIC DA AGONIST)	↓ ↓	↓ ↓
3. S-ADENOSYLHOMOCYSTEINE (METHYLTRANSFERASE INHIBITOR)	↑ ↑	NO CHANGE

Table 1: Summary of effects of dopamine (DA) agonist, antagonist, and PCM inhibitors on the release and synthesis of dopamine in striatal slices.

DISCUSSION

The results presented in this manuscript have suggested possible functions for PCM in the nervous system. More conclusive proof is needed to firmly establish such a role, however. The specific cellular localization of PCM in neurons, and the fact that regions such as the substantia nigra, locus coeruleus, and paraventricular neucleus have particularly high levels of PCM (Billingsley and Balaban, 1985) is consistent with the concept that PCM plays an important role in these brain regions. The relative paucity of the enzyme in glial cells, particularly oligodendrocytes, is not consistent with the idea that PCM is exclusively a repair enzyme, since myelin, a relatively long-lived protein is made by oligodendrocytes and all cells would be expected to have need for repair of damaged proteins. It is possible that an isozymic form of PCM is responsible for repair functions, however (Aswad and Deight, 1984; O'Connor, et al., 1984).

Calcineurin, a potentially important protein phosphatase (Stewart, et al., 1982) was found to be a good substrate for PCM in vitro, exhibiting stoichiometric incorporation of methyl groups consistent with a regulatory function. When calcineurin was carboxylmethylated to the extent of 1 mol CH_3/mol, calmodulin-stimulated, but not basal phosphatase activity was inhibited. This suggests that PCM may regulate the calmodulin-stimulated activation of this enzyme. Immunocytochemical studies have indicated that calcineurin and PCM are co-localized in similar populations of neurons, but that they may be compartmentalized in different subcellular regions. We need to conclusively demonstrate that calcineurin can be carboxylmethylated in vivo, and are attempting to use high performance chromatography to rapidly isolate calmodulin binding proteins to avoid the decay of labile methylesters. It is possible that the carboxylmethylation of calcineurin is occurring on a unique residue which resembles either an isoaspartyl or a racemized asparate (Aswad, 1984; Murray and Clarke, 1984; O'Connor, et al., 1984). Since the sequence of calcineurin is not known, this speculation remains a possibility.

Studies using purified PCM from human, rat and bovine sources have shown that although subtle differences in molecular weight exist between species, all forms share common antigenic determinants which allow for antibody recognition after SDS-PAGE and protein immunoblotting. Immunoblot studies also indicated that the antiserum against PCM did not show significant cross-reactivity with other brain cytosol proteins. When lectin columns were used to characterize potential glycosylation residues, we found that purified bovine brain PCM did not bind to any of the lectins, suggesting that alpha mannosides or N-acetylglucosamine-type residues were not a part of the molecule. Polastro and coworkers (1978) reported that equine erythrocyte PCM contained significant amounts (6%) of normal hexose sugars; thus there may be species and tissue-specific alterations in glycosylation.

Finally, in striatal slice preparations, treatment with AdoHcy resulted in a decreased rate of K^+-stimulated release of dopamine, but the same treatment did not affect DOPA accumulation, which is a measure of tyrosine hydroxylation in situ. It is possible that AdoHcy inhibited other methylation systems which lead to the enhanced dopamine release, since there is no specific inhibitor of PCM. However, previous studies on striatal slices suggested that dopamine autoreceptor agonists, which inhibit dopamine release (Roth, 1984), can increase methylester formation in striatal slices (Wolf and Roth, 1985). In addition, pretreatment of rats with 6-hydroxydopamine, a neurotoxin which destroys the nigrostriatal dopamine tract, inhibited the effects of dopamine autoreceptor agonists. Interestingly, we have found that PCM and calcineurin immunoreactivity is high in nigrostriatal neurons, again supportive of a role for PCM in these neurons. Future studies using paradigms which allow the simultaneous determination of functional methylation of a given tissue substrate and alteration in tissue function may clarify the regulatory potential of thie enigmatic enzyme.

REFERENCES

Aswad, D.W. and Deight, E.A. (1983) J. Neurochem. 40, 1718-1726.
Aswad, D.W. (1984) J. Biol. Chem. 259, 10714-10721.
Bradford, M.G. (1976) Analyt. Biochem. 42, 248-254.
Bannon, M.J., Michaud, R.L., and Roth, R.H. (1981) Mol. Pharmacol. 19, 270-275.
Billingsley, M.L., Kuhn, D.M., Velletri, P.A., Kincaid, R.L., and Lovenberg, W. (1984) J. Biol. Chem. 259, 6630-6635.
Billingsley, M.L., and Lovenberg, W. (1985) Neurochem. Int. (in press).
Billingsley, M.L., Kim, S., and Kuhn, D.M. (1985a) Neuroscience 15, 159-171.

Billingsley, M.L., and Balaban, C.D. (1985) Brain Res. (in press).

Billingsley, M.L., Kincaid, R.L., and Kuhn, D.M. (1985b) Proc. Natl. Acad. Sci. USA (in press).

Gagnon, C. (1983) Can. J. Biochem. Cell Biol., 61, 921-926.

Kim, S., Nochimson, S., Chin, W., and Paik, W.K. (1978) Analyt. Biochem. 84, 415-422.

Kincaid, R.L., and Vaughan, M. (1979) Proc. Natl. Acad. Sci. USA, 76, 4903-4907.

Kincaid, R.L., Manganiello, V.C., Odya, C.E., Osbourne, J.C. Jr., Sitth-Coleman, I.E., Daniello, M.A., and Vaughan, M. (1984) J. Biol. Chem. 259, 5150-5166.

Kincaid, R.L., Balaban, C.D., and Billingsley, M.L. (1985) Fed. Proc. 44, 697.

Klee, C.B., Crouch, T.H., and Krinks, M.H. (1979) Proc. Natl. Acad. Sci. USA 76, 6270-6273.

McFadden, P.N., and Clarke, S. (1982) Proc. Natl. Acad. Sci. USA, 79, 2460-2464.

Murray, E.D., and Clarke, S. (1984) J. Biol. Chem., 259, 10722-10732.

O'Connor, C.M., Aswad, D.W., and Clarke, S.E. (1984) Proc. Natl. Acad. Sci. USA

Pallen, C.J., and Wang, J.H. (1983) J. Biol. Chem. 258, 8550-8553.

Stewart, A.A., Ingebritsen, T.S., Manalan, A., Klee, C.B., and Cohen, P. (1982) FEBS Lett. 137, 80-84.

Terwilliger, T.C., and Clarke, S. (1981) J. Biol. Chem. 256, 3067-3076.

Towbin, H., Staehlin, T. and Gordon, J. (1979) Proc. Natl. Acad. Sci. USA, 76, 4350-4354.

Wolf, M.E., and Roth, R.H. 91985) J. Neurochem. 44, 291-298.

METHYL-ACCEPTING CHEMOTAXIS PROTEINS IN BACTERIA

Gerald L. Hazelbauer*[†] , John Bollinger*,
Chankyu Park[†], Dawn Nowlin* and Maqsudul Alam*

Biochemistry/Biophysics Program* and Program
in Genetics and Cell Biology[†], Washington
State University, Pullman, WA 99164-4660

The sensory transducers of Escherichia coli and
Salmonella typhimurium are the most extensively
characterized of any methyl-accepting proteins. Their
functions as central components in the chemotactic system
of these species have been well defined and recent work has
provided substantial information about structure of the
proteins. In this report, we review current understanding
of methyl-accepting transducer proteins, discuss evidence
that homologous proteins occur throughout the entire
spectrum of bacterial species, and consider specific
mutational alterations that affect covalent modification of
transducers.

FUNCTION AND STRUCTURE OF TRANSDUCER PROTEINS

Current understanding of bacterial chemotaxis is
the result of work from a number of laboratories. References
to the original publications can be found in Springer, et
al. (1979), Koshland (1981), Boyd and Simon (1982) and
Hazelbauer and Harayama (1983). Only references not
contained in those reviews will be cited.

An E. coli cell makes net progress along chemical
gradients by biasing a random walk consisting of straight-
line, smooth swimming punctuated by episodes of
uncoordination, called tumbles, that reorient the cell in a

new direction.   The cell continually monitors the
concentration of certain chemicals in its environment and
compares those values to records of the concentration a few
seconds previously. A difference between a past and current
value results in the appropriate bias by altering the
balance between counterclockwise and clockwise rotation of
the bacterial flagella, corresponding to smooth swimming and
tumbling, respectively.   Thus E. coli has a rudimentary
"memory" system of information storage and processing.
Information about past concentrations appears to be stored
in covalent modifications of transmembrane receptor
proteins, called transducers.   In an unchanging chemical
environment, the degree to which a receptor site is occupied
is reflected in the extent of carboxyl methylation of
several, specific glutamyl residues in the transducer.   An
increase or decrease in the concentration of an attractant
compound results almost immediately in a corresponding
change in occupancy of the binding site.   In contrast, the
linked increase or decrease in methylation, catalyzed by a
specific methyl transferase or a specific demethylase,
respectively, is relatively slow.   Both binding site
occupancy and methylation affect the excitatory domain of a
transducer protein.   This domain initiates a signal along an
excitatory pathway linking transducers to flagellar motors.
The nature of the pathway is unknown, but appears to involve
diffusion of protein-sized molecules through the cytoplasm
(Segall et al., 1985). The relatively slow rates of covalent
modification mean that in a changing chemical environment
the extent of transducer methylation does not correspond to
the current level of ligand binding but instead to the level
just previous; hence, the extent of methylation is a record
of a past chemical environment. When the level of ligand
binding and the extent of methylation are unbalanced, i.e.,
the current and past environments differ, the excitatory
domain is induced to send the appropriate excitatory signal.
However, the extent of modification is gradually adjusted to
balance binding site occupancy. When the balance is achieved
no further excitatory signal is generated and the
unstimulated behavioral pattern is restored; hence, E. coli,
like most other sensory cells, adapts to the continued
presence of stimulation.

        There are four different transducers in E. coli.   The
nucleotide sequences of the corresponding genes and the
respective deduced amino acid sequences (Boyd et al., 1983;
Krikos et al., 1983; Russo and Koshland, 1983; Bollinger et

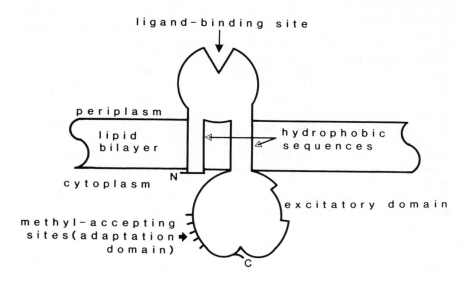

Figure 1.   Model for Disposition of Transducer Domains
Across the Cytoplasmic Membrane

al., 1984) reveal a transducer gene family that codes for
four homologous proteins all of approximately 60,000
daltons.   The Tsr transducer binds serine and the Tar
protein recognizes aspartate.   In addition, Tar also
interacts with ligand-occupied, maltose-binding protein.
Galactose- and ribose-binding proteins are linked in an
analogous manner to the Trg transducer.   No ligand has yet
been identified for the fourth transducer, Tap (Parkinson
et al., 1983).   A number of lines of genetic and biochemical evidence lend strong support to a simple model for
disposition of the transducer protein across the cytoplasmic
membrane (Fig. 1).   The model suggests that the protein
spans the membrane twice, once with a short, hydrophobic
sequence near the amino-terminus and again with a short,
hydrophobic stretch 40% of the way along the polypeptide
chain.   This places an amino-terminal, ligand-binding domain
on the extra-cytoplasmic face of the membrane and a
carboxy-terminal, covalent modification domain on the
cytoplasmic face.   The specific methyl-accepting glutamyl
residues have been located in two clusters.   Three or four
sites (depending on the protein) in a region just past the

middle of the protein and one or two sites in a region close
to the carboxy-terminus (Kehry and Dahlquist, 1982a, b;
Terwilliger et al., 1983; Terwilliger and Koshland, 1984).
One or two of the glutamyl residues in the first region
(again depending on the specific protein) are the result of
hydrolysis of the NH_2 moiety of a glutaminyl residue (a
reaction we will call amidolysis) to create a carboxyl group
that subsequently serves as a methyl-accepting site (Kehry
et al., 1983, Terwilliger and Koshland, 1984). The reaction
is catalyzed by the CheB demethylase and the rate of
reaction is influenced by tactic stimuli in the same way as
demethylation. The basis for this unusual sequence of
events may be a requirement that newly synthesized
transducers contain a balance at their modification sites
between negative charge and neutral residues so that the
modification domain is not at one extreme of its signaling
spectrum.

TRANSDUCER PROTEINS OCCUR THROUGHOUT THE BACTERIAL KINDGOMS

        Methyl-accepting proteins have been identified in a
number of bacterial species in addition to the enterics as
components of the respective sensory systems (see Nowlin et
al., 1985 for references). We have shown that methyl-
accepting chemotaxis proteins of Bacillus subtilis and of
Spirochaeta aurantia exhibit distinct homologies with the
transducers of E. coli (Nowlin et al., 1985). The
experiments involved direct immunoprecipitation of methyl-
^{3}H-labeled proteins from those species by antiserum raised
to a transducer from E. coli as well as comparison of
methylated tryptic peptides by high-pressure liquid chromatography. The observations imply that methyl-accepting
proteins in the three contemporary species were derived from
a protein that was contained in the common ancestor of these
distantly related bacteria. A scheme of bacterial evolution
based on analysis of ribosomal RNA (Fox et al, 1980;
Stackebrandt and Woese, 1982) identifies those species as
representatives of three of eight major lines of decent for
what are termed eubacteria (essentially all conventional
bacterial species, see below). Divergence of these major
groups is estimated to have occurred 3.5 to 3.8 billion
years ago (Stackebrandt and Woese, 1982). Thus methyl-
accepting transducers have ancient origins and we predicted
that the sensory systems of all flagellated eubacteria would
include homologous methyl-accepting proteins.

We have begun to test this prediction by examining a variety of bacterial species for proteins that are recognized by antibodies in our anti-transducer serum. Using immunoblotting techniques for cellular proteins displayed by SDS-polyacrylamide gel electrophoresis and signal amplification provided by biotinylated second antibody combined with an avidin:biotinylated horseradish peroxidase complex, we have found specific polypeptide bands that react with the anti-transducer serum in a number of species, including Salmonella typhimurium, Proteus vulgaris, Chromatium vinosum, S. aurantia and Halobacterium halobium. These clusters of multiple bands are in the range of 60 to 115 kilodaltons. In E. coli the multiplicity of transducer bands is due to both the several different gene products and the alteration in electrophoretic mobility of a single type of polypeptide chain that occurs upon covalent modification. We expect that the presence of multiple antibody-reactive bands in other species reflects both factors. For S. aurantia, the reactive bands correspond to the homologous methyl-accepting proteins (Kathariou and Greenberg, 1983) as demonstrated by our previous work (Nowlin et al., 1985). For S. typhimurium, homology with methyl-accepting protein of E. coli has already been well-documented, even at the level of deduced amino acid sequences (Russo and Koshland, 1983). For P. vulgaris and C. vinosum methyl-accepting chemotaxis proteins have not yet been described but it seems quite likely that the polypeptides visible are in fact methyl-accepting transducer proteins of the respective species. Of particular interest is Halobacterium halobium. This species is a member of an unusual group of organisms termed archaebacteria (Fox et al., 1980) that are distinctly different from all other bacteria and thus appear to represent a very early evolutionary divergence. In fact, analysis of rRNA suggests that three lines of descent emerged from the common ancestor of all living organisms (Fox et al., 1980). These lines are represented today by eukaryotic cells (minus colonizing organelles), by conventional bacteria (eubacteria) and by archaebacteria. Preliminary reports provided evidence for methyl-accepting chemotaxis proteins in H. halobium (Schimz, 1981). Intensive study of these proteins is in progress in our laboratory, and parallels with transducers in the enterics is striking (M. Alam, unpublished results). Methyl-accepting proteins in H. halobium appear on an SDS-polyacrylamide gel as two series of methyl-^{3}H-labeled bonds, one with apparent molecular weights in the range of 90,000 to 110,000 and the other in the region of 25,000. The relationship of these polypeptides to bands stained by anti-transducer antibody is not yet clear. If components related to methyl-accepting transducer proteins were present in H. halobium it would then appear that homologous proteins existed in the common ancestor to all living things. The related implication, that homologous proteins could exist in contemporary eukaryotes is being investigated.

MUTATIONS THAT ALTER TRANSDUCER MODIFICATION

Transducers perform several distinct functions. They bind ligands, transduce informational signals across the membrane, serve as substrates for covalent modification, and detect temporal gradients by comparing the degree of ligand occupancy to the extent of modification. We would like to relate these various functions to distinct domains, regions and residues within the structure of a transducer molecule. With this goal in mind, we are isolating transducer mutants that are defective in only a subset of transducer functions. We hope that characterization of the mutations found in such strains will allow dissection of the complexities of transducer structure and function.

MUTATIONS AT A METHYL-ACCEPTING SITE

We have utilized synthetic oligonucleotides to introduce single base changes into the codon corresponding to a methyl-accepting glutamyl residue of the Trg transducer protein of E. coli. The residue, Glu-509, is near the end of the 535 amino acid protein (Bollinger et al., 1984). Substitution of an alanine at position 509, thus eliminating the possibility of carboxyl methylation at that single site, has a subtle but significant effect on Trg-mediated tactic response to ribose. As shown in Table 1, a cell containing the mutant protein required a longer time to adapt to a saturating stimulus of the Trg-linked attractant, as if elimination of one potential methyl-accepting site has reduced the concentration of "substrate" for the enzymatic methylation reaction and thus reduced the apparent velocity of adaptation. Substitution of a glutamine or an aspartate at position 509 had no significant effect on adaptative behavior, nor on the pattern of methyl-^{3}H-labeled bands of Trg viewed after fluorography of SDS-polyacrylamide gels.

Preliminary characterization of the tryptic peptide containing residue 509 by high-pressure liquid chromatography is consistent with the conclusions that the substituted gln-509 undergoes amidolysis to yield a methyl-accepting glutamyl residue and that asp-509 can serve, at least to some extent, as a methyl-accepting residue. Experiments in progress will establish the validity of these possibilities. The observations are particularly interesting because they imply that the specificity of both the CheR methyltransferase and the CheB demethylase/amidehydrolase is determined to a substantial extent by groups other than the residue actually modified.

A MUTATION WITH COPY NUMBER-DEPENDENT DOMINANCE

We have been studying trg mutations, induced by random mutagenesis, that eliminate some, but not all, Trg functions with the hope of identifying parts of the protein that are crucial for specific transducer functions. One mutation, trg-21, confers a tactic phenotype that varies with the number of gene copies in the cell. A single copy of the mutant gene in place of the normal chromosomal copy creates a cell that has a reduced ability to respond to stimuli of ribose or galactose yet is otherwise normal in swimming behavior and tactic response to other attractants. Addition of a wild-type version of trg elsewhere on the chromosome restores normal response to the sugars. Thus, when present on the chromosome, trg-21 has the properties of

TABLE 1.   Effect of Amino Acid Substitution at Methyl-
           Accepting Site Glu-509 on Tactic Behavior[1]

Residue Position 509	Adaptation Time after 1mM Ribose Stimulus (sec.)
Glu (wild-type)	52 ± 7[2]
Ala	74 ± 18
Gln	48 ± 8
Asp	48 ± 10

1. Cells contained a single chromosomal copy of wild-type or mutant trg.
2. Values are averages of at least 20 cells with standard deviations indicated.

a leaky, recessive mutation. In striking contrast, amplification of the number of cellular copies of trg-21 results in a pervasive defect in tactic behavior. Otherwise wild-type cells that harbor a multicopy pUC13-trg-21 almost never tumble and thus are defective in chemotaxis to all compounds. This means that amplification of trg-21 creates a dominant, chemotaxis-negative phenotype. The cell can no longer respond appropriately to external chemical signals because the flagellar "gearshift" has been pushed far to the counterclockwise mode. This pattern has interesting parallels in the changes correlated with transformation of eukaryotic cells to neoplastic growth. Both specific mutations and gene amplification have been implicated in oncogenesis (Bishop, 1983) and some oncogenes code for proteins homologous to cell surface receptors (Heldin and Westermark, 1984). Transformed cells no longer respond to extracellular signals that normally limit growth and are locked into a mode of ceaseless division. E. coli cells containing multiple copies of trg-21 are unable to respond to chemical stimuli because their flagella are locked in a single direction of rotation.

Both eukaryotic receptors related to products of oncogenes and bacterial transducers are covalently modified at residues in a cytoplasmic domain. Thus, it is particularly interesting that the Trg-21 protein is defective in covalent modification. Two methyl-accepting sites on Trg are the result of amidolysis to create glutamyl from glutaminyl residues. That modification is essentially absent from the Trg-21 protein and thus two methyl-accepting sites are eliminated. It is not clear whether this defect is the cause or effect of the dominant, chemotaxis-negative phenotype. In any case methylation and demethylation at the remaining available sites is not substantially affected.

The trg-21 mutation substitutes threonine for alanine-419 in the transducer protein. This residue is in a part of the cytoplasmic domain, midway between the separate methyl-accepting regions, that is highly conserved among all four transducers of E. coli. All these proteins contain an alanine at this position. Replacement by threonine has profound effects since distant sites of covalent modification are blocked and the overall behavioral balance of the cell is deranged. It is plausible that the mutant defect is in some aspect of the signaling domain or of the linkage between the adaptation and signaling domains. This implies that the highly conserved region within which the mutational change occurs is involved in excitatory signaling to the flagella. Dominant, chemotaxis-negative mutations also occur in the tsr gene (Callahan and Parkinson, 1985). These mutations, called cheD, eliminate tumbling. However, no affect on amidolysis is apparent but instead, demethylation activity is greatly reduced (Kehry, et al., 1985). It may be that CheD proteins are permanently locked in a positive excitatory mode while the Trg-21 protein is incapable of attaining a negative excitatory mode.

CONCLUSIONS

As primary structures of more and more receptor proteins are deduced from nucleotide sequences, a few common structural motifs have emerged. One class of receptors, including bacterial transducers and eukaryotic receptors for insulin, epidermal growth factor and other polypeptide hormones (Heldin and Westermark, 1984; Ebina et al., 1985) appears to be organized with two large domains, one extra-cytoplasmic and the other cytoplasmic, connected by a short stretch of membrane spanning sequence. Ligand binding at the extra-cytoplasmic domain results in signal generation and covalent modification at the cytoplasmic domain. The issue of how information is transferred within the proteins and across the membranes is not yet resolved. The study of bacterial transducers promises to contribute to the resolution. It is particularly interesting, in light of data discussed here, that the detailed knowledge gained about the sensory transducers of E. coli will be directly applicable to the understanding of homologous components of sensory systems throughout the diversity of bacterial species.

ACKNOWLEDGEMENTS

Unpublished work cited here was supported by grants to GLH from the U.S. Public Health Service (GM-29863) and the McKnight Foundation.

REFERENCES

Bishop, J. M. (1983) Cell 32, 1018-1020.

Bollinger, J., Park, C., Harayama, S. and   Hazelbauer, G.
L. (1984) Proc. Natl. Acad. Sci. U.S.A. 81,
3287-3291.

Boyd, A. and Simon, M. I. (1982) Annu. Rev. Physiol. 44,
501-517.

Boyd, A., Kendall, K. and Simon, M. I. (1983) Nature
(London) 301, 623-625.

Callahan, A. M., and Parkinson, J. S. (1985) J. Bacteriol.
162, 96-104.

Ebina, Y., Ellis, L., Jarnagin, K., Edery, M., Graf, L.,
Clauser, E., Ou, J., Masiarz, F., Kan, Y. W., Goldfine, I.
D., Roth, R. A. and Rutter, W. J. (1985) Cell 40,
747-758.

Fox, G. ., Stackebrandt, E., Hespell, R. B., Gibson, J.,
Moniloff, J., Dyer, T. A.,, Wolfe, R. S., Balch, W. E.,
Tanner, R. S., Magrum, L. J., Zablen, L. B., Blakemore,
R.,Gupta, R., Bonen, L., Lewis, B. J., Stahl, D. A.,
Luehrsen, K. R., Chen, K. N. and Woese, C. R. (1980)
Science. 209, 457-463.

Hazelbauer, G. L. and Harayama, S. (1983) Int. Rev. Cytol.
81, 33-70.

Heldin, C. H. and Westermark, B. (1984) Cell 37, 9-20.

Kathariou, S. and Greenberg, E. P. (1983) J. Bacteriol. 156,
95-100.

Kehry, M. R. and Dahlquist, F. W. (1982a) Cell 29, 761-772.

Kehry, M. R. and Dahlquist, F. W. (1982b) J. Biol. Chem 257,
10378-10386.

Kehry, M. R., Bond, M. W., Hunkapiller, M. W. and Dahlquist,
F. W. (1983) Proc. Natl. Acad. Sci. USA 80, 3599-3603.

Kehry, M. R., Doak, T. G. and Dahlquist, F. W. (1985) J. Bacteriol. 161, 105-112.

Koshland, D. E., Jr. (1981) Annu. Rev. Biochem. 50, 765-782.

Krikos, A., Mutoh, N., Boyd, A. and Simon, M. I. (1983). Cell 33, 615-622.

Nowlin, D. M., Nettleton, D. O., Ordal, G. W. and Hazelbauer, G. L. (1985) J. Bacteriol. 163, in press.

Parkinson, J. S., Slocum, M. K., Callahan, A. M., Sherris, D. and Houts, S. E. (1983) in Mobility and Recognition in Cell Biology (Sund, H. and Veeger, C., Eds.) pp. 563-576, Walter de Gruyter and Co., Berlin.

Russo, A. F. and Koshland, D. E., Jr. (1983) Science 220, 1016-1020.

Schimz, A (1981) FEBS Letts. 125, 205-207.

Segall, J. A. Ishihara, A. and Berg, H. C. (1985) J. Bacteriol. 161, 51-59.

Springer, M. S., Goy, M. F. and Adler, J. (1979) Nature London 208, 2799-284.

Stackebrandt, E. and Woese, C. R. (1982) Molecular and Cellular Aspects of Microbial Evolution. (Carlile, M. J., Collins, J. F. and Moseley, B. E. B., Eds.) pp. 1-30. Cambridge U. Press, Cambridge.

Terwilliger, T. C. and Koshland, D. E., Jr. (1984) J. Biol. Chem. 259, 7719-7725.

Terwilliger, T. C., Bogonez, E., Wang, E. A. and Koshland, D. E., Jr. (1983) J. Biol. Chem. 258, 9608-9611.

BIOCHEMISTRY OF METHYLATED PHOSPHOLIPIDS

Jon Bremer, Kaare Norum and Pål Bjørnstad

Institute of Medical Biochemistry

University of Oslo, Oslo, Norway

Methylated phospholipids are widespread in nature, both in microorganisms, plants, and animals. The quantitative most important and widespread ones are phosphatidylcholine and sphingomyeline which contain phosphorycholine. However, a series of other methylated phospholipids have been detected in less commonly analyzed microorganisms, sea animals, and insects. The biosynthesis and breakdown of the choline-containing phospholipids have been extensively investigated while less is known about the metabolism of the other methylated phospholipids. In the following we will give a short surway on the less common methylated phospholipids followed by a discussion of the biosynthesis of phosphatidylcholine by the methylation of phosphatidylethanolamine.

UNCOMMON METHYLATED PHOSPHOLIPIDS

Fig. 1 shows the structure of methylated phospholipids isolated from different organisms.
Phosphatidylmethylcholine. Methylcholine ((+)trimethylaminoisopropanol) has been detected in the phospholipids of some choline-requiring insect larvae (housfly and blowfly) when they are reared on a choline-free diet supplied with methylcholine, trimethylaminoacetone, carnitine or γ-

55

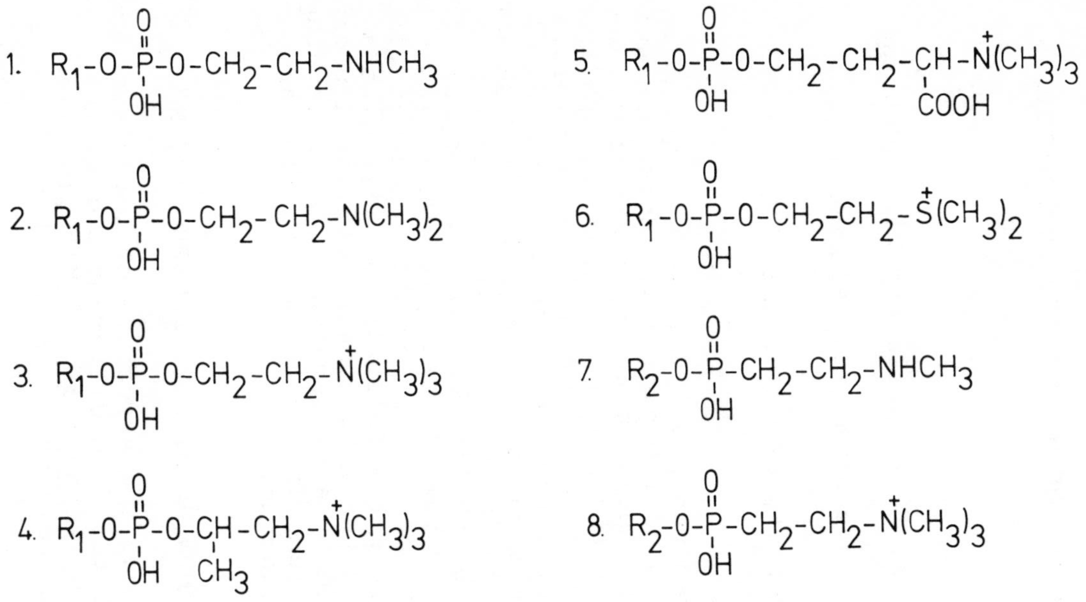

1. $R_1-O-\overset{\overset{O}{\parallel}}{\underset{\underset{OH}{\mid}}{P}}-O-CH_2-CH_2-NHCH_3$

2. $R_1-O-\overset{\overset{O}{\parallel}}{\underset{\underset{OH}{\mid}}{P}}-O-CH_2-CH_2-N(CH_3)_2$

3. $R_1-O-\overset{\overset{O}{\parallel}}{\underset{\underset{OH}{\mid}}{P}}-O-CH_2-CH_2-\overset{+}{N}(CH_3)_3$

4. $R_1-O-\overset{\overset{O}{\parallel}}{\underset{\underset{OH}{\mid}}{P}}-O-CH-CH_2-\overset{+}{N}(CH_3)_3$
   $\qquad\qquad\quad \overset{\mid}{CH_3}$

5. $R_1-O-\overset{\overset{O}{\parallel}}{\underset{\underset{OH}{\mid}}{P}}-O-CH_2-CH_2-CH-\overset{+}{N}(CH_3)_3$
   $\qquad\qquad\qquad\qquad\quad \overset{\mid}{COOH}$

6. $R_1-O-\overset{\overset{O}{\parallel}}{\underset{\underset{OH}{\mid}}{P}}-O-CH_2-CH_2-\overset{+}{S}(CH_3)_2$

7. $R_2-O-\overset{\overset{O}{\parallel}}{\underset{\underset{OH}{\mid}}{P}}-CH_2-CH_2-NHCH_3$

8. $R_2-O-\overset{\overset{O}{\parallel}}{\underset{\underset{OH}{\mid}}{P}}-CH_2-CH_2-\overset{+}{N}(CH_3)_3$

Fig. 1. Methylated phospholipids isolated from different organisms.
1) Phosphatidyl-(N-methyl)ethanolamine; 2) Phosphatidyl-(N-dimethyl)-
ethanolamine; 3) Phosphatidylcholine; 4) Phosphatidylmethylcholine;
5) Phosphatidyl-O-(N-trimethyl)homoserine; 6) Phosphatidyl-O-(S-dimethyl)-
mercaptoethanol; 7) Ceramide-(N-methyl)aminoethylphosphonate; 8) Ceramide-
(N-trimethyl)aminoethylphosphonate. (R_1= phosphatidyl-, R_2= ceramide)

butyrobetaine (Bieber et al. 1969). Both (+)- and
(-)carnitine are converted to (+)methylcholine.
It is likely therefore that both optical isomers
of carnitine is dehydrogenated to dehydrocarnitine
followed by decarboxylation to trimethylaminoacetone which is reduced to (+)methylcholine.

Phosphatidyl-0-(N-trimethyl)homoserine. This
trimethylamino acid has been detected in the phospholipids of some algae, a phytoflagellate, and a
pathogenic fungus (Evans et al. 1982). It is speculated that this phospholipid has a function in
photosynthesis. No studies on its biosynthesis
have appeared.

Phosphatidylsulfocholine. This sulfonium
analog (phosphatidyl-0-(S-dimethyl)mercaptoetha-
nol) of phosphatidylcholine is the major phospholipid of a marine diatome (Nitzschia alba). This
organism contains no nitrogenous base-containing
lipids (Anderson et al. 1979). Both the sulfur
and the methyl groups of this unusual phospholipid
are derived from methionine, possibly with dime-
thyl-β-propiothetine as an intermediate, but the
details of the biosynthetic pathway has not been
elucidated.

N-methylated aminoethylphosphono sphingolipids.
Phospholipids containing 2-aminoethylphosphonic
acid are relatively widespread in microorganisms
(Tetrahymena and rumen bacteria) and in many sea
animals. Both diacylglycerol- and ceramid derivatives are found. The corresponding N-methylated
ceramid aminoethylphosphonates have been isolated
from sea animals (Kittredge 1967, Hayashi et al.
1969) and Tetrahymena pyriformis (Viswanathan and
Rosenberg 1973). The corresponding diacylglycerol
derivatives have not been found. The biosynthetic
pathway for the methylated derivatives is not
known. The trimethylaminoethylphosphonic acid can
be incorporated into the phospholipids of housfly
larvae (Bieber 1968) and in the rat (Bjerve 1972),
although much more slowly than phosphorylcholine.
The cytidine monophosphate derivative seems to be
an intermediate in this incorporation.

METHYLATION OF PHOSPHATIDYLETHANOLAMINE

Lecithin (phosphatidylcholine) is synthesized either from preformed choline (Kennedy and Weiss 1956) or by methylation of phosphatidylethanolamine (Bremer et al. 1960). Both pathways are widespread in microorganisms, plants (Willemot and Boll 1967), and animals (Pelech and Vance 1984). Only the methylation pathway has been found in bacteria (Kaneshiro and Law 1964). Beside being a pathway of lecithin synthesis methylation of phosphatidylethanolamine represents the only known mechanism for the biosynthesis of choline. Reincorporation of choline into phospholipids therefore represents a salvage pathway for choline, although in most organisms and tissues this reincorporation is quantitatively the more important mechanism for lecithin synthesis. In the larvae of some insects (housfly, blowfly) the methylation pathway seems to be absent (Bieber and Newburg 1963).

In most organisms only minute amounts of the mono- and dimethylphosphatidylethanolamine are found as intermediates in the biosynthesis of lecithin. However, in clostridium strains (Goldfine 1962, Johnson and Goldfine 1983) and in a mutant strain of Neurospora crassa (Scarborough and Nyc 1967) the monomethyl derivative is the end product of the methylation.

It is still discussed whether more than one enzyme take part in the incorporation of the three methyl groups of lecithin. In Agrobacterium tumefaciens the methylating system has been separated in a partially purified soluble enzyme incorporating only the first methyl group, and a particulate system which incorporates all three methyl groups (Kaneshiro and Law 1964). This observation and the studies on mutants of Neurospora crassa (Scarborough and Nyc 1967) and saccharomyces cerevisiae (Yamashita et al. 1982) suggest that at least two enzymes coded for by two different genes are involved in the methylation of phosphatidylethanolamine in microorganisms. However, in animal preparations no such separation of enzyme activities have been obtained (Mato et al. 1984).

Methylation in Animals and Man

   The synthesis of lecithin by methylation is
localized mainly in the liver where about 20% of
the total lecithin synthesis takes place by
methylation of phosphatidylethanolamine in the
female rat and about half as much in the male rat
(Bjørnstad and Bremer 1966, Lyman et al. 1967).
However, the methylation pathway is present in
most animal tissues, but it is usually of minor
quantitative importance.
   In the liver it is mainly polyunsaturated
phosphatidylethanolamines which are methylated
while preformed choline is incorporated mainly
into mono- and diene phosphatidylcholines
(Arvidson 1968). Both pathways are localized in
the endoplasmetic reticulum. It is no major difference in the fate of the lecithins formed by
the two pathways. Both mitochondrial lecithin and
plasma lipoproteins are rapidly labeled by both
pathways (Bjørnstad and Bremer 1966) as is bile
lecithin, although lecithin formed from free
choline is preferentially excreted in the bile
when compared with lecithin formed by methylation
(Balint et al. 1967). Thus, lecithins formed by
the two pathways seem to behave essentially as
one pool, at least they are relatively rapidly
equilibrated. Thus, in the rat the specific activity of plasma lecithin reaches about 80% of the
specific activity of liver lecithin after 4 hours,
both after administration of labeled choline and
after administration of methyl-labeled methionine
(Bjørnstad and Bremer 1966).
   Fig. 2 shows a similar experiment on man.
Three men (aged 26, 40 and 41 years) were given
500 uCi [^{3}H-CH$_3$]-methionine per os, and the labeling of plasma phospholipids was followed. In one
case the main serum lipoproteins were also isolated.
   Fig.2A shows that the maximum specific activity of lecithin and lysolecithin was reached
after 24 hours and then the specific activity declined with a halflife of about 2-3 days. The
specific activity of spingomyeline probably reached
its maximum a little later than lecithin. This is
to be expected since sphingomyeline can be labeled

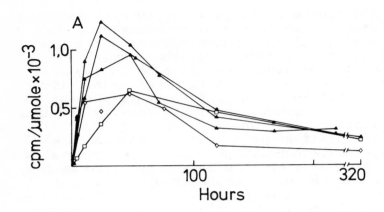

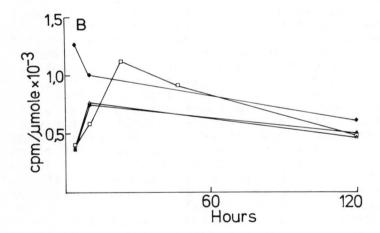

Fig. 2. Labeling of plasma licithin in man after
oral administration of 500 μCi of [^{3}H-CH$_3$]-methi-
onine.
A. ▲, total plasma lecithin (three different indi-
viduals).   , plasma lysolecithin; □ , plasma
sphingomyeline.
B. ◆ , lecithin of VLDL; Δ, lecithin of LDL; ▲,
lecithin of HDL. □ , total plasma lecithin.

only from labeled choline liberated from lecithin
labeled by methylation.

Fig. 2B shows that the lecithin of VLDL was
labeled earlier than LDL and HDL. This result
agrees with the rapid turnover of VLDL in plasma
and its conversion to LDL, and with exchange of
phospholipids between the different plasma lipoproteins.

If we assume that 1.5 kg of human liver contains 1% of lecithin, and that this lecithin is
in equilibrium with plasma lecithin after 24 hours
when the plasma lecithin (2 g/l) had reached its
maximum specific activity, we can calculate   that
at least 15% of the administrated methionine
methyl groups were used for lecithin synthesis in
the liver. In earlier experiments with rats we
found that 30% of an injected dose of methyl-
labeled methionine was recovered in liver lecithin
(Bjørnstad and Bremer 1966). It is reasonable to
conclude therefore that lecithin synthesis by the
methylation pathway is quantitative important also
in human liver.

The labeling of lysolecithin of plasma is
noteworthy. In rat experiments we found that
lecithin of extrahepatic tissues increased its
specific activity for a long time after injection
of methyl-labeled methionine. It is unlikely that
this phenomenon can be explained by a prolonged
"survival" of labeled methionine in these tissues,
thus making prolonged labeling by methylation possible. We also could exclude transport of free
labeled choline from the liver to extrahepatic
tissues. We concluded therefore that a transfer
of phospholipids from the liver to other tissues
took place (Bjørnstad and Bremer 1966). It is
known that LDL is taken up by extrahepatic tissues,
and it is also shown that lysolecithin in the
plasma is taken up by extrahepatic tissues (Stein
and Stein 1966). These mechanisms may be of quantitative importance in furnishing the extrahepatic
tissues with choline and choline-containing phospholipids.

Specificity of the Adenosylmethionine
Phosphatidylethanolamine Methyl Transferase(s)

The methyl transferase shows a certain preference for phosphatidyl-ethanolamine containing
palmitate as compared to stearate as saturated
fatty acid, and particularly for the palmitoyl-
docosahexanoyl derivative (Arvidson 1968). Also,
the phosphatidylethanolamine usually contains
more polyunsaturated fatty acids than lecithin.
Therefore the methylation pathway represents a
mechanism for enrichment of lecithin with polyunsaturated fatty acids. It has been found that
this may be important in blood platelets. In
trombin activation of platelets arachidonic acid
is liberated from lecithin by stimulation of a
phospholipase (Kanagi et al. 1980).
Mono- and dimethylphosphatidylethanolamine
are more rapidly methylated than phosphatidylethanolamine i.e. the incorporation of the first
methyl group is rate limiting (Bremer and
Greenberg 1961). Total methyl transfer is stimulated in hepatocytes incubated with mono- and
dimethylethanolamine. Phospholipid methylation is
also stimulated by incubation of the hepatocytes
with ethylethanolamine suggesting that the corresponding phosphatidyl derivative is active as
methyl acceptor. Diethylethanolamine also had
some effect (Åkeson 1977).
Adenosylselenomethionine is as efficient as
methyl donor as is adenosylmethionine (Bremer and
Natori 1960). Adenosylethionine gave no or neglible
transethylation (Bremer and Greenberg 1961).

Inhibitors and Competing Methyl Acceptors

Adenosylhomocysteine is an inhibitor of the
methyltransferase and probably takes part in the
regulation of lecithin biosynthesis by product
inhibition (Kaneshiro and Law 1964). 3-Deazadeno-
sine inhibits choline biosynthesis. It is converted
to deazaadenosylhomocysteine which is an inhibitor
both of the phosphatidylethanolamine methyltransferase and the adenosylhomocysteine hydrolase
(Pritchard et al. 1982). Adenosylhomocysteine

therefore also accumulates and contributes to the inhibition of lecithin biosynthesis.

Ethionine is converted to adenosylethionine which is an competitive inhibitor of the phosphatidylethanolamine methyl transferase (Bremer and Greenberg 1960). Ethionine inhibits lecithin biosynthesis by methylation in vivo. It also delays the equilibration of liver- and plasma lecithin (Bjørnstad and Bremer 1963), presumably by inhibiting the synthesis of apolipoproteins in the liver.

Guanidoacetic acid is methylated to creatine in the liver. When fed to rats in combination with a choline and methionine deficient diet, the activity of phosphatidylethanolamine methyltransferase increases and the activity of choline phosphotransferase (rate limiting in the incorporation of choline in lecithin) decreases. In spite of these changes the conversion of ethanolamine to choline is decrease, evidently due to a lack of the methyldonating methionine and adenosylmethionine (Hoffman et al. 1981).

Foreign sulfhydryl compounds like mercaptoethanol are strong inhibitors of phosphatidylethanolamine methylation in isolated microsomes of liver (Bremer and Greenberg 1961), evidently because of a relatively active sulfhydryl methyltransferase in the microsomes (Bremer and Greenberg 1961 B). It has not been investigated whether foreign sulfhydryl compounds can cause a deficiency of methyl groups in vivo.

The biosynthesis of choline is inhibited in vivo by 2-amino-2-methyl propanol. Apparently this inhibitor is incorporated into the phospholipids, and the abnormal phospholipid formed (presumably the phosphatidyl derivative) is an inhibitor of the methyltransferase (Wells and Remy 1961).

Rat liver cytosol is reported to contain an inhibitor, presumably a low molecular weight peptide, of the phosphatidylethanolamine methyltransferase (Chiva and Mato 1984). Its regulatory function is unknown.

Regulation of lecithin biosynthesis

Excellent reviews on phospholipid methylation and its possible functions have appeared (Mato and Alemany 1983, Pelech and Vance 1984). A series of studies have shown that the two main pathways for lecithin synthesis are under mutual control by hormones. The hormonal control seems to take place by means of Ca^{++}-stimulated protein kinases which phosphorylate the rate limiting enzymes of both pathways. The synthesis of lecithin from preformed choline is inhibited by phosphorylation of the phosphorylcholine citidyltransferase, and simultaneously the enzyme is translocated from the endoplasmatic reticulum to the cytosol where it appears to be inactive (Vance and Pelech 1984). The phosphatidylethanolamine methyltransferase of the methylation pathway is activated by phosphorylation (Varela et al. 1984).

References

Åkeson, B. (1977) Biochem. J. 168, 401-408.
Anderson, R., Kates, M. and Volcani, B.E. (1979) Biochim. Biophys. Acta 573, 557-561.
Arvidson, G.A.E. (1968) Eur. J. Biochem. 5, 415-421.
Batint, J.A., Beeler, D.A., Treble, D.H. and Spitzer, H.L. (1967) J. Lipid. Res. 8, 486-493.
Bieber, L.L. (1968) Biochim. Biophys. Acta 152, 778-780.
Bieber, L.L. and Newburgh, R.W. (1963) J. Lipid. Res. 4, 397-401.
Bieber, L.L., Sellers, L.G. and Kumar, S.S. (1969) J. Biol. Chem. 244, 630-636.
Bjerve, K.S. (1972) Biochim. Biophys. Acta 270, 348-363.
Bjørnstad, P. and Bremer, J. (1963) Acta Chem. Scand. 17, 903-904.
Bjørnstad, P. and Bremer, J. (1966) J. Lipid. Res. 7, 38-45.
Bremer, J., Figard, P.H. and Greenberg, D.M. (1960) Biochim. Biophys. Acta 43, 477-488.
Bremer, J. and Greenberg, D.M. (1961a) Biochim. Biophys. Acta 46, 205-216.

Bremer, J. and Greenberg, D.M. (1961b) Biochim. Biophys. Acta 46, 217-224.

Bremer, J. and Natori, Y. (1960) Biochim. Biophys. Acta 44, 367-370.

Chiva, A. and Mato, J.M. (1984) Biochem. J. 218, 637-639.

Evans, R.W., Kates, M., Ginzburg, M. and Ginzburg, B.-Z. (1982) Biochim. Biophys. Acta 712, 186-195.

Goldfine, H. (1962) Biochim. Biophys. Acta 59, 504-506.

Hayashi, A., Matsuura, F. and Matsubara, T. (1969) Biochim. Biophys. Acta 176, 208-210.

Hoffman, D.R., Haning, J.A. and Cornatzer, W.E. (1981) Can. J. Biochem. 59, 543-550.

Johnson, N.C. and Goldfine, H. (1983) J. Gen. Microbiol. 129, 1075-1081.

Kaneshiro, T. and Law, J.H. (1964) J. Biol. Chem. 239, 1705-1713.

Kanagi, R., Koizumi, K., Hata-Tanone and Masuda, T. (1980) Biochem. Biophys. Res. Commun. 96, 711-718.

Kennedy, E.R. and Weiss, S.B. (1956) J. Biol. Chem. 222, 193-214.

Kittredge, J.S. (1967) in Abstracts 7th International Congress of Biochemistry, Tokyo pp. 453-454.

Lyman, R.L., Tinoco, J., Bauchard, P., Sheehan, G., Ostwald, R. and Miljanich (1967) Biochim. Biophys. Acta 137, 107-114.

Mato, J.M. and Alemany, S. (1983) Biochem. J. 213, 1-10.

Mato, J.M., Pajares, A. and Varela, I. (1984) Trends Biochem. Sci. 9, 471-472.

Pelech, S.L. and Vance, D.E. (1984) Biochim. Biophys. Acta 779, 217-251.

Pritchard, P.H., Chiang, P.K., Cantoni, G.L. and Vance, D.E. (1982) J. Biol. Chem. 257, 6362-6367.

Scarborough, G.A. and Nyc, J.F. (1967) J. Biol. Chem. 242, 238-242.

Stein, Y and Stein, O. (1966) Biochim. Biophys. Acta 116, 95-107.

Vance, D.E. and Pelech, S.L. (1984) Trends Biochem. Sci. 9, 17-20.

Varela, I., Merida, I., Pajares, M., Villalba, M. and Mato, J.M. (1984) Biochem. Biophys. Res. Commun. 122, 1065-1070.

Viswanathan, C.V. and Rosenberg, H. (1973)
J. Lipid Res. 14, 327-330.
Wells, I.C. and Remy, C.N. (1961) Arch. Biochem.
Biophys. 95, 389-399.
Willemot, C. and Boll, W.G. (1967) Can. J. Botany
45, 1863-1876.
Yamashita, S., Oshima, A., Nikawa, J. and
Hosaka, K. (1982) Eur. J. Biochem. 128, 589-595.

PHOSPHOLIPID METHYLATION AND CELLULAR DIFFERENTIATION

Fusao Hirata[§], Masakazu Hatanaka[†], Yuji Wano[§] and Keiichi Matsuda[§]

Laboratory of Cell Biology, National Institute of Mental Health, Bethesda, Maryland 20205 U.S.A. [§] and Institute of Virus Research, Kyoto University, Kyoto 606 Japan [†]

Phospholipid methylation is a reaction in which phosphatidylethanolamine (PtdEtn) and its alkyl and alkenyl analogues are converted to phosphatidylcholine (PtdCho) and its analogues with S-adenosyl methionine (S-AdoMet) as a methyl donor (Hirata, 1984). The highest specific activity of enzyme(s)(PtdEtn methyltransferase) that catalyzes this reaction is generally found in the plasma membranes of most tissues and cells, except for in the liver and lung where this enzyme activity appears to be highest in the microsomes. In the latter two tissues, PtdEtn methyltransferase(s) is supposed to be involved in the synthesis of biles and surfactants, respectively. We have previously proposed that at least two enzymes are involved in this reaction (Hirata and Axelrod, 1980). Recently, Makishima, et al.(1985) highly purified these enzymes from the plasma membranes of murine lymphocytes and characterized some properties of two different enzymes. The first enzyme mainly methylates PtdEtn and the other enzyme forms PtdCho by adding two more methyl groups to monomethyl-PtdEtn. These enzymes have different kinetic parameters with respects to affinities for S-AdoMet, metal dependency and optimal pH.

Although phospholipid methylation is a minor pathway of PtdCho synthesis, it is now known to increase and/or decrease after stimulation of various receptors, suggesting its association with the signal transduction across the membranes (Hirata and Axelrod, 1980; Mato et al., 1984). In addition, the activities of PtdEtn methyltrans-

ferases alter as cells and tissues differentiate or develop (Hitzmann, 1982; Cimazierre et al., 1981; Honma et
al., 1981). These observations indicate that phospholipid
methylation and subsequent turnover of methylated lipids
in the plasma membranes might be related to initiating
programs of the cellular differentiation. Furthermore, 3-
deazaadenosine (3-deaza-Ado), a compound which intracellularly transforms to S-3-deazaadenosylhomocystein (S-3-
deaza-AdoHcy) to inhibit various transmethylations
(Cantoni et al., 1979), can induce the cellular differentiation of 3T3/6 fibroblasts towards adipocytes (Chiang,
1980). Thus, we were interested in the biochemical mechanism as to how phospholipid metabolism occurring in the
plasma membranes can regulate expression of the genes for
cellular differentiation. Here, we present several line
of evidences suggesting that the turnover of PtdCho synthesized by the transmethylation can change such gene
expression, mediating through altering cellular levels of
S-AdoMet and S-AdoHcy.

Phospholipid metabolism in transformed and differentiated cells

To study the turnover of phospholipid metabolism
during the differentiation-transformation period, we employed two cell lines of murine fibroblasts, Balb/3T3-A31
(Aaronson and Todaro, 1968a) and Balb/3T12-3 (Aaronson and
Todaro, 1968b). The former cells are nontumorgenic and
sensitive to contact-inhibition. On the other hand, the
latter cells derived from Balb/3T3-A31 are tumorgenic and
insensitive to contact-inhibition. The both cell lines
were found to contain PtdEtn methyltransferase as measured
by the incorporation of [^{3}H-methyl] group from methionine
into the phospholipid fraction. Under the culture conditions where these cells were confluent, activities of [^{3}H-
methyl] incorporation were 2 and 13 pmol/mg protein/hr in
3T3 and 3T12-3 cells, respectively. Upon the two dimensional thin layer chromatography (Niwa et al., 1984), 10%,
15% and 65% of the radioactivity were found in monomethyl-
and dimethyl- PtdEtn and PtdCho, respectively. PtdCho was
further identified as glycerophosphorylcholine after alkaline hydrolysis in 1N NaOH according to the method described (Ansell et al., 1971). The remainings of radioactivity were not identified. Interestingly, the rates of
the synthesis of PtdCho as measured by the incorporation

of [methyl-^{14}C] choline were 91 and 18 pmol/mg/hr, respectively. These observations suggest that PtdCho syntheses by the transmethylation and CDP-choline pathway are inversely regulated; in the malignant cells, the transmethylation can synthesize approximately 20% of the total PtdCho, while it does only 1% in the beneign cells.   To confirm that such alteration of the synthetic routes of PtdCho synthesis is a result of cellular transformation and/or differentiation,   3T3 and 3T12-3 cells were transformed by murine sarcoma virus (MSV).   The infection of MSV caused enhancement of the transmethylation pathway in the PtdCho synthesis in 3T3 cells but not in 3T12-3 cells.   Furthermore, the treatment with 0.3% dimethylsulfoxide, a cellular differentiation inducer, resulted in decreasing the transmethylation pathway in 3T12-3 cells.

Although the difference between the transmethylation pathway in 3T3 and 3T12 cells was 6 fold in intact cells, that of PtdEtn methyltransferase activity was only 2 fold in the isolated particulate (membrane) fractions from these cells, as measured with S-AdoMet as a substrate. These results suggest that the increase of incorporation of [^{3}H-methyl] group into the PtdCho fraction in intact cells is attributed not only to the increased activity of PtdEtn methyltransferase but also to the increased supply of methylated phospholipids to the pools which turnover rapidly.   When 3T3 and 3T12-3 cells were labelled with [1 - ^{14}C] arachidonic acid, the rate of arachidonic acid incorporation into the phospholipid fraction was 3 fold higher in 3T12-3 cells.   It was also the case with the rate of arachidonic acid release from the membrane phospholipids. Since the species of PtdCho synthesized by the transmethylation but not by the CDP-choline pathway contains more arachidonic acid in its side chain (Crews et al., 1981; Toccani et al., 1985), we concluded that phospholipase A$_2$ activity is also stimulated in the transformed cells and that the transmethylation pathway is secondarily enhanced to supply the substrate for this phospholipase A$_2$.

Basal level of phospholipase A$_2$ and cellular differentiation

To study the role of phospholipase A$_2$ in the cellular differentiation, we employed HL60 cells, a promyeloleukemia cell line, because this cell line is often used as a

model system to study the mechanism of cellular differentiation (Breitman et al., 1980; Elias et al., 1980). The
basal level of phospholipase A_2 in promyeloleukemia cells
is also proposed to be associated with the cellular compe-
tence by which cellular differentiation is initiated
(Simantov and Sachs, 1982). HL60 cells are developmental-
ly bipotential to acquire the characteristics of macrophages or granulocytes, depending upon kinds of chemical
inducers. When this cell line was treated with phorbol
esters, the incorporation and release of $[1 - {}^{14}C]$ arachidonic acid into and from phospholipids, respectively, were
stimulated. On the other hand, retinoic acids inhibited
such turnover of phospholipids. Since arachidonic acid
was mainly incorporated into and released from the PtdCho
fraction under the present conditions, we thought that
phospholipase A_2 plays an important role in the metabolism
of PtdCho. Since phorbol esters have been reported to
enhance the turnover of PtdCho synthesized by the transmethylation (Hoffman and Herberman, 1982), these observations suggest that phospholipid methylation occurs in the
sites close to phospholipase A_2. Phorbol esters directed
HL60 cells towards macrophages, while retinoids promote
the differentiation of HL60 cells to granulocytes. These
findings implicate that the basal level of phospholipase
A_2 determines the direction of differentiation. This interpretation was further supported by the observations
that melittin, a phospholipase A_2 activator, directed HL60
cells to acquire the macrophage properties, while the C-MT
peptide, a newly synthesized peptidic inhibitor of phospholipase A_2 (Notsu et al., 1985), stimulated HL60 cells
to obtain the characteristics of granulocytes (Hirata et
al., 1985).

Effects of 3-deazaadenosine and 5-azacytidine on cellular
differentiation

        3-Deazaadenosine (3-deaza-Ado) is often used to
inhibit various transmethylations in intact cells (Cantoni
et al., 1979) and is reported to induce the cellular differentiation of 3T6-fibroblast (Chiang, 1980). To determine the involvement of phospholipid methylation and other
methylation reactions in cellular differentiation, we
treated HL-60 cells with varying concentrations of 3-
deazaadenosine. At 0.3 µM of 3-deaza-Ado, HL60 cells
expressed LeuM₃, an antigen of macrophages, while at 10 µM

of 3-deaza-Ado, they had LeuM$_4$, an antigen of granulocytes, on the cell surfaces. In fact, the turnover of arachidonic acid in HL60 cells as measured by its incorporation and release was inhibited at 10 μM but not at 0.3 μM of 3-deaza-Ado. To examine which methylation reaction is associated with this cellular differentiation, we measured phospholipid methylation, protein methylation, and DNA and RNA methylation by incubating the cells with [^{3}H-methyl]-methionine, a precursor of S-AdoMet. The inhibition of DNA methylation appeared to be more closely associated with the direction of cellular differentiation. To obtain further evidence, we treated HL60 cells with 5-azacytidine, a specific inhibitor of DNA methylation. At 0.3 μM of 5-azacytidine, HL60 cells expressed Leu M$_3$, while at 10 μM, they did Leu M$_4$. 5-Azacytidine inhibited not only DNA methylation but also phospholipid methylation, because this compound decreased S-AdoMet level probably due to inhibition of S-AdoMet synthetase.

To confirm that phorbol esters and retinoic acids change the DNA methylation by altering ratios of S-AdoHcy/S-AdoMet, we measured the cellular levels of these compounds using ^{35}S-methionine. HL60 cells were cultured in RPMI 1640 medium containing 10 μCi/ml ^{35}S-methionine for 2 days and then treated with various compounds for 12 hrs. Phorbol myristearic acid (PMA) increased S-AdoMet as well as S-AdoHcy. Accordingly, the ratio of S-AdoHcy to S-AdoMet in these cells increased to 0.05, compared with 0.01 in the nontreated cells. On the other hand, retinoic acid increased S-AdoHcy level without changing S-AdoMet level: thus, the ratio raised up to 0.2. DNA Methylation was less inhibited in the PMA treated cell than in the retinoic acid treated cells. Since hypomethylation of DNA is now proposed to be associated with certain types of active genes (Doerfler, 1983), such difference in the methylation of DNA might play an important, if not primary, role in the determination of direction of cellular differentiation. However, it remains unclear why genes for macrophages are easily hypomethylated rather than genes for neutrophils. This difference might be based upon difference in structures of genes or their association with histones (Groudin and Corkin, 1985), because many genes are now reported to be methylated in different sites during the developmental periods (Boenvensity et al., 1985).

Mechanism on regulation of S-AdoMet level

How basal level of phospholipase A_2 in the plasma membranes can change cellular level of S-AdoMet and S-AdoHcy remains to be elucidated. Since phospholipase A_2 activity is directly related to Na+/H+ - antiport coupled to epidermal growth factor receptors (Kicentini et. al., 1984), we measured ^{22}Na+ influx in the chemical inducer-treated and non-treated cells. The influx of ^{22}Na+ increased in the PMA-treated cells, whereas it decreased in the retinoic acid-treated cells. The increase in ^{22}Na+ influx appeared to be attributed to that in Na+/H+ - antiport, because this was blocked by amiloride. On the other hand, the decrease of ^{22}Na+ influx in the retinoid-treated cells were attributed to the stimulation of Na+, K+ - ATPase as well as inhibition of Na+/H+ - antiport, because ouabain could partially restore it. Amiloride and ouabain inhibited PMA - and retinoid-induced differentiation, respectively. The importance of intracellular Na+ sequestration in cellular differentiation was further supported by the findings that monensin and gramicidin, Na+ ionophores, were able to induce the differentiation of HL60 cells to macrophages (Hirata et al., 1985). In addition, these ionophores also changed the ratio of S-AdoHcy/S-AdoMet as seen with phorbol esters and melittin. The stimulation of Na+/H+ - antiport usually accompany with intracellular alkalization. PMA and melittin increased intracellular pH, but retinoic acid and C-MT peptide decreased it. In fact, when HL60 cells were cultured in acidic pH (pH 7.0), they obtained neutrophilic characteristics and had increased S-AdoHcy level. From these results, we assumed that S-AdoHcy hydrolase and S-AdoMet synthetase are regulated by intracellular Na+ concentrations or intracellular pH or both.

Summary

Phospholipid methylation supplies the species of Ptd-Cho which contain more arachidonic acid. This species of PtdCho is rapidly metabolized by phospholipase A_2. Such metabolism of phospholipids occuring in the plasma membranes accompany alteration in the Na+/H+ - antiport activity followed by changes in intracellular pH. These intracellular changes affect the metabolism of S-AdoMet as well as S-AdoHcy. The increased ratio of S-AdoHcy to S-AdoMet inside cells inhibits various methylations, especially DNA methylation. Hypomethylation of DNAs at certain sites results in expressing these DNAs or modifying their expression, which are necessary for determination of directions of cellular differentiation.

References

Aaronson, S. A. and Todaro, G. T. (1968a) J. Cell Physiol. 72, 141–148.

Aaronson, S. A. and Todaro, G. T. (1968b) Science 162, 1024–1026.

Ansell, G. B., and Spanner, S. (1971) Biochem. J. 122, 741–750.

Boenvensity, N., Mencher, D., Meynhas, O., Razin, A. and Reshef, L. (1985) Proc. Nat. Acad. Sci. U.S.A. 82, 267–271.

Breitman, T. R., Selonick, S. E. and Collins, S. J. (1980) Proc. Nat. Acad. Sci. U.S.A. 77, 2936–2940.

Camazierre, C., Maziere, J. C., Mora, L. and Polonovski, J. (1981) FEBS Lett. 129, 67–69.

Cantoni, G. L., Richards, H. H. and Chiang, P. K., (1979) in Transmethylation (Usdin, E., Borchardt, R. T. and Creveling, C. R., Eds.) pp. 155–165, Elsevier, Amsterdam.

Chiang, P. K. (1980) Science, 211, 1164–1166.

Crews, F., Morita,Y., McGivney,A., Hirata, F., Siraganian, R. P. and Axelrod, J. (1981) Arch. Biophys. Biochem. 212, 561–571.

Doerfler, W. (1983) Ann. Rev. Biochem. 52, 93–124.

Elias, L., Wogenrich, F. J., Wallace, J. M. and Longmire, J. (1980) Leukemia Res. 4, 301–307.

Groudin, M. and Corkin, K.F. (1985) Science 228, 1061–1068.

Hirata, F. (1984) in Handbook of Neurochemistry (Lajtha, A., Ed.) 6, pp. 527–539, Plenum Press, New York.

Hirata, F. and Axelrod, J. (1980) Science 209, 1082–1090.

Hirata, F., Hattori, T., Notsu, Y., Wano, Y. and Hattori, T. (1985) Int. J. Immunopharmacol., in press.

Hitzemann, R. (1982) Life Sci. 30, 1297–1303.

Hoffman, D. R. and Herberman, E. (1982) Carcinogenesis 3, 875–880.

Honma, Y., Kasukabe, T. and Hozumi, M. (1981) Biochim. Biophys. Acta. 664, 441–444.

Kicentini, L. M., Miller, R. J. and Villereal, M. L. (1984) J. Biol. Chem., 259, 6912–6916.

Makishima, F., Toyoshima, S. and Osawa, T. (1985) Arch.

Biophys. Biochem. 238, 315–324.

Mato, J. M. and Alemany, S. (1983) Biochem. J. 213, 1–10.

Niwa, Y., Sakane, T. and Taniguchi, S. (1984) Arch. Biophys. Biochem. 234, 7–14.

Notsu, Y., Namiuchi, S. Hattori, T., Matsuda, K. and Hirata, F. (1985) Arch. Biophys. Biochem. 236, 195–204.

Simantov, R., and Sachs, L. (1982) Biochim. Biophys. Acta. 720, 111–119.

Toccani, M. and Wurtzman, R. J. (1985) Proc. Nat. Acad. Sci. U.S.A. in press.

METHYLATION OF PHOSPHATIDYLETHANOLAMINE: ENZYME

CHARACTERIZATION, REGULATION AND PHYSIOLOGICAL FUNCTION

Dennis E. Vance and Neale Ridgway

Department of Biochemistry

University of British Columbia

Vancouver, British Columbia V6T 1W5 Canada

In this article we review the major developments in the conversion of phosphatidylethanolamine (PE) to phosphatidylcholine (PC) during the past four years. An introduction to the topic and its relationship to phospholipid metabolism has been published (Vance, 1985). A summary of the field until 1981 was published in the book originating from the 1981 Transmethylation Conference (Vance et al. 1982).

In 1981 the PE methylation field was embroiled in several controversies. Open questions included how many enzymes were involved in the conversion of PE to PC? Was PE methylation involved in biological signal transmission? Although there is still no agreement on the number of enzymes involved in the formation of PC from PE, the weight of evidence now suggests that PE methylation is not involved in biological signal transmission. A new area of discussion is whether the PE-methyltransferase is regulated by reversible phosphorylation? The current status of these questions are discussed in this article.

ENZYME CHARACTERIZATION

An understanding of the N-methylation pathway of PC biosynthesis has been plagued by an inability to purify the enzyme(s) involved. Available data on enzyme characterization were derived from membrane associated

75

enzyme(s) or highly unstable solubilized preparations.
Hence, conclusions are tentative due to the possible
presence of factors that affect enzyme activity, ill-
defined endogenous substrate levels or the labile nature
of the partially purified enzyme.

Purification of the methyltransferase(s) has lagged
owing to the lack of a suitable detergent for solubili-
zation. Original attempts (Schneider & Vance, 1979;
Tanaka et al., 1979) were partially successful with 0.2%
Triton X-100. However, after solubilizing the methyltransferase, the detergent rapidly denatured the enzyme.
Recently Pajares et al. (1984) reported a 32-fold purification of methyltransferase from solubilized rat liver
microsomes. In their partial purification they used
CHAPS, a zwitterionic cholate derivative. We have
confirmed that CHAPS will release methyltransferase from
rat liver microsomes in good yield and in relatively
stable state. Using optimal conditions, we have prepared
a solubilized enzyme with a specific activity of 2.5 and
6.1 nmoles/min/mg using exogenous PE and PME, respectively.

Using partially purified methyltransferase, Pajares et
al. (1984) photoaffinity labeled (with 8-azido-S-
adenosylmethionine) a protein of 25 Kdal. Treatment of
the same preparation with Mg-ATP and cAMP-dependent
protein kinase resulted in ^{32}p incorporation into a
protein of 50 Kdal and a 4-fold activation of the methyltransferase (Varela et al., 1984). The conclusion that
the methyltransferase is composed of two subunits, one
catalytic (25 Kdal) and one regulatory (50 Kdal), is
enticing. However, it should be cautioned that the enzyme
was not pure. Indeed, the authors conceeded that the
enzyme was part of a large (300,000 dal) complex of
detergent, PE, PC, free fatty acids and other contaminating
proteins, some of which may be phosphorylated or use
AdoMet in some catalytic function. A phospholipid/protein
ratio of 0.4 in this complex is claimed to negate the
requirement for exogenous PE in the assay. Unpublished
data from our lab indicate that methyltransferase
solubilized with CHAPS and partially purified on DE 52
cellulose has a nearly absolute requirement for exogenous
PE and PME, in agreement with the lipid requirement by the
Trition solubilized and partially purified enzyme
(Schneider and Vance, 1979).

Most efforts on purification have centered on liver microsomes as a source of methyltransferase. The obvious reason is the specific activity of the methyltransferase on liver microsomes is on the average 10-1000 fold higher than other sources. However, Makishima et al. (1985) have partially purified and separated two methyltransferases from mouse thymocyte microsomes. Deoxycholate solubilized methyltransferase was resolved into two distinct activities by affinity chromatography on AdoHcy-Sepharose. One activity converted PE to PME and eluted at high salt. The second activity converted PME to PC and was eluted by reducing the pH of the elution buffer. There was considerable cross-contamination of both activities. Possibly, two enzymes exist possessing both activities, but with reciprocal Km's for the two separate methylation reactions. Alternatively, the kinetics may vary as a function of the physical state of the enzyme. Thus, PME synthesizing activity may exist primarily in the higher molecular weight aggregated form, while PC synthesizing activity is associated with a lower molecular weight fraction.

The preparation by Makishima et al. (1985) contained significant phospholipase A_2 activity. The extremely high content of free fatty acids in the enzyme isolated by Mato's group (Pajares et al., 1984) may, in part, be explained by the presence of an active phospholipase A_2 in their preparations. Methylation of this endogenous fatty acid accounts for approximately one-third of the methylated products produced by this partially purified enzyme. This is an anomalous observation considering that liver is low in fatty acid methylation activity relative to PE methylation when compared to lung (Zatz et al., 1981).

Elucidation of the number of enzymes involved in the PE methylation reaction has been probed based on Km's, pH-activity profiles and cation dependency of the three reactions. Such studies have led Hirata and Axelrod (1980) to propose the existence of 2 separate enzyme activities. The first converts PE to PME and the second PME to PC. However, it seems that evidence for two enzymes based on kinetic studies may be unfounded (Audubert & Vance, 1983). Most Km estimates for the formation of PME have not taken into account the subsequent conversion of PME to PDE and PC. True estimates of PME,

PDE and PC synthesis are gained by taking into account radioactivity in products distal to the intermediates. Detailed formulas have been described (Audubert & Vance, 1983).

The pH dependency of PE methylation is equally misunderstood. Sastry et al. (1981), for rat liver microsomes, reported that the first methylation of PE has an apparent pH optimum of 8.0, a Km for AdoMet of 0.83 μM, and PME production of 83 fmoles/μg/10 min. How this low production of PME from PE provides enough intermediates to produce the 20-fold accumulation of PC at higher pH's was not explained. An alternative is that the results represent an optimization of the accumulation of PME in a steady state. The first reaction would occur but owing to suboptimal pH and AdoMet concentrations, subsequent steps would proceed slowly regardless of whether one or two enzymes were involved. Activity-pH profiles of two different partially purified preparations of methyltransferase from rat liver microsomes show a very distinct pH optimum at 9-9.5 for all three activities (Schneider & Vance, 1978; Pajares et al., 1984). The alkaline pH optimum of the liver methyltransferase seems to be a true value and not an artefact (Audubert & Vance, 1983).

Opinions on the topology of the methyltransferase(s) in cellular membranes are divided. Hirata and Axelrod (1980) claimed in rat erythrocytes that the first methylation step occurs on the cytoplasmic face of the plasma membrane. The subsequent two steps occur on the external face of the membrane. A similar report was made by Higgins (1981) for rat liver microsomes using Hirata and Axelrod's assay methods. In each instance, suboptimal pH and AdoMet concentrations were used. Under optimal conditions, Audubert and Vance (1984) reported that, in sealed microsomes, all three activities were susceptible to trypsin digestion, indicating a cytosolic orientation for the enzyme(s). Although the number of enzymes involved in the conversion of PE to PC is controversial in animal cells, genetic evidence for 2 enzymes in N. Crassa (Scarborough & Nyc, 1967) and S. cerevisiae (Greenburg et al., 1983) is clear.

Clearly a great deal of confusion and nonconsensus can be found in reports on the number of enzymes, cation requirements, pH optima and Km values for the steps in the methyltransferase reaction. Some of the confusion has been created by a misunderstanding of the steady state nature of the pathway. Reconciliation of these problems awaits the purification to homogeneity of the enzyme(s) involved in PE methylation.

REGULATION OF THE CONVERSION OF PHOSPHATIDYLETHANOLAMINE TO PHOSPHATIDYLCHOLINE

Influence of Substrates and Products

The rate of PE methylation can be influenced by the concentration of PE, AdoMet and AdoHcy. When Åkesson (1978) incubated cultured hepatocytes with 1 mM ethanolamine, the concentration of PE in the cells almost doubled. Concomitantly, [^{14}C]methionine incorporated into PC also doubled. In further experiments with microsomes, Åkesson (1983) showed that a decrease in PE reduced conversion of PE to PC without an effect on the amount of PE methyltransferase. It is not clear that such fluctuations of PE in the liver are normally important for regulation of conversion of PE to PC.

The concentration of AdoMet and AdoHcy seem important for the rate of PE methylation. Hoffman et al. (1980) achieved high levels of AdoMet (300 nmoles/g liver) in livers perfused with methionine with no effect on AdoHcy concentration (8-20 nmol/g liver). Unfortunately, they did not evaluate the rate of PE methylation. However, hepatocytes in culture (Sundler & Åkesson, 1975) showed a doubling of PC formation from PE when incubated with 100 µM methionine. Thus, it seems likely that the supply of methionine could limit PE methylation.

In related experiments, Hoffman et al. (1980) perfused rat livers with Hcy (3.4 mM) and adenosine (4.0 mM) and dramatically increased the concentration of AdoMet (45 to 1250 nmol/g) and AdoHcy (8 to 4000 nmol/g) and reduced the AdoMet/AdoHcy ratio from 5.6 to 0.3. Under these conditions, the methylation of PE decreased by at least 99%. Although their results do not take into account isotope dilution of [^{14}C]methionine by increased AdoMet, it seems likely that PE methylation was severely retarded. Since AdoHcy is a potent competitive inhibitor of PE

methyltransferase (Pelech & Vance, 1984), the AdoMet/AdoHcy
ratio seems a potential control point. This is further
substantiated by studies of AdoHcy analogues in cultured
hepatocytes (Schanche et al., 1982; Pritchard et al.,
1982). Whether this ratio is important under normal
physiological variations remains to be demonstrated.

Hormones and cAMP Effects in Hepatocytes

There is disagreement as to the effect of cAMP
analogues and hormones that induce cAMP on the rate of PE
methylation. One group have proposed that increased levels
of cAMP promote PE methylation (Mato & Alemany, 1983).
Whereas, with a cAMP analogue or glucagon, we have observed
a decrease in conversion of PE to PC (Pritchard et al.,
1981; Pelech et al., 1984). We believe experiments on
hormone effects are best done with an initial preincubation
(∿30 min) of cells with [³H]ethanolamine which labels
PE extensively. Subsequent incubations + hormone allow
for measurement of the formation of PC from labeled PE,
without possible effects of the hormones on the specific
radioactivity of PE. Unfortunately, many studies have not
used this approach. However, a recent study with hepatocytes from adrenalectomized rats correlated isoprenaline
treatment with increased conversion of [³H]PE to PC and
higher cellular cAMP and PE methyltransferase activity
assayed in vitro (Marin-Cao et al., 1983). Such treatment
of normal hepatocytes had no effect on PE methyltransferase
activity assayed in vitro. Whether or not the adrenalectomized rat model has a relevance to normal physiological
systems is a valid question. We, therefore, conclude that
the most unambiguous experiments suggest that PE methylation in cultured hepatocytes is partially inhibited by
cAMP analogues and glucagon.

Does Phosphorylation/Dephosphorylation Alter
PE Methyltransferase Activity In Vitro?

In evaluating this question, we should be aware that
the PE methyltransferase assay is complex and varies
considerably among laboratories. Normally, enzymes are
assayed at the optimal pH. The PE methyltransferase has a
pH optimum of 10.2 (Audubert & Vance, 1983), yet it is
commonly believed that pH in the cytosol is ∿7.4. We

recommend that measurements of enzyme activity be done at
both pHs. Secondly, unless evaluating the effect of
AdoMet concentration, PE methyltransferase assays should
be done at saturating concentrations of AdoMet under
conditions that are linear with time and protein concentration. Perhaps variations in assay conditions might
account for some of the differences noted below.

Mato and coworkers report that PE methyltransferase is
activated by a cAMP-dependent protein kinase (Varela et
al., 1984; Mato & Alemany, 1983). They report increased
PE methyltransferase activity recovered from hepatocytes
treated with glucagon or isoprenaline. Secondly,
treatment of microsomes with cAMP and ATP caused a 2-fold
activation of the enzyme activities. More recently they
have reported a 4-fold stimulation of the partially
purified enzyme by incubation with the catalytic subunit
of cAMP-dependent protein kinase. The assays were not
done near the optimum pH and whether they were using
sufficient concentrations of AdoMet is unclear.

We have been unable to duplicate many of the above
effects. Treatment of hepatocytes with glucagon had no
effect on PE methyltransferase assayed in vitro under
optimal conditions (Pelech et al., 1984). Secondly, when
assayed at pH 7.0 or 9.2, microsomal PE methyltransferase
was unaffected by pure preparations of cAMP-dependent
protein kinase, calmodulin- dependent protein kinase or
casein kinase-2 (Pelech et al., 1985, unpublished experiments). Consistent with this finding, we saw no effect on
methyltransferase activity by purified catalytic subunits
of protein phosphatase-1 or -2A. While our studies argue
against the involvement of cAMP-dependent protein kinase
and two other kinases in activation of the PE methyltransferase, rat liver cytosol plus Mg·ATP and NaF produced a
1.6-fold stimulation of the microsomal enzyme activity.
GTP could substitute for ATP, but the nonhydrolyzable 5'
adenylylimidodiphosphate would not. The reasons for the
discrepancies between our data and those of Mato's
laboratory are presently unexplained.

Other Regulatory Studies

Several reports (Hashizume et al., 1983; Alvarez Chiva
& Mato, 1984; Pelech et al., unpublished experiments)

implicate several factors in cytosol which inhibit PE methyltransferase. Further analysis of these reports awaits purification and characterization of the inhibitors and determination of the specificity of inhibition.

Audubert et al. (1984) showed an inhibition of PE methylation by free fatty acids both in cultured rat hepatocytes and with microsomes. Unsaturated fatty acids or acyl-CoAs were much better inhibitors than saturated fatty acids. The inhibition could be easily reversed. Since fatty acid levels in serum fluctuate between 0.2 and 1.0 mM, these results may have physiological relevance. It is noteworthy that fatty acids stimulate the CDP-choline pathway for PC biosynthesis (Pelech and Vance 1984).

There is a small stimulation of PE methyltransferase in hepatocytes from juvenile and mature partially hepatectomized rats by epidermal growth factor (Alvarez Chiva et al., 1983). The increase was 1.6-fold (maximum), eliminated after 12 min. and dependent on Ca^{2+}. Mato's laboratory (Alemany et al., 1981) previously reported an activation of the methyltransferase in hepatocytes by the cationophore A23187 or hormones whose actions are mediated by Ca^{2+}. Also, Alemany et al. (1982) provided evidence for a calmodulin-Ca^{2+} mediated activation of rat liver microsomal PE methyltransferase. Inconsistent with this report is our finding that Ca^{2+}-calmodulin or purified calmodulin-dependent protein kinase had no effect on microsomal PE methyltransferase (Pelech, et al., 1985, unpublished data) even though the same kinase preparation readily phosphorylated glycogen synthase (site 2).

In summary, PE methylation in rat hepatocytes can be regulated by the supply of PE and fluctuations of the AdoMet/AdoHcy ratio, but the physiological importance remains to be determined. Whether hormones, cAMP or Ca^{2+} have any significant effect on the PE methyltransferase is an open question. The inhibition of PE methylation in vitro and in vivo by fatty acid is the one reported effect which definitely appears to have physiological relevance.

PHYSIOLOGICAL FUNCTION OF PE METHYLATION

PE methylation is 10- to 1000-fold higher in liver

than reported for other tissues (Vance et al., 1982) and accounts for ∿20% of PC made in rat hepatocytes (Sundler & Akesson, 1975). Thus, a clear function of PE methylation is to make PC in liver. This is also the only reported pathway in animals and plants for the synthesis of choline as shown below.

$$\text{Serine} \longrightarrow \text{PS} \searrow$$
$$\text{Ethanolamine} \longrightarrow \text{PE} \longrightarrow \text{PC} \begin{array}{c} \nearrow \text{choline-PO}_4 \longrightarrow \text{choline} \\ \searrow \text{Diglyceride} \end{array}$$

Since PC is secreted from liver as a component of lipoproteins (Vance & Vance, 1985), we wondered if PC from the methylation pathway was required for lipoprotein secretion. This question was tested in rat hepatocytes in which the methylaton of [^{3}H]ethanolamine-labeled PE was blocked by greater than 90% by 3-deazaadenosine. The results unambiguously demonstrated no effect on lipoprotein secretion for over 18 h (Vance, J.E., Nguyen, T. and Vance, D.E. (1985), unpublished experiments). Possibly, the compensation for the blockage of PE methylation by increased PC synthesis via CDP-choline (Pritchard et al., 1982) was sufficient for lipoprotein secretion.

Although PE methylation activity is low in non-hepatic tissues, some activity is clearly present. This is demonstrated by the 1548-fold purification of PE methyltransferase activity from mouse thymus (Makishima et al., 1985). After such extensive purification, the specific activity of the thymus enzyme was still 30-fold less than found in rat liver microsomes. The intriguing discovery by Bansal & Kanfer (1985), that PE methylation will occur in the absence of enzyme activity, could not account for the mouse thymus activity.

Hirata and Axelrod (1980) proposed that PE methylation occurs as an integral part of biological signal transmission. Their hypothesis would provide an excellent rationale for low activity of PE methyltransferase in various cells. Although a stimulating proposal, many laboratories have now eliminated a linkage of PE methylation with transmission of biological signals at the cell surface. Table I lists the experiments in the recent literature which contradict the Hirata and Axelrod hypothesis.

TABLE I

Lack of Correlation Between PE Methylation
and Biological Response

Cells	Hormone or Activator	Biological Response	Reference
Platelets	Thrombin	Serotonin Release	Shattil et al., 1981
Platelets	Collagen	Platelet Aggregation	Randon et al., 1981
Parotid Acini	Isoprenaline, Carbamoyl-choline	Amylase secretion	Padel et al. 1982
Hepatocytes	Glucagon, Adrenaline	cAMP increase	Schanche et al., 1982
Macrophage Cell Line	Endotoxin-Activated Serum	Chemotaxis	Askamit et al., 1983
Myogenic Cells	Isoproterenol	cAMP increase	Koch et al., 1983
Mast Cells	Anti-Immuno-globulin E	Histamine release	Boam et al., 1984
2H3 Leukemic Cells	Aggregated Ovalbumin	Histamine release	Moore et al. 1984
Mast Cells	Concanavalin A	Histamine release	Moore et al. 1984
Thymocytes	Concanavalin A	Histamine release	Moore et al. 1984
Macrophages	IgG-coated Erythrocytes, Zymosan	Phagocytosis	Sung & Silverstein, 1985

The enigma remains. What, if any, is the function of low levels of PE methyltransferase in non-hepatic cells? Is there significance in the report that ACTH stimulates and insulin inhibits the methyltransferase in rat adipocytes (Kelly et al., 1985)? Why does the same laboratory report that insulin stimulates the methyltransferase in isolated adipocyte plasma membranes (Kelly et al., 1984)? Clearly, there is a need for innovative research on this problem.

ACKNOWLEDGEMENT

Research on PE methylation in this laboratory is supported by grants from the Medical Research Council of Canada and British Columbia Heart Foundation. Neale Ridgway is supported by a Studentship from the Canadian Heart Foundation.

REFERENCES

Akesson, B (1978) FEBS Lett. 92, 177–180

Akesson, B (1983) Biochim. Biophys. Acta 752, 460–466.

Aksamit, R.R., Backlund Jr., P.S. and Cantoni, G.L. (1983) J. Biol. Chem. 258, 20–23.

Alemany, S., Varela, I., Harper, J.F. and Mato, J.M. (1982) J. Biol. Chem. 257, 9249–9251.

Alemany, S., Varela, I. and Mato, J.M. (1981) FEBS Lett. 135, 111–114

Audubert, F. and Vance, D.E. (1983) J. Biol. Chem. 258, 10695–10701.

Audubert, F. and Vance, D.E. (1984) Biochem. Biophys. Acta. 792, 359–362.

Audubert, F., Pelech, S.L. and Vance, D.E. (1984) Biochim. Biophys. Acta 792, 348–357.

Alvarez Chiva, V., Marin Cao, D. and Mato, J.M. (1983) FEBS. Lett. 160, 101–104.

Alvarez Chiva, V. and Mato, J.M. (1984) Biochem. J. 218, 637-639.

Bansal, V.S. and Kanfer, J.N. (1985) Biochem. Biophys. Res. Comm. 128, 411-416.

Boam, D.S.W., Stanworth, D.R., Spanner, S.G. and Ansell, G.B. (1984) Biochem. Soc. Trans. 12, 782-783.

Greenburg, M.L., Kleg, L.S., Letts, V.A., Loewry, R.S. and Henry, S.A. (1983) J. Bacteriology 153, 791-799.

Higgins, J.A. (1981) Biochem. Biophys. Acta. 640, 1-15.

Hirata, F. and Axelrod, J. (1980) Science 209, 1082-1090.

Hashizume, K., Kobayashi, M., Yamauchi, K., Ichikawa, K., Haraguchi, K. and Yamada, T. (1983) Biochem. Biophys. Res. Comm. 112, 108-114.

Hoffman, D.R., Marion, D.W., Cornatzer, W.E. and Duerre, J.A. (1980) J. Biol. Chem. 255, 10822-10827.

Kelly, K.L., Kiechle, F.L. and Jarett, L. (1984) Proc. Natl. Acad. Sci. USA 81, 1089-1092.

Kelly, K.L., Wong, E.H.-A. and Jarett, L. (1985) J. Biol. Chem. 260, 3640-3644.

Koch, T.K., Gordon, A.S. and Diamond, I. (1983) Bioc. Biophys. Res. Comm. 114, 339-347.

Makishima, F., Toyoshima, S. and Osawa, T. (1985) Arch. Bioc. Biophys. 238, 315-324.

Marin-Cao, D., Alvarez Chiva, V. and Mato, J.M. (1983) Biochem. J. 216, 675-680.

Mato, J.M. and Alemany, S. (1983) Biochem. J. 213, 1-10.

Moore, J.P., Johannsson, A., Hesketh, T.R., Smith, G.A. and Metcalfe, J.C. (1984) Biochem. J. 221, 675-684.

Padel, U., Unger, C. and Söling, H-D (1982) Biochem. J. 208, 205-210.

Pajares, M.A., Alemany, S., Varela, I., Marin Coa, D. and Mato, J.M. (1984) Biochem. J. 223, 61-66.

Pelech, S.L., Pritchard, P.H., Sommerman, E.F., Percival-Smith, A. and Vance, D.E. (1984) Can. J. Biochem. Cell Biol. 62, 196-202.

Pelech, S.L. and Vance, D.E. (1984) Biochim. Biophys. Acta 779, 217-251.

Pritchard, P.H., Chiang, P.K., Cantoni, G.L. and Vance, D.E. (1982) J. Biol. Chem. 257, 6362-6367.

Pritchard, P.H., Pelech, S.L. and Vance, D.E. (1981) Biochim. Biophys. Acta 666, 301-306.

Randon, J., Lecompte, T., Chignard, M., Siess, W., Marlas, G., Dray, F. and Vargaftig, B.B. (1981) Nature 293, 660-662.

Sastry, B.V.R., Statham, C.N., Axelrod, J. and Hirata, F. (1981) Arch. Biochem. Biophys. 217, 762-773.

Scarborough, G.A. and Nyc, J.F. (1967) J. Biol. Chem. 242, 238-242.

Schanche, J.S., Ogreid, D., Doskeland, S.O., Pefsnes, M., Sand, T.E., Ueland, P.M. and Christoffersen, T. (1982) FEBS Lett. 138, 167-172.

Schanche, J.S., Schanche, T. and Ueland, P.M. (1982) Biochim. Biophys. Acta 721, 399-407.

Schneider, W.J. and Vance, D.E. (1978) J. Biol. Chem. 254, 3886-3991.

Shattil, S.J., McDonough, M. and Burch, J.W. (1981) Blood 57, 537-544.

Sundler, R. and Akesson, B. (1975) J. Biol. Chem. 250, 3359-3367.

Sung, S-S.J. and Silverstein, S.C. (1985) J. Biol. Chem. 260, 546-554.

Tanaka, Y., Doi, O. and Akamatsu, Y. (1979) Biochem. Biophys. Res. Comm. 87, 1109-1115.

Vance, D.E. (1985) In Biochemistry of Lipids and Membranes (D.E. Vance & J.E. Vance, eds.) Benjamin Cummings Pub. Co., Menlo Park, CA, 242-270.

Vance, D.E., Audubert, F. and Pritchard, P.H. (1982) In Biochem. of S. Adenosylmethionine and Related Compounds (E. Usdin, R.T. Borchardt, C.R. Creveling, eds.) MacMillan Press, Ltd., 119-128.

Vance, J.E. and Vance, D.E. (1985) Can. J. Biochem. Cell Biol. 63, In Press.

Varela, I., Mérida, I., Pajares, M., Villalba, M. and Mato, J.M. (1984) Biochem. Biophys. Res. Comm. 122, 1065-1070.

Zatz, M., Dudley, P.A., Kloog, Y. and Markey, S.P. (1981) J. Biol. Chem. 256, 10028-10032.

REGULATION OF PHOSPHOLIPID METHYLATION BY REVERSIBLE PHOSPHORYLATION.

I. VARELA, M. PAJARES, I. MERIDA, M. VILLALBA,

C. CABRERO, P. ORTIZ, J. TRAVER and J.M. MATO.

METABOLISMO, NUTRICION Y HORMONAS. FUNDACION
JIMENEZ DIAZ. REYES CATOLICOS 2. 28040 MADRID.
SPAIN.

INTRODUCTION

At physiological doses, glucagon produces a fast and transient activation of phospholipid methyltransferase activity in isolated rat hepatocytes (Castaño et al., 1980). Similarly, glucagon produces a transient accumulation of radioactivity into phospholipids in rat hepatocytes prelabeled with (methyl-3H)-methionine (Schuller et al., 1985). Exogenous cyclic AMP (Castaño et al., 1980) or chlorophenyl thio-cyclic AMP (Pritchard et al., 1981), added to isolated rat hepatocytes, mimic the effect of glucagon on phospholipid methyltransferase. These results suggested that the activation of phospholipid methyltransferase by glucagon is a cyclic AMP-dependent process. Further evidence about this hypothesis was obtained with isolated rat liver microsomes. Cyclic AMP, in the presence of ATP, produces an activation of phospholipid methyltransferase in isolated rat liver microsomes (Mato et al., 1982). Phospholipid methyltransferase has now been purified some 300-fold from rat liver (Pajares et al., 1983). The purified enzyme is activated by incubation with ATP and the catalytic subunit of cyclic AMP dependent protein kinase (cAMP-PK) (Varela et al., 1984). Under these conditions, only one protein of Mr about 50K and pI 4.75 is phosphorylated at serine residues (Vare-

la et al., 1984). The time course of phosphorylation of
this protein correlates well with the time course of activa
tion of the enzyme (Varela et al., 1984). These results indicate that this 50K protein modulates phospholipid methyltransferase activity. The present paper shows new data on
the regulation of the phosphorylation of the 50K protein
of phospholipid methyltransferase both, using a purified
preparation of the enzyme and with intact rat hepatocytes.

METHODS

Phosphorylation of Phospholipid Methyltransferase

Phospholipid methyltransferase was purified as previously described (Pajares et al., 1984) and phosphorylated
during 5 min in the presence of cAMP-PK and (gamma-32P)-ATP
as mentioned by Varela et al. (1984). After phosphorylation,
proteins were separated by SDS-PAGE and the phosphorylated
proteins identified by autoradiography using intensifier
screens. Under these conditions only one phosphoprotein
with Mr of about 50K was identified.

Analysis of 32P-labeled Tryptic Peptides of Phospholipid
Methyltransferase

Phosphorylated phospholipid methyltransferase was precipitated with acetone at -20°C. Acetone was then removed
and the pellet dried with a stream of N2. After drying, the
pellet was resuspended into 50 mM ammonium bicarbonate, pH
7.7, and dialysed overnight against the same buffer. After
dialysis trypsin was added (1 part trypsin/20 parts protein)
and incubated 1h at 37°C. After trypsinization, the solution
was concentrated by lyophilization, dissolved into 0.1 ml
10 mM ammonium acetate pH 6.5 and applied on a Nucleosil
C18 HPLC column. Tryptic peptides were eluted from the column with a linear gradient starting with 100% 10 mM ammonium acetate pH 6.5 to 70% ammonium acetate and 30% acetoni-
trile. The flow rate was 1.5 ml/min. Chromatographic fractions were collected directly into scintillation vials at
1.5 min intervals and the Cherenkov radiation determined.
After HPLC, 32P-labeled samples were concentrated and dissolved into 0.01 ml water, centrifuged and applied to a
TLC-cellulose plate. The plate was developed with 1-butanol/
pyridine/water/acetic acid (65:50:40:10). 32P-labeled pep-

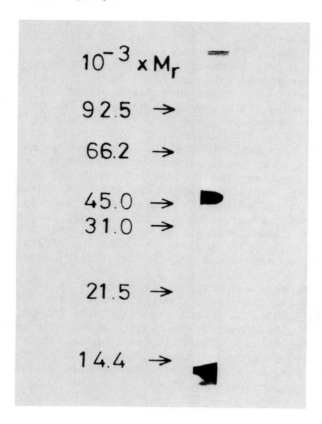

Figure 1. Phosphorylation of the 50K protein of phospholipid methyltransferase by the cAMP-PK. Conditions were
as described under Methods.

tides were localyzed by autoradiography.

Phospholipid Methyltransferase Phosphorylation by Intact
        Rat Hepatocytes: Effect of Glucagon.

        Anti-phospholipid methyltransferase serum was obtained
in rabbits by i.m. injection of the purified enzyme. The
gamma fraction of this antiserum was purified and coupled
to CNBr-activated Sepharose 4B and used to immunoprecipita-

te lysates of rat hepatocytes. Isolated rat hepatocytes, preincubated with 0.1 mM (32P)-phosphate (0.2 mCi/ml, Amersham) (Garrison, 1983), were exposed for 10 min to 0.001 μM glucagon or to the dissolvent of glucagon before lysis with acetone (4 ml acetone/ml cells) and incubated at -20°C for 20 min. Samples were then centrifuged, dried and treated with 0.5 ml of a mixture of detergents (1% Triton X-100, 0.1% sodium deoxycholate and 0.1% SDS) containing 10 mM Tris-HCl, pH 7.0, 20 mM sucrose, 150 mM KF, 15 mM EDTA, 2 mM EGTA, 50 mM beta-mercaptoethanol, 1 mM phenylmethanesulphonyl fluoride, 1 mM benzamidine, 50 μg/ml leupeptine and 1 mM nitrophenyl-4-phosphate. The anti-phospholipid methyltransferase serum, coupled to Sepharose, was then added. After 20 min incubation at 4°C the immunoprecipitate was centrifuged and extensively washed. After washing, the immunoprecipitate was dissociated at 100°C for 2 min in 2% SDS and 100 μl of each sample analysed by SDS-PAGE (10% acrylamide). After electrophoresis the gel was dried and autoradiographed.

For the analysis of phosphoaminoacids, after staining the gel weakly, the piece of gel containing the 50K protein was cut and subjected to acid hydrolysis in 6N HCl during 2h at 110°C. After hydrolysis, phosphoaminoacids were separated by high voltage electrophoresis on cellulose plates by the procedure of Hunter and Sefton (1980) as previously described (Varela et al., 1984). Phosphoaminoacids were localyzed by autoradiography.

RESULTS

Phosphorylation of partially purified phospholipid methyltransferase by the cAMP-PK results in the incorporation of 32P into one single protein with Mr of about 50K (Figure 1). Digestion of the phosphorylated enzyme with trypsin, followed by analysis of the tryptic peptides by HPLC, indicates the presence of one single site of phosphorylation which we have named P1 (Figure 2). After its isolation by HPLC, P1 was concentrated and further purified by TLC on a cellulose plate. After chromatography, the TLC plate was autoradiographed. Only one 32P-labeled spot was visualized by this procedure (Figure 2). The amino acid composition of P1 purified by HPLC and TLC, is: (Asx)2, Thr, Ser, (Glx)2, Pro, (Gly)2, Ala, Val, Ile, Leu, Tyr, Phe, His, Lys and Arg.

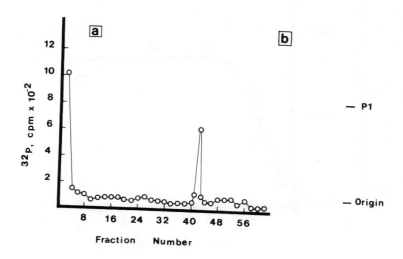

Figure 2. Analysis of 32P-labeled tryptic peptides of phosphorylated phospholipid methyltransferase by HPLC (a) and TLC (b). Conditions were as described under Methods.

Phosphorylation of phospholipid methyltransferase in the presence of 50 uM S-adenosylmethionine (AdoMet) followed by tryptic digestion and HPLC analysis reveals that under these conditions phosphorylation of P1 is enhanced about 2.5 fold. No other peptides besides P1 were found to be phosphorylated in the presence of 50 μM AdoMet (not shown). AdoMet-dependent phosphorylation occurs only on serine residues. S-adenosylhomocysteine (AdoHcy) has no effect on phospholipid methyltransferase phosphorylation but inhibits, in a dose-dependent manner, AdoMet-dependent phosphorylation of P1 (Figure 3).

We have obtained a rabbit antiserum specific for rat liver phospholipid methyltransferase. The gamma fraction of this antiserum recognizes the 50K and 25K proteins of phospholipid methyltransferase, using immunoblotting techniques. This gamma fraction was coupled to activated Sepha-

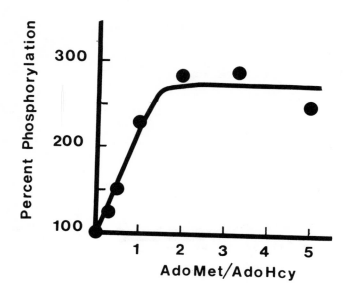

Figure 3. Effect of the ratio AdoMet/AdoHcy on phospholipid methyltransferase phosphorylation. Conditions
were as described under Methods. The concentration of Ado-
Met was 50 μM and the concentration of AdoHcy was varied
to obtain the desired ratio of AdoMet/AdoHcy.

rose and used to immunoprecipitate detergent solubilized
acetone pellets obtained from isolated rat hepatocytes.
Analysis by SDS-polyacrylamide gel electrophoresis of the
immunoprecipitate reveals two main proteins with Mr of
respectively about 50K and 25K (not shown). Isolated rat
hepatocytes were preincubated with (32P)-phosphate and exposed to 0.001 μM glucagon for 10 min before homogenization.
The 50K protein of phospholipid methyltransferase was then
purified by immunoprecipitation and analyzed by SDS-polyacrylamide gel electrophoresis. Exposure of isolated rat
hepatocytes to glucagon enhances the phosphorylation of
the 50K protein (Figure 4). Treatment of isolated rat hepatocytes with a saturating doses of glucagon (1 μM) produces a time-dependent stimulation of phospholipid methyl-

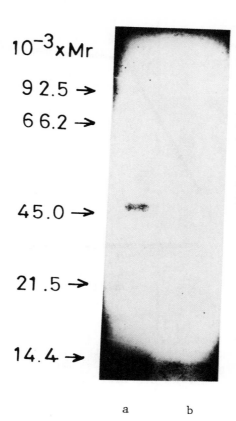

Figure 4. Autoradiogram showing the effect of glucagon on the phosphorylation of the 50K protein of phospholipid methyltransferase by intact hepatocytes. (a) glucagon 0.001 μM; (b) dissolvent of glucagon. Conditions were as described under Methods.

transferase phosphorylation (Figure 5). Maximal phosphory-lation is attained about 10 min and sustained for at least 30 min after the addition of the hormone.

Autoradiograms of high-voltage cellulose electrophore-sis of an acidic hydrolysate of the 50K protein of phospho-lipid methyltransferase isolated from rat hepatocytes pre-

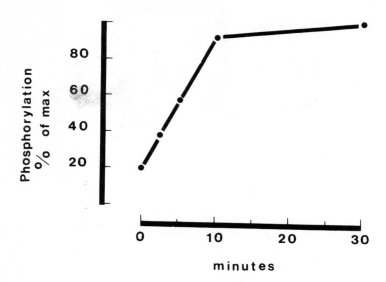

Figure 5. Effect of glucagon on the time–course of phosphorylation of phospholipid methyltransferase by intact hepatocytes. At time zero cells were stimulated with 1 μM glucagon. Conditions were as described under Methods.

incubated with (32P)-phosphate and treated with 1 μM glucagon
showed only phosphoserine (Figure 6). The incorporation of
32P into the 50K protein of non-stimulated hepatocytes was
also on phosphoserine (not shown).

DISCUSSION

The present results show that the 50K protein of rat
liver phospholipid methyltransferase is phosphorylated by
the cAMP-PK at one single serine residue (P1). AdoMet enhances, in a time- and dose-dependent manner, P1 phosphorylation. Since AdoMet stimulates P1 phosphorylation at micromolar concentrations, which are believed to be physiological (Duerre, 1982), these results suggest that this effect

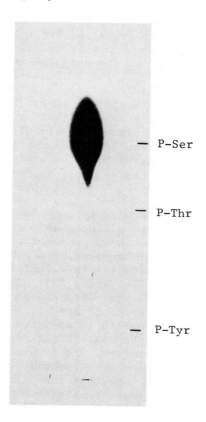

Figure 6. Autoradiogram showing that serine is the only aminoacid of the 50K protein of phospholipid methyltransferase phosphorylated by intact rat hepatocytes exposed to glucagon. Conditions were as described under Methods. Hepatocytes were stimulated with 1 µM glucagon for 10 min. P-Ser, phosphoserine; P-Thr, phosphothreonine; P-Tyr, phosphotyrosine.

of AdoMet might also occur <u>in vivo</u>. AdoHcy alone has no effect on Pl-phosphorylation but inhibits AdoMet-dependent Pl-phosphorylation. The present results indicate that the ratio AdoMet/AdoHcy modulates Pl-phosphorylation in a dose-dependent manner. In these experiments the concentration of AdoMet was .fixed at 50 µM, which is thought to be physiolo-

gical for the liver (Duerre, 1982), and the amount of Ado-
Hcy was varied to obtain AdoMet/AdoHcy ratios varying from
0.25 to 5. This range is of physiological interest since
the ratio AdoMet/AdoHcy in the normally fed adult rat liver
is about 1.5 (Miura et al., 1984). These results suggest
that the ratio AdoMet/AdoHcy might be an important factor
in modulating the phosphorylation of Pl. Since phosphorylation of the 50K protein of phospholipid methyltransferase
stimulates its transmethylase activity (Varela et al.,
1984), the ratio AdoMet/AdoHcy might control this methylation reaction by regulating both the state of phosphorylation of the enzime and the availabitity of the substrate
AdoMet.

From the present results it can also be concluded that
in intact rat hepatocytes glucagon stimulates the phosphorylation of the 50K protein of phospholipid methyltransferase at serine residues. Glucagon, and other conditions
which are known to elevate the intracellular levels of
cyclic AMP (Castaño et al., 1980; Pritchard et al., 1981;
Marin Cao et al., 1983), activates phospholipid methyltransferase in rat hepatocytes. Furthermore, phosphorylation of
the 50K protein in the partially purified enzyme at one
single serine residue enhances its methylating activity (Varela et al., 1984). Therefore, the available evidence indicates that phosphorylation of phospholipid methyltransferase in hepatocytes is an important mechanism for the short-
term hormonal control of the synthesis of phosphatidylcholine by the transmethylation pathway. It remains to be determined whether phospholipid methyltransferase in cells
other than hepatocytes is also phosphorylated and whether
in these enzymes phosphorylation modulates the enzyme activity.

ACKNOWLEDGEMENTS

We thank Paloma Bellod for reading the manuscript. IV
and MV are fellows of the Plan Nacional del Síndrome Tóxi-
co. MP and IM are fellows of the Fundación Conchita Rábago
and JT is a fellow of the CAICYT. This work was supported
by grants from CAICYT, FISS and Europharma.

REFERENCES

Castaño, J. G., Alemany, S., Nieto, A. and Mato, J. M. (1980) J. Biol. Chem. 255, 9041-9043.

Duerre, J. A. (1982) in Biochemistry of S-adenosylmethionine and Related Compounds (Usdin, E., Borchardt, R. T. and Creveling, C. R.; Eds.) pp. 595-602, McMillan Press, London.

Garrison, J. C. (1983)   Methods in Enzymology 99, 20-36.

Hunter, T. and Sefton, B. (1980) Proc. Nat. Acad. Sci. U. S.A. 77, 1311-1315.

Marin Cao, D., Alvarez Chiva, V. and Mato, J. M. (1983) Biochem. J. 216, 675-680.

Mato, J. M., Alemany, S., Garcia Gil, M., Marin Cao, D., Varela, I. and Castaño, J. G. (1982) in Biochemistry of S-adenosylmethionine and Related Compounds (Usdin, E., Borchardt, R. T. and Creveling, C. R.; Eds.) pp 187-198, McMillan Press, London.

Miura, G. A., Santangelo, J. R., Gordon, R. K. and Chiang, P. K. (1984) Anal. Biochem. 141, 161-167.

Pajares, M. A., Alemany, S., Varela, I., Marin Cao, D. and Mato, J. M. (1984) Biochem. J. 223, 61-66.

Pritchard, P. H., Pellech, S. L. and Vance, D. E. (1981) Biochim. Biophys. Acta 666, 301-306.

Schuller, A., Moscat, J., Diez, E., Fernandez Checa, J. C., Gavilanes, F. and Municio, A. M. (1985) Hepatology.   In Press.

Varela, I., Merida, I., Pajares, M. A., Villalba, M. and Mato, J. M. (1984) Biochim. Biophys. Res. Commun. 122, 1065-1070.

BRAIN PHOSPHATIDYLCHOLINE POOLS AS POSSIBLE SOURCES OF FREE CHOLINE FOR ACETYLCHOLINE SYNTHESIS.

M. Lakher, R.J. Wurtman, J. Blusztajn,
P. Holbrook, J-C. Maire, C. Mauron and
M. Tacconi

Massachusetts Institute of Technology,
Cambridge, Massachusetts, 02139, USA

HYPOTHESIS: PRODUCTION OF FREE CHOLINE IN BRAIN.

Choline in cholinergic neurons has two fates: it is a constituent of phosphatidylcholine (PC) and other phospholipids (sphingomyelin, choline plasmalogens, lysophosphatidylcholine) and is used as a precursor for synthesis of a neurotransmitter, acetylcholine (ACh). The pool of PC in the brain (about 16 μmol/g tissue) is several orders of magnitude larger than the pools of free choline and ACh. A number of experimental observations support the hypothesis that at least a portion of this lipid-bound choline can provide free choline for ACh formation. Firstly, more choline molecules leave the brain than enter it (i.e., there is a negative arteriovenous difference) (Dross & Kewitz, 1972; Aquilonius et al., 1975; Choi et al., 1975; Spanner et al., 1976), even though lipid-bound circulating PC apparently does not enter the brain (Pardridge et al., 1979), indicating that brain cells both produce choline-containing compounds (like PC) de novo, and liberate free choline from these larger molecules. Secondly, when labelled choline was infused intravenously into rats, specific radioactivities of free choline in the brain were found to be lower than those in the blood or liver, suggesting that unlabelled choline, produced within the brain, was diluting the material taken up from the blood (Choi et al., 1975; Kewitz & Pleul, 1976; Spanner et al., 1976). Thirdly, consumption of a choline-deficient diet had no effect on the striatal levels of choline and ACh in rats, even though blood cho-

line concentrations were markedly decreased (Millington &
Wurtman, 1982).

Consistent with the view that neuronal PC is a reser-
voir of choline for ACh synthesis, levels of PC in the cat's
superior cervical ganglion fell by 31% when preganglionic
trunk was stimulated electrically in the presence of hemi-
cholinium, i.e., when more choline was needed for ACh synthesis (Parducz et al., 1976). We have also observed a
25-50% decrease in the PC content of electrically stimulated
(30 V, 15 Hz, 30 min.) rat striatal slices superfused with
Krebs buffer (pH=7.4) lacking exogenous choline (Mauron &
Wurtman, unpublished experiments). At the same time, ACh
release from slices increases from 7.5 ± 1.3 pmol/mg protein x min. (mean ± S.D.) to 25.6 ± 5.9 pmol/mg protein x
min., and tissue choline and ACh were not depleted, in
parallel. (The combined decrease in choline+ACh within the
tissue was 16 pmol/mg protein x min., compared with a total
efflux of 75 pmol/mg protein x min. into the superfusate
(Maire et al., 1983).) These data, again suggest that cholinergic neurons might utilize choline liberated from all
or part of the endogenous PC in brain to sustain ACh synthesis.

POOLS OF PHOSPHATIDYLCHOLINE IN BRAIN.

There are a variety of "pools" of PC in the brain, defined by their biochemical pathway of synthesis, fatty acid
composition, subcellular localization, and turnover rates.
Three pathways of PC biosynthesis are known to exist: the
CDP-choline pathway (the Kennedy cycle), in which PC is
synthesized from diacylglycerol and activated choline (cytidine diphosphate choline); the "base exchange" pathway,
in which PC is formed by exhanging pre-existing free choline with the ethanolamine in phosphatidylethanolamine (PE)
or the serine in phosphatidylserine (PS); and the transmethylation pathway, in which PC is formed by the stepwise
methylation of PE, using S-adenosylmethionine (SAM) as a
donor of methyl groups. Only this pathway synthesizes
"new" choline moieties. Choline must, otherwise, be transported to the brain through the blood-brain barrier (Pardridge et al., 1979). Even though it is widely believed
that most of the PC in the brain is synthesized by the CDP-
choline pathway, i.e., by the incorporation of pre-existing

choline (Ansell & Spanner, 1971), the transmethylation pathway might produce a functionally-distinct pool of PC, perhaps related to membrane fluidity, asymmetry, or remodelling,
or even a source of free choline, as proposed above. It is
of particular interest that choline deficiency led to activation of the phospholipid methylation pathway in the liver
(Glenn & Austin, 1971; Schneider & Vance, 1978) and in neuroblastoma x glioma hybrid cells (Blusztajn et al., 1985).
In our preliminary experiments PE methylation was increased
when rat striatal slices superfused in the absence of choline were stimulated electrically (a treatment which concur-
rently reduced the total PC content of the slices) (Lakher &
Wurtman, unpublished experiments).

The fatty acid composition of a particular PC molecule,
or the average composition of a PC "pool", is determined by
its mode of synthesis (i.e., from the glycerol backbone in
diacylglycerol, PE, or PS) and by postsynthetic modification
by reacylation. This latter process involves coordinated
actions of the enzymes phospholipase A2, which releases a
fatty acid from the 2 position of a phospholipid (forming a
lysophospholipid), and of lysophospholipid:acylCoA acyl-
transferase, which then adds a free fatty acid. We have
determined that the PC's formed in vitro in rat brain synaptosomes by any of the three pathways contain much larger
proportions of polyunsaturated fatty acids (PUFA) than
unlabelled synaptosomal PC (Table 1). (We assume that the
labelled PC synthesized in our experiments was not modified
by reacylation since our preparations did not contain exogenous cofactors (Mg^{++}, ATP, and CoA) necessary for reacylation activity (Sun et al., 1983). It is not known whether
reacylation equally affects PC's formed by each of the three
synthetic pathways.) This suggests that newly-synthesized
PC in synaptosomes, regardless of its pathway of synthesis,
is rich in PUFA. One might speculate that the fatty acid
composition of such PC is being modified within the membrane
by the reacylation process while its molecules diffuse away
from their site of synthesis. As a result of this process,
this PC pool loses PUFA and gains more saturated fatty acids
becoming similar to the "bulk" PC pool. Alternatively, and
perhaps additionally, the difference between the fatty acid
composition of newly-synthesized and bulk synaptosomal PC
could reflect the rapid irreversible destruction of more-
unsaturated molecules soon after their formation.

Table 1, Molecular species of phosphatidylcholine
synthesized in synaptosomes by PE methylation, base
exchange, or cholinephosphotransferase: comparison
with the "bulk" pool,

MOLECULAR SPECIES	PC (phosphate)	DISTRIBUTION OF RADIOACTIVITY		
		PE METHYLATION	BASE EXCHANGE	CHOLINE-PHOSPHO-TRANSFERASE
		% of total		
SATURATES, MONO- AND DIENES	77.1	3.2	34.4	38.0
TETRAENES	15.8	34.6	28.7	36.9
PENTA- AND HEXAENES	7.1	62.2	37.0	25.0

Rat brain synaptosomes were incubated in the presence of
0.01 mM [3H-methyl]-SAM for 30 min.(PE methylation) (Tacconi & Wurtman, unpublished experiments); or 0.05 mM
[14C]-choline for 20 min. (base exchange); or 0.5 mM
CDP-[14C]-choline for 20 min, (cholinephosphotransferase
assay) (Holbrook & Wurtman, unpublished experiments).
Phospholipid fractions were subjected to TLC on silica gel
plates. Segments of silica gel corresponding to the ra-
diolabelled PC were extracted with methanol and PC molecular species were resolved using chromatography on argen-
tated silica gel plates, The identity of molecular species was verified by detecting the fatty acid composition
in each band using gas chromatography,

It is conceivable that there might exist, besides a
larger pool of "structural" PC, smaller, more metabolically
active PC pools, Free choline could originate from such
pools. Although the exact pathways that liberate free choline from synaptosomal PC are not known, one can outline

two mechanisms that seem likely to mediate this process.
Firstly, part of the lysoPC produced by phospholipase A2
can be catabolized to glycerophosphocholine (GPCh) by lyso-
phospholipase. GPCh-diesterase, an enzyme widely distributed throughout the brain (Mann, 1975; Ansell & Spanner,
1981), can metabolize the GPCh further to form glycero-
phosphate and free choline. Secondly, free choline can be
released from PC directly by phospholipase D, a Ca^{++}-depen-
dent enzyme (Kanfer, 1972). Our studies suggest the existence of a short-lived PC pool, formed in synaptosomes
in vitro via the transmethylation pathway. In these experiments 30% of the PC molecules synthesized by the transmethylation pathway are converted to free choline within
30 min. (Blusztajn & Wurtman, 1980).

PC SYNTHESIS VIA TRANSMETHYLATION IN RAT BRAIN IN VIVO.

Quantitative aspects of the N-methylation of PE have
not previously been investigated thoroughly in brain. In
vivo studies (Chida & Arakawa, 1971; Morganstern & Abdel-
Latif, 1974) revealed that brain PC was labelled shortly
after injection of radioactive methionine into rats, and
that this labelling was greater after intracranial than
after systemic injections. These studies, however, did not
allow quantitative conclusions since the specific radioactivities of the methyl donor (SAM) were not measured. An
additional problem confronting researchers attempting to
quantitate PE methylation in brain has been the lack of an
established mathematical approach for estimating the kinetic parameters of PE methylation in brain without knowing
the size of the PC pool that is being synthesized by methylation (Zawad & Brown, 1985).

We have characterized the synthesis of PC via the
transmethylation pathway in vivo, infusing [3H]-methionine
(10-25 µCi) into the rat's lateral cerebral ventricle (via
a plastic cannula implanted 3-5 days earlier) and following
the time-course of radioactivities in brain SAM and PC.
Brains were homogenized in 0.4 N perchloric acid. SAM was
determined by HPLC (Gharib et al., 1982). Phospholipid
fractions were extracted into chloroform:methanol (2:1)
mixture according to the method of Folch (Folch et al.,
1957) and purified on silica columns. PC was isolated by
TLC, hydrolyzed by 6 N HCl, and the resulting choline was

then rechromatographed in another TLC system. Brain extracts contained very small amounts (compared with [3H]-PC)
of labelled phosphatidyl nomo- and di- methylethanolamines,
two intermediates of the PE methylation pathway. The same
was true for liver extracts, analyzed as controls, from
animals receiving systemic or intracerebral [3H]-methio-
nine.

To affirm that the [3H]-SAM and [3H]-PC measured in
brain tissue after intracerebroventricular (i.c.v.) [3H]-
methionine were synthesized within this tissue, we injected
a bolus of [3H]-methionine (10 μCi) into the rat's jugular
vein and measured the specific radioactivities (S.R.A.'s)
of SAM and PC in the brain and in the liver. The S.R.A.'s
of brain SAM 15-45 minutes after intravenous [3H]-methio-
nine were 25-55 dpm/nmol, as compared with 3000-6250 dpm/
nmol following i.c.v. injections of the same amount of
[3H]-methionine. Since SAM poorly penetrates the blood-
brain barrier, it is likely that even the small amounts of
radioactive SAM detected in brains of rats receiving peripheral [3H]-methionine were made within the brain (from
transported [3H]-methionine). The S.R.A.'s of SAM in the
liver did not differ following the two routes of [3H]-me-
thionine administration and were 10-40 dpm/nmol SAM. Only
traces of radioactive PC could be detected in rat brain
after intravenous [3H]-methionine whereas after i.c.v. administrations the S.R.A.'s of brain PC were 170-400 dpm/
μmol PC. At the same time, the S.R.A.'s of liver PC were
comparable following two routes of [3H]-methionine administration (1000-3000 dpm/μmol PC). These observations strongly
support the central origin of the [3H]-PC detected in the
brain after i.c.v. [3H]-methionine.

QUANTITATIVE ANALYSIS OF THE CONVERSION OF SAM TO PC IN VIVO.

The experimental data for the disappearance of the
[3H]-SAM synthesized from [3H]-methionine in rat brain
(Fig. 1) were fitted to an exponential function; the best
fit corresponded to a rate constant (K_{sam}) of 0.01 min.$^{-1}$.
The synthesis rate of SAM calculated using the actual concentrations of brain SAM (17.6 nmol/g) was 176 pmol/g x min.
and the half-life of the SAM was 68.7 min. An estimate of
the PC synthesis rate (64 $\pm$ 6 pmol/g x min.) was than obtained applying the following equation (derived from one
proposed by Neff et al., 1974) to values of [3H]-SAM and

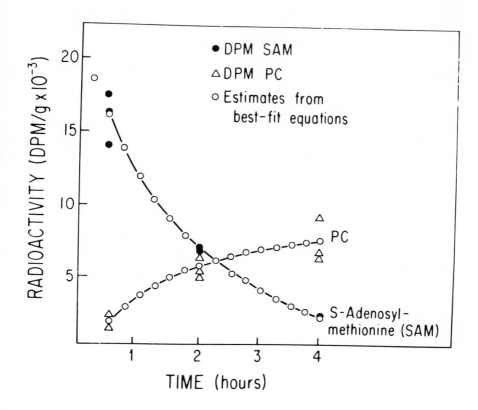

Figure 1. Time-course of [3H]-SAM and [3H]-PC present in rat brain after intracerebroventricular injections of [3H]-methionine.

Injections of [3H]-methionine and determinations of [3H]-SAM and [3H]-PC were performed as described in the text. Values are given as dpm per 1,000,000 dpm of tritium present in the brain. Each point represents an individual rat. The curves are interpolations of experimental points. Open circles are points obtained by fitting the experimental data as described in the text.

[3H]-PC that were interpolated from the experimental data
for 14 consecutive 15-minute-intervals of the time-course,
and averaging the 14 calculated values.

$$K_{pc} \times [PC] = 2 \times (PC_2 - PC_1) \times [SAM]/(SAM_1 + SAM_2) \times (t_2 - t_1)$$

(K_{pc} is the rate constant of PC synthesis by the transmethylation pathway; [PC] is the metabolic pool of PC formed by
methylation of PE in rat brain; $K_{pc} \times [PC]$ is the synthesis
rate of PC formed by the transmethylation pathway; PC_1, PC_2,
SAM_1, and SAM_2 are radioactivies in PC and SAM, respectively, at two different times, t_1 and t_2, after [3H]-me-
thionine injection; [SAM] is the pool of SAM in rat brain.)

Since the size of the PC pool formed by methylation of
brain PE ([PC]) is not known, and calculation of the rate
constant for PC (K_{pc}) thus could not be performed directly
using the same procedure, we had to utilize a fitting procedure in which two parameters, K_{pc} and [PC], were fitted
simultaneously. A model curve for [3H]-PC accumulation has
been constructed using the following equation:

$$PC_2 = PC_1 \times [2 - K_{pc} \times (t_2 - t_1)]/[2 + K_{pc} \times (t_2 - t_1)] +$$
$$+ K_{pc} \times [PC] \times (t_2 - t_1) \times (SAM_1 + SAM_2)/[SAM] \times [2 + K_{pc} \times (t_2 - t_1)]$$

where the designations are the same as above.

The optimal value of K_{pc} was estimated to be 0.0004
min.$^{-1}$ and of [PC] - 167 nmol/g. Thus, the pool of PC
formed by the transmethylation represents about 1% of total
brain PC (16 μmol/g as determined by assaying phosphorus).
The time to replace half of this pool is 18.3 hr, - which is
considerably less than literature values for the half-lifes
of brain PC obtained using choline, glycerol, or phosphorus
as tracers (up to 52 days) (Porcellati et al., 1983). By
comparing the calculated synthesis rates of the SAM and PC,
we draw the tentative conclusion that about 40% of SAM synthesized in brain from methionine is used for the production
of PC via transmethylation. This finding implies that changing the activity of the PE methylation pathway may affect
the availability of SAM for other transmethylation reactions
in the brain.

SUMMARY,

The hypothesis is presented that the brain generates free choline for acetylcholine synthesis from endogenous PC, and that a particular "pool" of PC - perhaps that formed by PE methylation - turns over rapidly and is used as a choline source. Our observations show that this pool - which probably accounts for about 1% of brain PC, and may or may not be quantitatively more significant within cholinergic terminals, is highly enriched with polyunsaturated fatty acids when synthesized, does turn over rapidly, and its synthesis may be activated when neuronal firing is accelerated. Moreover, the fraction of total brain SAM used for PE methylation is very great, suggesting that changes in the rate of this process may influence the amounts of SAM available for methylating other acceptors.

ACKNOWLEDGEMENTS.

These studies were supported in part by research and training grants from the National Institute of Mental Health (MH-28783; MH-15761), and fellowships from the Center for Brain Sciences and Metabolism Charitable Trust. Mr.Lakher and Ms.Holbrook hold pre-doctoral fellowships (MH-08854 and MH-09199) from the National Institute of Mental Health.

REFERENCES.

Aquilonius, S.M., Cedar, G., Lying-Tunell, U., Malmund, H.O. and Schubert, J. (1975) Brain Res. 99, 430-433

Ansell, G.B. and Spanner, S. (1971) Biochem.J. 122, 741-750

Ansell, G.B. and Spanner, S. (1981) in Advances in Behavioral Biology 25, Cholinergic Mechanisms (Pepeu, G. and Ladinsky, H., Eds.) pp.393-403, Plenum Press, New York

Blusztajn, J.K. and Wurtman, R.J. (1980) Nature 290, 417-418

Blusztajn, J.K., Chapman Lingham, C., Richardson, U.I. and Wurtman, R.J. (1985) Int.Soc.Neurochem., Satellite Meeting, Abstract P18, 66

Chida, N. and Arakawa, T. (1971) Tohoku J.exp.Med. 104, 359-371

Choi, R.L., Freeman, J.J. and Jenden, D.J. (1975) J.Neu-
rochem. 24, 735-741
Dross, K. and Kewitz, H. (1972) Naunyn-Scmiedberg's Arch.
Pharmacol. 274, 91-106
Folch, J., Lees, M. and Sloanne-Stanley, G.H. (1957)
J.Biol.Chem. 226, 497-509
Gharib, A., Sarda, N., Chabannes, B., Cronenberger, L. and
Pacheco, H. (1982) J.Neurochem. 38, 810-815
Glenn, J.L. and Austin, W. (1971) Biochim.Biophys.Acta 231,
153-160
Kanfer, J.N. (1972) J.Lipid Res. 13, 468-477
Kewitz, H. and Pleul, O. (1976) Proc.Natl.Acad.Sci.USA 73,
2181-2185
Maire, J-C., Tacconi, M. and Wurtman, R.J. (1983) Soc.
Neurosci. 9, Abstract 283.8
Mann, S.P. (1975) Experientia 31, 1256-1257
Millington, W.R. and Wurtman, R.J. (1982) J.Neurochem. 38,
1748-1752
Morganstern, R.D. and Abdel-Latif, A.A. (1974) J.Neurobiol.
5, 393-411
Neff, N.H., Spano, P.F., Gropetti, A., Wang, C.T. and
Costa, E. (1974) J.Pharm.Exp.Ther. 176, 701-710
Pardridge, W.M., Cornford, E.M., Braun, L.D. and Olden-
dorf, W.H. (1979) in Nutrition and Brain 5, Choline and
Lecithin in Brain Disorders (Barbeau, A., Growdon, J.H.
and Wurtman, R.J., Eds.) pp.25-34, Raven Press, New York
Parducz, A., Kiss, Z. and Joo, F. (1976) Experientia 32,
1520-1521
Porcellati, G., Goracci, G. and Arienti, G. (1983) in
Handbook of Neurochemistry 5, Metabolic Turnover in the
Nervous System (Lajtha, A., Ed.) pp.277-294, Plenum
Press, New York and London
Schneider, W.J. and Vance, D.E. (1978) Eur.J.Biochem. 85,
181-187
Spanner, S., Hall, R.C. and Ansell, G.B. (1976) Biochem.J.
154, 133-140
Sun, G.Y., Tang, W., Majewska, M.D., Hallett, D.W., Foudin,
L. and Huang, S. (1983) in Neural Membranes (Sun, G.Y.,
Bazan, N., Wu, J-Y., Porcellati, G. and Sun, A.Y., Eds.)
pp.67-95, Humana Press, Clifton, New Jersey
Zawad, J.S. and Brown, F.C. (1985) J.Neurochem. 44, 808-
811

B. Nucleic Acid Methylations

DNA METHYLATION: OVERVIEW AND PROSPECTIVES

Thomas W. Sneider

Department of Biochemistry, Colorado State

University, Fort Collins, CO 80523 USA

INTRODUCTION

"Epicytosine" or 5-methylcytosine was first noted as a component of calf thymus DNA in 1948 (Hotchkiss, 1948). The non-random distribution of 5-methylcytosine in DNA led to the suggestion that this minor base derived from post-replication modification of DNA (Kornberg et al., 1959). Subsequent studies showed that DNA modification in prokaryotes is part of the host range restriction system (Arber, 1968) and is also involved in strand selection in mismatch repair of DNA (Radman and Wagner, 1984). Although DNA methylation may serve other functions in prokaryotes, attention has recently focused on DNA methylation in eukaryotic systems. Application of molecular biological techniques to analyses of eukaryotic DNA methylation has led to explosive growth of this field; almost 300 papers were published just in 1984. This paper will present an overview of only selected recent analyses of eukaryotic DNA methylation.

DNA METHYLATION AND REGULATION OF GENE EXPRESSION

Evidence for linkage of DNA methylation and gene expression has come primarily from three experimental approaches: in vitro methylation of viral or cellular DNAs followed by analyses of transcription in oocytes or animal cells; analyses of the general or site-specific methylation patterns of genes in transcriptionally-active versus - inactive cells;

and, treatment of cells with 5-azacytidine, an inhibitor of
DNA methylation. Results from such studies have been extensively reviewed (Doerfler, 1984; Jaenisch and Jähner,
1984; Razin and Cedar, 1984; Razin and Szyf, 1984; THIS
VOLUME) and will not be repeated here. In many instances,
site-specific methylation clearly does suppress expression
and site-specific hypomethylations do correlate well with
gene expression. What are not yet clear are the molecular
mechanisms involved in, and the control of, these two processes.

Methylation-mediated suppression of gene expression
could be effected by altering interactions of modified tem-
plate with components of the transcriptional machinery. If
so, then differences in transcription of methylated versus
nonmethylated DNAs might be seen in vitro using soluble
transcription assays as well as in structured Xenopus oocyte
or animal cell systems. However, Jove et al. (1984) detected no effect of in vitro methylation (Hha I methylase) of
poly d(GC):d(GC) blocks inserted adjacent to transcriptional
control regions in SV40 or adenovirus-2 plasmid constructs
when using a HeLa whole cell lysate system. Methylation of
naturally-occurring CpGs in the viral:plasmid constructs
also had no effect on in vitro transcription. These results
are especially interesting since in vitro methylation of the
single Hpa II site in SV40 does inhibit late gene transcription in the Xenopus oocyte system (Fradin et al., 1982) but
has no effect on SV40 late gene expression studied in vivo
(Graessman et al., 1984) or in vitro (Fradin et al., 1982).
Hence, DNA packaging into chromatin may be important in
methylation-mediated gene suppression since exogenous DNA
injected into oocytes assembles into chromatin (Laskey et
al., 1977) whereas no assembly occurs in the HeLa whole cell
lysate system (Hough et al., 1982). The disparate results
using the same DNA in several biological systems also suggest the possibility that cell/tissue-specific regulatory
factors may govern the ability of methylation to silence gene
expression. But it is not yet known at a molecular level
how chromatin configuration, putative regulatory factors,
and methylation state of gene control regions precisely in-
terrelate.

Similarly, mechanisms for generating hypomethylated
sites in DNA which often, but not always, correlate with
gene expression are not yet worked out. Such sites could be
generated by an active demethylase or by interference with
maintainence-type methylase activity. Only a few reports
support the former concept. Nucleoplasm from DMSO-induced

murine erythroleukemia cells apparently catalyzed in vitro
removal of (^{3}H-methyl)-groups from labeled DNA CCGG sites
(Gjerset and Martin, 1982) but no additional information on
this activity has appeared. The most accepted model of
hypomethylation involves interference with methylase action
at hemimethylated sites such that, after two rounds of replication, a fully nonmethylated site is generated. Hence,
replication is required. However, specific Hpa II sites in
the chick lens delta-crystalline gene and in the chicken
vitellogenin II gene became non-methylated in biological
systems that naturally (former case) or artificially (latter
case) had ceased DNA replication leading the authors to suggest the presence of active demethylase activity (Sullivan
and Grainger, 1984; Wilks et al., 1984). Factors that might
influence the fidelity of maintainence-type methylase and
thus generate hypomethylated sites are considered in the
next section.

Finally, the mechanisms by which hypomethylated sites
might make a gene more accessible for transcription are not
understood. The initial supposition that specific methylation and hypomethylation might be an off/on switch has given
way to the concept that hypomethylation might be a necessary
but not sufficient condition for gene expression. For example, a cloned (unmethylated) human globin gene introduced
into murine erythroleukemia cells was only expressed after
treatment of the cells with the inducer DMSO (Chao et al.,
1983; Wright et al., 1983); mere absence of site-specific
methylation in the transfected gene was not sufficient for
its expression. Similarly, chickens treated with phenyl-
hydrazine then 5-azacytidine showed only low levels of embryonic rho-globin mRNA even though this gene underwent nearly complete demethylation. However, if the inducer sodium
butyrate was given after 5-azacytidine treatment, a 5 to 10-
fold increase in embryonic rho-globin mRNA was seen but only
if the rho-globin gene was first demethylated by azacytidine
treatment (Ginder et al., 1984).

There is, however, evidence that the "necessary but not
sufficient" concept can not be universally applied. Full
methylation of putatively critical CpG sites in the spacer
of rDNA from Xenopus sperm was not at all inimical to transcription in an oocyte system (Macleod and Bird, 1983). More
recently, no hypomethylation (at testable sites) was noted
upon induction of rearranged or nonrearranged kappa immuno-
globin genes in a B-cell lympoma line (Nelson et al., 1984),
upon activation of the chicken alpha-2(I) collagen gene
(McKeon et al., 1984), or the estrogen-inducible vitellogenin

VA1 and VA2 genes in Xenopus (Gerber-Huber et al., 1983).
Perhaps the most extreme example is found with retinoic acid
induced activation of the H-2K transplantation antigen gene
in embryonal carcinoma cells. In this system two cell
clones from retinoic acid treated cells showed site-specific
hypomethylation of albumin, insulin, and endogenous mammary
tumor virus DNAs (compared to their methylation state in untreated F9 cells) but no detectable transcription from these
genes. The H-2K gene is not expressed in the parental F9
cell yet is hypomethylated compared to the genes mentioned
above. However, a cloned line derived from retinoic acid
treated F9 cells shows increased methylation of H-2K at Hpa
II, Hha I, Ava I, and FnuDII sites and strong expression of
the H-2K gene. Moreover, treatment of this clone with 5-
azacytidine results in H-2K hypomethylation and silencing of
expression (Tanaka et al., 1983).

        This recent evidence suggests that some genes tran-
scribed by RNA polymerases I and II (see above) and III
(Brown and Gurdon, 1977; Jove et al., 1984) may not be modulated by methylation. What, then, is to be made of the
many studies which do show a correlation of methylation state
of a gene and transcriptional activity and of the more direct
experiments demonstrating silencing of expression by site-
specific in vitro methylations? Perhaps some of the former
studies might be explained "... as an accidental consequence
of an interaction whose real function lies elsewhere" as
stated by Macleod and Bird (1983). That is, hypomethylated
sites could be footprints of regulatory factors (proteins
and/or RNAs) that need to interact at those sites in order
to activate expression. Whether or not the methylation pattern per se or alterations in chromatin structure that it
might facilitate are important in modulating such interactions may vary from case to case.

                            Prospectives

        There are clearly many unanswered questions about
eukaryotic DNA methylation and modulation of gene expression.
Does methylation per se act as a signal for repressor-like
factors that silence expression? There is one recent report
of a DNA binding protein that preferentially bound to double-
stranded methylated DNA (Huang et al., 1984) but more work
is needed to identify and characterize such factors in well-
defined systems that can be functionally assayed vis a vis
transcription. The role of chromatin configuration and its
relationship to methylation also requires more intensive

analyses with respect to both silencing gene expression and
relationship to hypomethylated sites. CpG clusters at the
5'-end of the hypoxanthine phosphoribosyl transferase gene
and the 3'-end of the glucose-6-phosphate dehydrogenase gene
are hypomethylated and DNAase-I hypersensitive on the transcriptionally active X-chromosome but not the inactive X-
chromosome (Wolf and Migeon, 1985) but other results
(Gerber-Huber et al., 1983; Nelson et al., 1984; McKeon et
al., 1984) do not support a correlation between active
chromatin configuration [DNAase I hypersensitivity (Weisbrod,
1982)] and methylation state. However, Costlow et al. (1985)
recently showed that, in Drosophila heat shock protein 70
gene, sequences outside the DNAase I hypersensitive site are
involved in generating the site and suggest that the crea-
tion of the site might result from interaction of the external sequences with some protein factor (see also Emerson and
Felsenfeld, 1984). A role for Z-type DNA has also been suggested in establishing DNAase I hypersensitive sites
(Groudine and Weintraub, 1984). The demonstrated in vitro
involvement of DNA methylation in facilitating a B to Z
transition (Behe and Felsenfeld, 1981) therefore demands
further study. Further progress in characterizing tissue-
specific transcription-initiation factors and the sites and
modes of their interaction with gene control regions will
also be crucial for understanding the role of DNA methylation.

EUKARYOTIC DNA METHYLTRANSFERASES

     The establishment and maintainence of eukaryotic DNA
methylation patterns are functions of de novo and maintainence-type DNA methylases, respectively. The de novo activity
symmetrically methylates cytosine residues at a site in both
strands of DNA and the maintainence-type activity methylates
the cytosine residue in one strand of DNA at a hemimethylated
site. Recently developed molecular biological approaches
permit the construction of specific DNA fragments in non-
methylated (cloned DNA) or half-methylated states. The
availability of these defined substrates has revealed a relationship between de novo and maintenance methylase activities.
     Two DNA methylases, purified to near-homogeneity from
nuclei of uninduced Friend erythroleukemia cells, methylated
hemimethylated sites in poly d(meCG):d(CG) much more readily
than fully nonmodified poly d(CG:d(CG) but activity towards

the nonmethylated copolymer duplex did occur at significant
levels (Bestor and Ingram, 1983). DNA methylases from human
placenta (Pfeifer et al., 1983; Wang et al., 1984), calf
thymus cells (Sano et al., 1983), and mouse mastocytoma cells
(Grünwald and Drahovsky, 1984) also show significant de novo
methylase activity. In the cases of the placental and mastocytoma cell enzymes, both de novo and maintainence-type
activities copurified at all stages of purification to near-
homogeneity suggesting that a single enzyme may be responsible for both activities. De novo methylase activity can
also be elicited from a predominantly maintainence-type
methylase by limited proteolytic cleavage of DNA methylase
partially purified from Krebs II ascites tumor cells (Adams
et al., 1983).

Regulation of DNA Methylase Activities

DNA methylases interact with DNA at single-stranded
regions followed by a process of one-dimensional facilitated
transfer along duplex DNA. Both de novo and maintainence-
type DNA methylase activities apparently use this mechanism
(Bestor and Ingram, 1983). However, the regulation of
methylase activities is not well studied. No experimental
support exists for regulation of methylase activities directly at the enzyme level. Instead, observed patterns of
methylation have recently been suggested to arise from an
interplay between intracellular levels of DNA methylase(s)
and differing affinities of various DNA sites for the en-
zyme(s) (Razin and Syzf, 1984). Variations in DNA methylase
activities have been reported with the cell cycle (Sneider,
1977), during DNA repair in proliferating versus nonprolif-
erating cells (Kastan et al., 1982), and in regenerating rat
liver (Razin and Szyf, 1984). Differing affinities of various DNA sites for DNA methylase could be related to DNA
type or chromatin structure. In vitro, given DNA sequences
that can exist in either B or Z configurations, are about
equally well methylated de novo in either configuration when
using mammalian DNA methylases (Pfeifer et al., 1983; Bestor
and Ingram, 1983; Bolden et al., 1984) whereas DNA methylase
from Haemophilus haemolyticus (M·Hha I) was unable to act on
poly d(GC):d(GC) tracts maintained in Z-configuration in
supercoiled plasmids (Vardimon and Rich, 1984; Zacharias et
al., 1984). The role of Z configuration in modulating mammalian DNA methylase:DNA interactions is not, therefore,
clear.

Mammalian DNA methylases predominantly methylate cytosines in CpG (Gruenbaum et al., 1982). However, the sequence context of the CpG dinucleotides does influence methylase activity in vitro. HeLa cell DNA methylase, which has both de novo and maintainence-type activities, is strongly inhibited vis a vis hemimethylated DNA if coincubated with poly d(G), poly d(G):d(C), or poly d(A):d(T)(Bolden et al., 1984). The authors suggest that stretches of A or T near a CpG methylation site could affect methylase binding and further note that the single undermethylated CpG upstream from the 5' end of the chicken vitellogenin gene is located in an AT-rich region (Geiser et al., 1983) and that T/ACGA/T sites are much less highly methylated than CCGG sites in bovine satellite DNA (Sano and Sager, 1982). Thus, at least for methylation of C in CpG, sequence context could help generate sites with differing methylation potentials.

The role of chromatin structure/DNA interaction with chromatin proteins in modulating the affinity of DNA methylases is not clear. A retrospective approach has been to analyze 5-methylcytosine distribution in DNA from staphylococcal-nuclease-sensitive versus nuclease-resistant chromatin but conflicting results were obtained. Most recently, Barr et al. (1985) showed 2 to 3-fold enrichment of 5-methylcytosine in staphylococcal nuclease-resistant chromatin and nuclease-resistant purified naked DNA from human dipold fibroblasts suggesting that the observed enrichment is not a function of association of the DNA with chromatin proteins but that the DNA is intrinsically resistant to digestion. A more direct approach involves analysis of DNA or chromatin isolated from mouse L1210 cells grown in the presence or absence of 5-azacytidine and incubated with partially purified mouse spleen DNA methylase. Naked hemimethylated DNA prepared from nucleosomes or DNAase II-resistant residual nuclei was an excellent substrate for the methylase whereas nucleosomes or residual nuclei from 5-azacytidine-treated cells were 10 to 100-fold poorer substrates. Trypsinization and salt extraction removed the block to in vitro methylation suggesting that the association of histones with DNA may play a role in modulating methylation patterns. In vitro methylation of DNA can also be influenced by RNA:DNA interactions: an as yet uncharacterized component of total HeLa cell RNA effected greater than 90% inhibition of HeLa cell DNA methylase acting on hemimethylated DNA sites (Bolden et al., 1984).

DNA Methylase Activity in Structured Systems

In _vitro_ studies using purified DNA methylases and DNA or chromatin substrates do not approximate the structured _in vivo_ conditions in which eukaryotic DNA methylases act in either a _de novo_ or maintainence mode. Fuller understanding of eukaryotic DNA methylation may require analyses of more structured systems. For example, the multi-enzyme complex for DNA synthesis isolatable from a calf thymus cell type also contained DNA methylase activity (Noguchi et al., 1983). The enzyme complex which contained nascent DNA was distinguishable from the nuclear matrix, nuclear cage, or scaffold but could be associated with those elements in intact cells. It is thus of interest that mouse L929 cell nuclei, extracted with 0.2M NaCl to remove "soluble" DNA methylase, retained greater than 80% of their ability to effect "delayed" methylation of DNA (i.e. methylation of DNA that occurs only significantly after the synthesis of that DNA)(Davis et al., 1985). This methylase activity is apparently bound to the nuclear matrix. A very recent study employed a structured _in vitro_ DNA synthesizing system from mouse fibroblasts to analyze relationships between DNA replication and DNA methylation. In this system newly replicated DNA had 50% of the 5-methylcytosine content found in the total DNA but the Okazaki fragments, which did chase into high molecular wieght DNA, did not become methyl-labeled. Hence delayed methylation might reflect the second of two forms of maintainence methylation in which a methylase (soluble?) acts on newly replicated and hemimethylated sites in the leading strand of DNA and another methylase (matrix-bound?) acts on newly replicated and hemimethylated sites in the lagging strand but only at some time after ligation of Okazaki fragments into higher molecular weight and assembly into chromatin (Grafstrom et al., 1985).

Prospectives

Although eukaryotic DNA methylases have been studied for 15 years, the recent results cited suggest that this area is only beginning to yield its secrets. Little information is available concerning the properties --and control-- of _de novo_ methylases of early development that are presumably crucial to establishment of methylation patterns. More extensive analyses of levels of maintainence methylases through the cell cycle and of substrate factors that influence maintainence enzyme activity could be helpful in understanding the genesis of hypomethylated sites. Newer techniques of enzyme purification and of defined substrate preparation should greatly facilitate these efforts. However, because DNA methylases may be part of structured replication complexes interacting with nuclear superstructures, progress in these areas may well depend upon advances in understanding the dynamic structure of chromatin as it undergoes replication.

DNA METHYLATION AND NEOPLASTIC TRANSFORMATION

Transformation is the heritable conversion of a normal mitotically quiescent cell into one which, among other things, has lost cellular replicative control. Transforming agents are presumed to induce mutations at one or more sites in the genome which are crucial to control of cell replication but the biochemical diversity of transformed cells (reflecting altered patterns of gene expression) is not explained by this hypothesis. The finding that DNA methylation patterns, which are clonally heritable (Stein et al., 1982), can be correlated with gene activity, has led to the concept that perturbations in DNA methylation might be part of the transformation process.

Methylation patterns have been analyzed in extant tumor cell lines, experimentally-induced neoplasms, and human tumors. The results of such analyses suggest that general and site specific hypomethylation of DNA is often found as part of the transformed phenotype (Hoffman, 1984; Goelz et al., 1985) including hypomethylation of cellular homologues of viral oncogenes (Feinberg and Vagelstein, 1983; Cheah et al., 1984; Chandler et al., 1985). Moreover, a variety of chemical transformation agents have been shown to directly interfer with DNA methylation. In in vitro DNA methylation systems, benzo(a)pyrene-adducted DNAs are significantly poorer methyl acceptors than their non-adducted DNA counterparts. Both fully unmodified as well as hemimethylated DNA are hypomethylated in proportion to their extent of adduction when using a human placental DNA methylase (Pfeifer et al., 1984) and with Hpa II or mouse spleen methylases (Wojciechowski and Meehan, 1984). The latter report is especially significant in that the extent of adduction of DNA shown to inhibit methylation was one modified residue per 20,000 to 40,000 nucleotides -- levels known to be able to initiate transformation but sufficiently low to avoid gross helix distortion.

The active form of benzo(a)pyrene also inactivated mouse spleen, rat liver, and Hpa II DNA methylases directly, presumably by covalent modification of critical regions of the enzyme required for catalysis but not for initial interaction with substrate (Wilson and Jones, 1983; Wojciechowski and Meehan, 1984). In vitro methylation of natural and/or artificial DNAs is also inhibited by adducts of DNA formed with acetylaminofluorene (AAF) and N-methyl-N-nitrosourea (NMU) (Pfohl-Leszkowicz et al., 1984a; Ruchirawat et al., 1984). These agents, as well as N-methyl-N'-nitro-N-nitrosoguanidine (MNNG) also direclty inhibit DNA methylases (Chan et al., 1983).

These studies present a pattern of hypomethylation of DNA induced by carcinogen-adduction of the DNA and/or by direct chemical inactivation of DNA methylases but exceptions have been reported. Treatment of mouse lymphoma cells, human lymphoblasts, or human diploid fibroblasts with UV irradiation, NMU, or N-acetoxy-AAF had no detectable effect on methylation levels of newly replicated DNA (Krawisz and Lieberman, 1984). Treatment of BALB/3T3 cells with chemical carcinogens known to transform this cell line did lead to genomic hypomethylation but treatment of C3H/10T½ cells with benzo(a)pyrene -- which does transform this cell line -- did not result in detectable genomic hypomethylation. Moreover, when BALB/3T3 cells were treated with hydrocarbons which do not transform this line, significant genomic hypomethylation was still observed (Wilson and Jones, 1983; 1984).

Chemical carcinogens can also induce hypermethylation of DNA. For example, in vitro methylation is significantly enhanced if the DNAs are covalently modified with 4-acetoxy-aminoquinoline-1-oxide or with 2-aminofluorene (Pfohl-Leszkowicz et al., 1983; 1984b). Poly d(CG):d(CG) which is ethylated at the N7 of G by ethylmethanesulfonate (EMS) is hypermethylated 2-fold over the non-adducted polymer when incubated with a rat spleen DNA methylase but in vitro methylation of EMS-treated hemimethylated copolymer is inhibited (Farrance and Ivarie, 1985). Space-filling models of CpG dinucleotides modified at the N7 of G or with the ethyl group esterified at a dioxyphosphate oxygen 5' to the cytosine show that the ethylated poly d(CG):d(CG) sites resembly a hemimethylated symmetrical site. Given the preference of maintainence-type DNA methylases for hemimethylated sites (Gruenbaum et al., 1982), the EMS-modified poly d(CG):d(CG) is apparently recognized by the rat spleen methylase as a hemimethylated substrate and so is hypermethylated compared to the nonmodified copolymer. These

results provide a plausible explanation for earlier studies
(Ivarie and Morris, 1982) showing that an EMS-induced pro-
lactin-deficient "mutant" derived from GH_3 cells could be
reverted at high frequency by treatment of the mutant line
with 5-azacytidine. Although other interpretations are
possible, the combined results might indicate that a heritable change in the genome was effected at the epigenetic
level of DNA modification and not at the level of the base
sequence in DNA.

Prospectives

The current studies cited do not address the question
of whether observed hypomethylations in transformed cells
are simply concomitants of the transformed state or whether
transforming agents initially perturb DNA methylation,
which perturbations set in motion transcriptional events
that ultimately yield the transformed state. Experiments
to distinguish between these two possibilities await development of transformation systems amenable to clonal isolation
of initiated cells at very early stages of transformation.
The results of Ivarie and colleagues do suggest, however,
that the concept of an epigenetic basis for transformation
is well worth pursuing.

FINAL COMMENTS

In the four years since the last conference on S-
adenosylmethionine, eukaryotic DNA methylation has been established as a probable element in control of expression of
some genes. Further studies over the next few years should
establish the molecular bases for such a control function
as well as the factors that govern DNA methylase activities.
Such information will be necessary before drugs targeted at
DNA methylation can be developed to manipulate gene expression.

LITERATURE CITED

Adams, R.L.P., Burdon, R.H., McKinnon, K. and Rinaldi, A.
    (1983) FEBS Letters 163, 194.
Arber, W. (1965) Ann. Rev. Microbiol. 19, 365.

Barr, F.G., Kastan, M.B. and Lieberman, M. (1985) Biochem-
    istry 24, 1424.
Behe, M. and Felsenfeld, G. (1981) Proc. Natl. Acad. Sci.
    U.S.A. 78, 1619.
Bestor, T.H. and Ingram, V.M. (1983) Proc. Natl. Acad. Sci.
    U.S.A. 80, 5559.
Bolden, A., Ward, C., Siedlecki, J.A. and Weissbach, A.
    (1984) J. Biol. Chem. 259, 12437.
Brown, D.D. and Gurdon, J.B. (1977) Proc. Natl. Acad. Sci.
    U.S.A. 74, 2064.
Chan, J.Y.H., Ruchirawat, M., Lapeyre, J.-N. and Becker, F.
    F. (1983) Carcinogenesis 4, 1097.
Chandler, L.A., Jones, P.A. and DeClerck, Y.A. (1985) Fed.
    Proc. 44, 1337.
Chao, M.V., Mellon, P., Charnay, P., Maniatis, T. and Axel,
    R. (1983) Cell 32, 483.
Chea, M.S.C., Wallace, C.D. and Hoffman, R.M. (1984) J. Natl.
    Cancer Inst. 73, 1057.
Costlow, N.A., Simon, J.A. and Lis, J.T. (1985) Nature 313,
    147.
Davis, T., Kirk, D., Rinaldi, A., Burdon, R.H. and Adams,
    R.L.P. (1985) Biochem. Biophys. Res. Comm. 126, 678.
Doerfler, W. (1984) Angew. Chem. Int. Eng. Ed. 23, 919.
Emerson, B.M. and Felsenfeld, G. (1984) Proc. Natl. Acad.
    Sci. U.S.A. 81, 95.
Farrance, I.K. and Ivarie, R. (1985) Proc. Natl. Acad. Sci.
    U.S.A. 82, 1045.
Feinberg, A.P. and Vogelstein, B. (1983) Biochem. Biophys.
    Res. Comm. 111, 47.
Fradin, A., Manley, J.L. and Prives, C.L. (1982) Proc. Natl.
    Acad. Sci. U.S.A. 79, 5142.
Geiser, M., Mattaj, I.W., Wilks, A.F., Seldran, M. and Jost,
    J.-P. (1983) J. Biol. Chem. 258, 9024.
Gerber-Huber, S., May, F.E.B., Westley, B.R., Felber, B.K.,
    Hosbach, H.A., Andres, A.-C. and Ryffel, G.U. (1983)
    Cell 33, 43.
Ginder, G.D., Whitters, M.J. and Pohlman, J.K. (1984) Proc.
    Natl. Acad. Sci. U.S.A. 81, 3954.
Gjerset, R.A. and Martin, D.W. (1982) J. Biol. Chem. 257,
    8581.
Goelz, S.E., Vogelstein, B., Hamilton, S.R. and Feinberg,
    A.P. (1985) Science 228, 187.
Graessmann,M., Ziechmann, C. and Graessmann, A. (1984) FEBS
    Letters 173, 151.
Grafstrom, R.H., Yuan, R. and Hamilton, D.L. (1985) Nucl.
    Acids Res. 13, 2827.

Groudine, M. and Weintraub, H. (1984) Cell 30, 131.

Gruenbaum, Y., Cedar, H. and Razin, A. (1982) Nature 295, 620.

Grünwald, S. and Drahovsky, D. (1984) Int. J. Biochem. 16, 883.

Hoffman, R.M. (1984) Biochim. Biophys. Acta 738, 49.

Hotchkiss, R.D. (1948) J. Biol. Chem. 175, 315.

Hough, P.V.C., Mastrangelo, I.A., Wall, J.S., Hainfield, J.F., Simon, M.N. and Manley, J.L. (1982). J. Mol. Biol. 160, 375.

Huang, L.-H., Wang, R., Gamma-Sosa, M.A., Shenoy, S. and Ehrlich, M. (1984) Nature 308, 293.

Ivarie, R.D. and Morris, J.A. (1982) Proc. Natl. Acad. Sci. U.S.A. 79, 2967.

Jaenisch, R. and Jähner, D. (1984) Biochim. Biophys. Acta 782, 1.

Jove, R., Sperber, D.E. and Manley, J.L. (1984) Nucl. Acids Res. 12, 4715.

Kastan, M.B., Gowans, B.J. and Lieberman, M. (1982) Cell 30, 509.

Kautiainen, T.L. and Jones, P.A. (1985) Biochemistry 24, 1193.

Kornberg, A., Zimmerman, S.B. and Kornberg, S.R. (1959) Proc. Natl. Acad. Sci. U.S.A. 45, 772.

Krawisz, B.R. and Lieberman, M. (1984) Carcinogenesis 5, 1141.

Laskey, R.A., Honda, B.M., Mills, A.D., Morris, N.R., Willie, A.H., Mertz, J.E., DeRobertis, E.M. and Gurdon, J.B. (1977) Cold Spring Harb. Symp. Quant. Biol. 42, 171.

Macleod, D. and Bird, A.P. (1983) Nature 306, 200.

McKeon, C., Pastan, I. and deCrombrugghe, B. (1984) Nucl. Acids Res. 12, 3491.

Nelson, K.J., Mather, E.L. and Perry, R.P. (1984) Nucl. Acids Res. 12, 1911.

Noguchi, H.H., Prem veer Reddy, G. and Pardee, A.B. (1983) Cell 32, 443.

Pfeifer, G.P., Grünwald, S., Boehm, T.L.J. and Drahovsky, D. (1983) Biochim. Biophys. Acta 740, 323.

Pfeifer, G., Grunberger, D. and Drahovsky, D. (1984) Carcinogenesis 5, 931.

Pfohl-Leszkowicz, A., Galiegue-Zouitina, S., Bailleul, B., Locheux-Lefebvre, M.H. and Dirheimer, G. (1983) FEBS Letters 163, 85.

Pfohl-Leszkowicz, A., Fuchs, R.P.P., Keith, G. and Dirheimer, G. (1984a) Recent Results Cancer Res. 84, 193.

Pfohl-Leszkowicz, A., Fuchs, R.P.P. and Dirheimer, G. (1984b) FEBS Letters 178, 59.

Radman, M. and Wagner, R. (1984) Current Topics Microbiol.
    Immunol. 108, 23.
Razin, A. and Cedar, H. (1984) Int. Rev. Cytol. 92, 159.
Razin, A. and Szyf, M. (1984) Biochim. Biophys. Acta 782,
    331.
Ruchirawat, M., Becker, F.F. and Lapeyre, J.-N. (1984)
    Nucl. Acids. Res. 12, 3357.
Sano, H. and Sager, R. (1982) Proc. Natl. Acad. Sci. U.S.A.
    79, 3584.
Sano, H., Noguchi, H., and Sager, R. (1983) Eur. J. Biochem.
    135, 181.
Sneider, T.W. (1977) in The Biochemistry of S-adenosylmeth-
    ionine (Salvatore, F., Borek, E., Zappia, V., Williams-
    Ashman, H.G. and Schlenk, F., Eds.) pp. 383-400,
    Columbia Univ. Press, New York.
Stein, R., Gruenbaum, Y., Pollack, Y., Razin, A. and Cedar,
    H. (1982) Proc. Natl. Acad. Sci. U.S.A. 79, 61.
Sullivan, C.H. and Grainger, R.M. (1984) J. Cell. Biol. 99,
    143a.
Tanaka, K., Appella, A. and Jay, G. (1983) Cell 35, 457.
Vardimon, L. and Rich, A. (1984) Proc. Natl. Acad. Sci.
    U.S.A. 81, 3268.
Wang, R.Y.-H., Huang, L.-H. and Ehrlich, M. (1984) Nucl.
    Acids Res. 12, 3473.
Weisbrod, S. (1982) Nature 297, 289.
Wilks, A., Seldran, M. and Jost, J.-P. (1984) Nucl. Acids
    Res. 12, 1163.
Wilson, V.L. and Jones, P.A. (1983) Cell 32, 239.
Wilson, V.L. and Jones, P.A. (1984) Carcinogenesis 5, 1027.
Wojciechowski, M.F. and Meehan, T. (1984) J. Biol. Chem.
    259, 9711.
Wolf, S. and Migeon, B.R. (1985) Nature 314, 467.
Wright, S., de Boer, E., Grosveld, F.G. and Flavell, R.A.
    (1983) Nature 305, 333.
Zacharias, W., Larsen, J.E., Kilpatrick, M.W. and Wells,
    R.D. (1984) Nucl. Acids Res. 12, 7677.

TISSUE SPECIFIC DNA METHYLATION PATTERNS:
BIOCHEMISTRY OF FORMATION AND POSSIBLE ROLE.

AHARON RAZIN

DEPARTMENT OF CELLULAR BIOCHEMISTRY,

THE HEBREW UNIVERSITY MEDICAL SCHOOL,

JERUSALEM ISRAEL 91010

It is now well established that tissue specific DNA methylation patterns exist in vertebrates. A long list of gene sequences exhibiting tissue specific expression have been studied in the past 8 years with respect to their methylation pattern (for recent review, see Razin and Szyf, 1984). Investigators took advantage of the restriction enzymes HpaII (CCGG) and HhaI (GCGC) that are inactive when the internal cytosine residue in their recognition site is methylated. Cleaving the genomic DNA with one of these enzymes, blotting and hybridizing with the appropriate labeled probes allowed the establishment of the state of methylation of each of these specific sites in a given gene sequence (Bird and Southern, 1978). The results of such an analysis represent the methylation pattern of the given sequence since methylation of higher eukaryotic DNA occurs exclusively at cytosine residues in CpG sequences. In most studies, when the pattern of methylation of a tissue specific gene has been correlated with the expression of the gene, an inverse correlation has been found (Yisraeli and Szyf, 1984). Many genes are under-methylated in the tissue of expression as compared to the extent of their methylation in

127

other tissues. It should, however, be noted that
in about 20% of the genes studied, no such
correlation is found. Keeping in mind that the
HpaII and Hha I recognition sequences constitute
a subset of the CpG sites in the DNA and represent only about 10% of the CpGs, it is not
altogether surprising that some exceptions are
found to the rule correlating gene expression
with undermethylation of the gene. In fact, the
correlation found in most genes is overwhelming
and indicates that patterns of methylation of
CCGG and GCGC sites represent quite faithfully
the pattern of methylation of CpGs. This
compilation of data strongly supports the ten
year old theory, independently put forward by
Riggs (1975) and Holliday and Pugh (1978), that
DNA methylation in higher organisms is associated
with differentiation.

The idea that methylation of cytosine
residues in CpG sequences marks a stage of
differentiation is very attractive. Two major
requirements should be fulfilled by a marker of a
differentiation state: (i) it should be capable
of changing during the process of differentiation. (ii) it should have intrinsic properties
that allow its clonal inheritance in the fully
differentiated cell lineage. The first requirement will be satisfied if demethylation and
de novo methylation of the DNA could be
demonstrated during differentiation. This
article will discuss recent data obtained by us
that shed some light on these biochemical processes. The clonal inhertiance of a methylation
pattern in a somatic cell line has been clearly
shown (Pollack et al., 1980; Wigler et al.,
1981). It has also been shown that the clonal
inheritance is accomplished by a maintenance
methylase that faithfully replicates the
methylation at CpG sequences in a semiconservative manner at the replication fork (Gruenbaum et
al., 1982; Stein et al., 1982; Gruenbaum et al.,
1983). The symmetry provided by the CpG sequence
serves the basis for this semiconservative process. It should be noted that in plants an
exception to the rule that methylation occurs

exclusively at CpG has been observed. However,
methylation at sequences other than CpG have been
shown to reside in the symmetric sequence CXG
where X can be A,T or C (Gruenbaum et al.,
1981b). This, again, allows the clonal inheritance of the methylation pattern by a maintenance type methylase.

CHANGES IN THE METHYLATION PATTERN DURING DIFFERENTIATION

The tissue-specific patterns of methylation
observed in many gene sequences (Yisraeli and
Szyf, 1984) clearly indicate that small changes
in the methylation topography have occurred
during early stages of development. In order to
understand the role played by DNA methylation in
the process of differentiation, it is not
sufficient to study only the inheritance of
methylation. It is extremely important to investigate the mechanisms which lead to the
alteration of the methylation patterns. The
analysis of many specific gene sequences indicates that some degree of specific demethylation must occur during differentiation, since
these sequences are generally heavily methylated
in germ line DNA and are undermethylated in the
specific tissue of expression (Razin and Cedar,
1984). Furthermore, there is some indication
that de novo methylation may occur during
early stages of development (Jahner and Jaenisch,
1984). By their very nature, these changes are
difficult to monitor since they occur in a very
small number of cells at highly specific sites.
Certain cell lines capable of differentiation
in vitro, such as teratocarcinoma and erythroleukemia cells may, however, provide model
systems for studying demethylation and de
novo methylation. The use of these cells by
several laboratories including ours revealed the
surprising phenomenon of genome-wide hypomethylation during differentiation (Razin et al.,
1984; Young and Tilghman, 1984; Bestor et al.,
1984).

About 30% of the methyl groups in the F9
mouse teratocarcinoma cell DNA is lost in response to treatment with retinoic acid. This agent
is known to induce differentiation in these
pleuripotent cells to parietal or visceral type
primitive endoderm (Strickland and Mahdavi,
1980). The fact that DNA from extraembryonic
tissues of the mouse; placenta and yolk sac,
which are derived from primitive endoderm, have
been found to be undermethylated (Razin et al.,
1984), suggests that the in vitro undermethylation of the teratocarcinoma cell DNA
mimics the process that takes place in vivo
during the differentiation of extraembryonic
tissues.

Although we do not understand the relationship between the differentiation of primitive
endoderm and the process of demethylation, it
appeared that there might be a general correlation between these two phenomena. In fact, other
differentiating systems are also associated with
massive variations in the DNA methylation state
(Bestor et al., 1984; Razin et al., 1985).

Mouse erythroleukemia cells, when treated
with one of several standard inducers, such as
DMSO, HMBA, butyrate, etc., undergo distinct
morphological changes and begin to produce hemoglobin by 5 days after induction. If the extent
of DNA methylation is analyzed at that time,
minor hypomethylation of the cellular genome is
observed (Christman, 1984). A careful kinetic
analysis of the genomic DNA of these cells during
the induction process showed that this DNA undergoes a dramatic (50-70%) demethylation
followed by a process of remethylation, returning
the methylation level close to that present
before induction (Razin et al., 1985). This
transient demethylation occurs within 2 days,
well ahead of the appearance of hemoglobin in
these cells. The fact that every known inducer
causes similar kinetic alterations, suggests that
this process is indeed an integral part of the
differentiation program (Table 1).

Inducer	% CpG methylated				B+ cells
	day 1	day 2	day 3	day 4	day 5
5-Azacytidine (4μM)	48	78	77	79	+
DMSO (200 mM)	78	65	78	80	+
TPA (10ng/ml)	72	76	80	80	−
Butyrate (1mM)	43	76	80	80	+
TPA+Butyrate	32	72	73	80	+
8Br-cAMP (10μM)	64	80	78	80	−
IBMX (1mM)	56	30	80	78	+
8Br-cAMP + IBMX	22	56	80	76	+
HMBA (5mM)	32	60	80	78	+
Insulin (1 μg/ml)	68	56	80	78	−
Dexamethasone (4μM)	75	72	54	80	−
Insulin + Dex	40	80	72	72	−
HMBA + Dex	80	60	72	80	−

Table 1: Various inducers of differentiation cause transient genome-wide hypomethylation. Friend murine erythroleukemia cells (clone 745) were grown in DMEM containing 10% FCS in the absence or presence of the inducers and at the concentrations indicated in the table. Cell samples were analyzed daily for the extent of DNA methylation at CpG sequences. The extent of methylation was analyzed by an extension of the standard nearest neighbor analysis (Gruenbaum et al., 1981a). The values presented in the Table represent averages of at least 3 determinations, the reproducibility being ±2%. The data has been obtained by integrating the radioactivity in the cytosine and 5 methylcytosine spots which were quantitated by densitometry. In non-treated cells the level of methylation of CpG sequences was 80±2% and persisted for long periods in culture. Hemoglobin containing cells (B+) were identified by benzidine staining (Orkin et al., 1975).

Examination of the results presented in the
table reveals a two stage mechanism for the
transient hypomethylation which constitutes
active demethylation and de novo methylation
of the DNA. Since these two biochemical processes
were found to operate during differentiation it
lends strong support to the idea that DNA methylation may serve as a marker of a differentiation state. It should be mentioned here, that
many of the agents listed in the table are known
inducers of cell messenger systems. It is
tempting to speculate that signals from outside
the cell affect genome expression by changing the
methylation pattern via second messenger systems.

The transient hypomethylation involved in
some cases (cAMP+IBMX, HMBA) a loss of about 75%
of the methyl groups. This implies that at least
50% of the sites must have lost the methyl groups
from both DNA strands. The generally accepted
mechanism for hypomethylation is based on a
possible loss of methyl groups during replication
in the absence of maintenance methylation. This
passive mechanism can account for the hypomethylation reported in the table, only if it occurred
during at least two rounds of replication. In a
more detailed kinetic experiment in which cells
were treated with HMBA the hypomethylation
occurred within a period of less than one cell
cycle (Razin et al., 1985). This result indicates
that during differentiation removal of the
methyl groups from the DNA takes place by an
active mechanism. This conclusion is supported
by recent observations made by us in another
system. Epstein-Barr virus (EBV) can be induced
in an EBV producer Burkitt lymphoma cell line,
P3HR-1, by the combination of phorbol ester
(TPA) and n-butyrate. This induction has been
found to be associated with a complete
demethylation of a region in the viral DNA
(BamH1-H region that codes for the EAR region of
the EA complex; Glaser et al., 1983). The
hypomethylation is completed by 24 hrs while the
onset of viral DNA amplification occurs at about

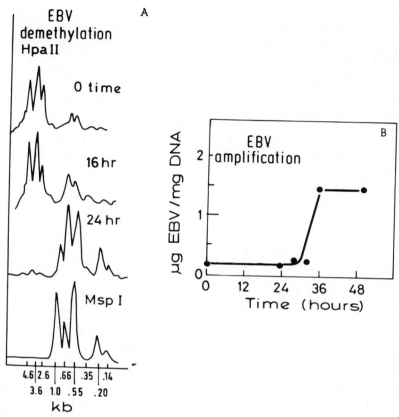

Fig. 1: <u>EBV DNA hypomethylation and amplification</u>. The EBV-producer line P3HR-1 has been treated with 10ng/ml TPA + 3mM n-butyrate. Cell samples were removed at various times after induction. A. total DNA was purified and digested with the combination of BamH1 and HpaII or MspI. The cleaved DNA was blotted and hybridized to ^{32}P labeled BamH1-H probe. Autoradiograms were scanned. Size markers were HindIII fragments of λDNA and HaeIII fragments of φXDNA. B. DNA samples (50ng) were dot blotted and hybridized to ^{32}P labeled probe. The concentration of EBV sequences were determined by measuring the intensity of the radioactive spots relative to the intensity of a BamH1-H standard and expressed as μg EBV/mg cell DNA.

32 hrs (Fig. 1). Since no increase in viral DNA
is observed during the period when hypomethylation takes place, it can be concluded that in
this case, as well, inducers of cell differentiation trigger an active biochemical mechanism
for the removal of methyl-groups from the DNA.
It should be noted that active hypomethylation
has been observed in one HpaII site located about
600 bp upstream of the chicken vittelogenin II
gene (Wilks et al., 1984). The type of mechanism
involved in this active demethylation is still
obscure.

A MODEL FOR MARKING A DIFFERENTIATION STAGE.

    We have presented here data supporting the
idea that DNA methylation may serve as a marker
of a differention state. It has been shown that
dramatic changes in DNA methylation take place in
cells induced to differentiate in vitro. This
property of DNA methylation together with its
built-in capacity of clonal inheritance strongly
suggest that DNA methylation is a good candidate
for serving a marker of a differentiation stage.
The association of changes in DNA methylation
patterns with changes in chromatin structure
(Groudine and Conklin, 1985) and the propagation
model of chromatin structure during development
(Groudine and Weintraub, 1982) prompted us to
propose a theoretical model for marking a
differentiated stage by DNA methylation (Fig. 2).

    The results presented here suggest that in
order to proceed from one stage of differentiation to the next the methylation pattern is
erased and rebuilt. We propose, therefore, that
removal of the methyl groups allows free movement
of the nucleosomes. Riggs and Jones (1983)
suggested that "determinator proteins" take part
in the establishment of specific methylation
patterns. We suggest that these proteins which
are specific to a given differentiation stage
determine the new nucleosomal structure of the
chromatin. This new structure is then locked by
de novo methylation and the determinator

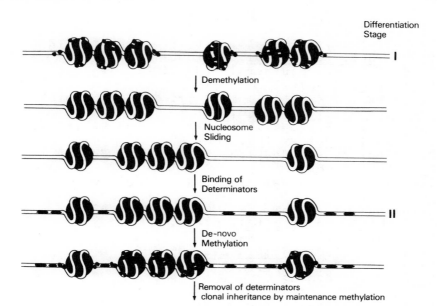

Differentiation
Stage

I

Demethylation

Nucleosome
Sliding

Binding of
Determinators

II

De-novo
Methylation

Removal of determinators
clonal inheritance by maintenance methylation

Fig. 2: A theoretical model for the
change and maintenance of cell specific
chromatin structure by DNA methylation.
Closed circles represent methyl groups. Closed
oval shapes represent determinator proteins. The
non-methylated sites remain unmethylated since
de novo methylase activity is transient and
restricted to the periods when determinator
proteins protect the regions covered by them from
de novo methylation.

proteins dissociate. The methylation pattern
will guarantee clonal-inheritance of the new
nucleosomal structure for many generations.

ACKNOWLEDGMENTS

    The work carried out in our laboratory was
supported by the Israel Cancer Association Grant
1/84 and NIH grant GM 20483. The help of Caroline
Gopin in preparing this manuscript is very much
acknowledged.

REFERENCES

Bestor, T.H., Hellewell, S.B. and Ingram, V.M.
(1984) Mol. Cell. Biol. 4, 1800-1806.
Bird, A.P. and Southern, E.M. (1978) J. Mol.
Biol. 118, 27-47.
Christman, J.K. (1984) in Curr. Top. Microbiol
and Immunol. 108, 49-58.
Glaser, R., Boyd, A., Soerker, J. and Holliday,
J. (1983) Virology 129, 188-195.
Groudine, M. and Conklin, K.F. (1985) Science
228, 1061-1068.
Groudine, M. and Weintraub, H. (1982) Cell
30, 131-139.
Gruenbaum, Y., Stein, R., Cedar, H. and Razin, A.
(1981a) FEBS Letters 124, 67-72.
Gruenbaum, Y., Naveh-Many, T., Cedar, H. and
Razin, A. (1981b) Nature 292, 860-862.
Gruenbaum, Y., Cedar, H. and Razin, A. (1982)
Nature 295, 620-622.
Gruenbaum, Y., Szyf, M., Cedar, H. and Razin, A.
(1983) Proc. Natl. Acad. Sci U.S.A. 80,
4919-4921.
Holliday, R. and Pugh, J.E. (1975) Science
187, 226-232.
Jahner, D. and Jaenisch, R. (1984) in DNA
methylation: Biochemistry and Biological
Significance (Razin, A., Cedar, H. and Riggs,
A.D., eds). pp. 189-219., Springer-Verlag Inc.
New York.
Orkin, S.H., Harosi, F.I. and Leder, P. (1975)
Proc. Natl. Acad. Sci. U.S.A. 72, 98-102.
Pollack, Y., Stein, R., Razin, A. and Cedar, H.
(1980) Proc. Natl. Acad. Sci. U.S.A. 77,
6463-6467.
Razin, A., Webb, C., Szyf, M., Yisraeli, J.,
Rosenthal, A., Naveh-Many, T. Sciaky-Gallili, N.
and Cedar, H. (1984) Proc. Natl. Acad. Sci.
U.S.A. 81, 2275-2279.
Razin, A. and Szyf, M. (1984) Biochim. Biophys.
Acta 782, 331-342.
Razin, A. and Cedar, H. (1984) Int. Rev. Cyt.
92, 159-185.
Razin, A., Feldmesser, E., Kafri, T. and Szyf, M.
(1985) in: Biochemistry and Biology of DNA
methylation (Razin, A. and Cantoni, G.L., eds.)
Alan R. Liss Inc., N.Y., in press.

Riggs, A.D. (1975) <u>Cytogenet Cell Genet</u> <u>14</u>,
9-11.
Riggs, A.D. and Jones, P. (1983) <u>Adv. Cancer
Res.</u> <u>40</u>, 1-40.
Stein, R., Gruenbaum, Y., Pollack, Y., Razin, A.
and Cedar, H. (1982) <u>Proc. Natl. Acad. Sci.
U.S.A.</u> <u>79</u>, 61-65.
Wigler, M., Levy, D. and Perucho, M. (1981)
<u>Cell</u>, <u>24</u>, 33-40.
Wilks, A., Seldran, M. and Jost, J.P. (1984)
<u>Nucleic Acids Res.</u> <u>12</u>, 1163-1177.
Yisraeli, J. and Szyf, M. (1984) in <u>DNA
methylation: Biochemistry and Biological
Significance</u> (Razin, A., Cedar, H. and Riggs,
A.D., eds). pp. 353-378, Springer-Verlag Inc.,
New York.
Young, P.R. and Tilghman, S.M. (1984) <u>Mol.
Cell. Biol.</u> <u>4</u>, 898-907.

REGULATION OF GENE EXPRESSION BY SITE-SPECIFIC PROMOTER METHYLATION

Walter Doerfler, Klaus-Dieter Langner, Dagmar Knebel, and Ulrike Weyer

Institute of Genetics, University of Cologne, Cologne, Germany

INTRODUCTION

It was established that the DNA encapsidated into purified adenovirions did not contain detectable levels of modified bases (Günthert et al., 1976; Sutter et al., 1978; Eick et al., 1983). Even the DNA of a symmetric recombinant (Deuring et al., 1981; Deuring & Doerfler, 1983) between the left terminus of adenovirus type 12 DNA and large amounts of human cell DNA, which was encapsidated into virus particles, was not methylated (Deuring et al., 1981). The very same cellular DNA sequences as part of the human chromosomal DNA were heavily methylated (Deuring et al., 1981). Similarly, free viral DNA in human cells productively infected by human adenovirus type 2 or in hamster cells abortively infected by adenovirus type 12 was apparently not methylated at 5'-CCGG-3' (HpaII), 5'-GCGC-3' (HhaI), 5'-GATC-3' (MboI), or 5'-TCGA-3' (TaqI) sequences (Vardimon et al., 1980; Wienhues & Doerfler, 1985). These latter results were based on an extensive hybridization analysis in which the free intranuclear DNA was cleaved with the appropriate restriction endonucleases. Obviously, this type of study, though widely used, is limited due to the fact that, e.g. in the 35,937 base pairs of adenovirus type 2 DNA, only 22.5 % of the potentially methylated 5'-CG-3' dinucleotide combinations reside in 5'-CCGG-3' or 5'-GCGC-3' sequences (Wienhues & Doerfler, 1985). Nevertheless, it

139

appears highly unlikely that free intracellular adenovirus DNA in infected human or hamster cells would be extensively methylated. We have initiated a study of the actual patterns of methylation particularly of the major late promoter sequence of free adenovirus DNA at early and late times after the infection of cells by using the genomic sequencing technique (Church & Gilbert, 1984).

In contrast to free intranuclear adenovirus DNA, adenovirus type 12 (Sutter et al., 1978; Sutter & Doerfler, 1979, 1980; Kruczek & Doerfler, 1982; Kuhlmann & Doerfler, 1982) or adenovirus type 2 DNA (Vardimon et al., 1980; Vardimon & Doerfler, 1981; Klimkait & Doerfler, 1985) integrated into the genomes of virus-transformed cells or of adenovirus type 12-induced tumors (Kuhlmann & Doerfler, 1982; Kuhlmann et al., 1982) is methylated in 5'-CCGG-3' and 5'-GCGC-3' sequences in highly specific patterns. In fact, these transformed cell systems were among the first functionally well defined ones (Sutter & Doerfler, 1979, 1980) to implement the notion that in eukaryotic cells inverse correlations existed between the extent of DNA methylation of integrated viral DNA sequences and the level at which these sequences were expressed into messenger RNA. This area of research has already been extensively reviewed (Razin & Riggs, 1980; Doerfler, 1981, 1983, 1984). It was soon recognized that the most convincing inverse correlations could be established in the promoter and 5' regions of integrated adenovirus genes (Kruczek & Doerfler 1982). This observation prompted and encouraged us to test the effect of sequence-specific **in vitro** promoter methylations after transfecting or microinjecting appropriate promoter constructs into mammalian cells or into oocytes of Xenopus laevis, respectively. The design and the results of some of these experiments will be discussed below.

From a functional point of view, and in particular with respect to the state of adenovirus DNA methylation, different compartments can be distinguished in the nuclei of adenovirus-infected or -transformed cells. Viral DNA incorporated into the "chromatin compartment" was subject to different rules of DNA methylation, probably similar to those that applied to cellular DNA. These findings also demonstrated unequivocally that adenovirus DNA was **de novo** methylated at some time between infection of the cell and the stable fixation of viral DNA in the host genome. However, the situation proved to be more complicated in that at relatively early times after integration of adenovirus type 12 DNA, e.g. in DNA directly extracted from adenovirus type 12-induced tumors, viral DNA was not methylated or was hypomethylated (Kuhlmann & Doerfler, 1982). Upon explantation of cells from these tumors and continued cell passage in culture, a gradual increase of viral DNA methylation was observed (Kuhlmann & Doerfler, 1982; Kuhlmann et al., 1982), and viral DNA sequences were then methylated in a non-random fashion (Kuhlmann & Doerfler, 1983). At present, we do not understand at all how levels of DNA methylation are regulated, nor how such shifts in specific viral DNA methylation can occur·or what their consequences may be. The adenovirus system and the study of levels of methylation of well characterized viral DNA sequences in different mammalian cell environments may help to elucidate some of the still enigmatic features of DNA methylation.

Increased levels of DNA methylation could have been the cause or the consequence of gene inactivation. A direct experimental approach had to be devised to decide between these alternatives. The most clear-cut inverse correlations in the adenovirus system were observed for the fourteen 5'-CCGG-3' (HpaII) sites in the E2A region of integrated adenovirus type 2 DNA in the cell lines HE1, HE2, and HE3 (Vardimon et al., 1980). In cell line HE1, the integrated E2A region was expressed (Johannson et al., 1978; Esche, 1982), and all 14 HpaII sites were unmethylated. In contrast, in cell lines HE2 and HE3 the E2A region was not expressed (Johannson et al., 1978; Esche 1982), and all 14 sites were methylated. These and other findings (Sutter & Doerfler, 1979, 1980; Kruczek & Doerfler, 1982) signaled that the levels of methylation at the 5'-CCGG-3' sequences had - at least at a correlative echelon - functional significance. We therefore decided to mimick this functional signal in the E2A region of adenovirus type 2 DNA by **in vitro** methylating all 5'-CCGG-3' sequences and by testing the biological activity of the methylated or unmethylated E2A construct. Fortunately, a prokaryotic DNA methyltransferase of that specificity was available from hemophilus parainfluenzae (Mann & Smith, 1977). The results of the experiments (Vardimon et al., 1981; Vardimon et al., 1982a; Vardimon et al., 1982b) demonstrated:

1. Upon injection into Xenopus laevis oocytes, the 5'-CCGG-3' methylated construct was transcriptionally inactive, the unmethylated DNA was transcribed into adenovirus type 2-specific RNA. At least some of the RNA was initiated at the authentic late promoter of the E2A region (Vardimon et al., 1981; Vardimon et al., 1982a).

2. Histone genes from sea urchin were coinjected in the unmethylated state with methylated E2A DNA. Histone genes were expressed, the E2A DNA was not. These data demonstrated that transcriptional inactivation of the E2A region of adenovirus type 2 DNA was not an artifact of the in vitro methylation reaction (Vardimon et al., 1982a).

3. In vitro methylation of the 5'-GGCC-3' (BsuRI) sites of the E2A region had no effect on the transcriptional activity of this gene in Xenopus laevis oocytes. This result further attested to the specificity of the methylation signal. In cell lines HE1, HE2, HE3, none of the 5'-GGCC-3' sites in the integrated E2A genes of adenovirus type 2 DNA was methylated (Vardimon et al., 1982b).

This experimental approach was further refined by selectively methylating **in vitro** the E1A promoter of adenovirus type 12 DNA (Kruczek & Doerfler 1983). This promoter was inserted into the pSVO-CAT plasmid (Gorman et al., 1982) in front of the prokaryotic chloramphenicol acetyl transferase (CAT) gene (pAd12E1A-CAT construct). After transfection into mouse cells, the unmethylated construct was expressed and CAT enzyme could be readily detected in transfected cells, whereas the methylated construct was not expressed. It could also be ascertained that methylations in the CAT gene itself had no effect on the expression of the construct: In the pSV2-CAT construct, the early SV40 promoter was responsible for the activation of the CAT gene. This promoter contained no 5'-CCGG-3' sites, the CAT gene carried four such sites, and methylation of the construct did not decrease its expression (Kruczek & Doerfler 1983). It was interesting to note that in the pAd12E1A-CAT construct the two methylatable 5'-CCGG-3' sites and many of the methylatable 5'-GCGC-3' sites lay upstream of the TATA signal of the promoter. The pIX gene promoter of adenovirus type 12 DNA carried one site each, downstream from the respective TATA signal, and in an appropriate pAd12pIX-CAT plasmid construct, methylation did not inactivate expression (Kruczek & Doerfler 1983). These data taken together suggested that for **in vitro** methylations to inactivate the promoter, the modified sites had to be located in highly specific positions and these positions might be different depending on the structure of individual promoters.

From the results of studies on viral and other eukaryotic promoters the concept emerges that at least for a certain group of genes specific promoter methylations cause gene inactivations. The methylation-sensitive sites may be different in different genes although the number of eukaryotic promoters investigated in sufficient detail is as yet too small to draw general conclusions. It is too early to report on the biochemical mechanisms involved in the recognition of methylated nucleotides representing signals in promoter sequences. It is conceivable, however, that these modifications can affect specific promoter-protein interactions or cause structural alterations of promoter DNA sequences. A combination of both effects is also possible. We shall now describe in detail recent results on the influence of promoter methylations in a number of experimental systems.

METHYLATIONS OF ONE OR A FEW SEQUENCES IN THE PROMOTER OF VIRAL OR CELLULAR GENES SUFFICE TO INACTIVATE THESE GENES.

We have designed experiments to methylate **in vitro** viral genes by restricting methylation to very few sequences, notably in the promoters of viral genes. Partly methylated clones of the E2A gene were constructed (Langner et al., 1984). In the promoter (5')-methylated construct, three 5'-CCGG-3' sequences at the 5' end of the subclone were methylated. One of these sites is

located 215 base pairs (bp) upstream (bp 26,169 of adenovirus type 2 DNA), and two sites are located 5 and 23 bp
downstream from the cap site (bp 25,931 and 25,949 of
adenovirus type 2 DNA), of the E2A gene. The bp numbers
refer to the nucleotide sequence of adenovirus type 2 DNA
(Roberts et al., 1986). The construct was transcriptionally inactive upon microinjection into nuclei of
Xenopus laevis oocytes. In the gene (3')-methylated
construct, eleven 5'-CCGG-3' sequences in the main part
of the transcribed gene region were methylated **in vitro.**
This construct was actively transcribed in Xenopus laevis
oocytes, and at least some of the adenovirus type 2-
specific RNA synthesized was initiated at the same sites
as in adenovirus type 2-infected human cells in culture
(Langner et al., 1984). Mock methylation experiments were
carried out similarly to methylation experiments, except
that the methyl donor (S-adenosylmethionine) was omitted.
Both mock-methylated constructs were transcribed into
Ad2-specific RNA in Xenopus laevis oocytes. These results
demonstrate that DNA methylations at or close to the
promoter and 5' end of the E2A gene cause transcriptional
inactivation. Perhaps only one methyl group would be
adequate for inactivation. The construct retained its
activity when it was grown on an E. coli strain deficient
in adenosine methylation (dam⁻) (Marinus & Morris, 1973)
and subsequently microinjected into Xenopus laevis
oocytes (Langner et al., 1984). These data indicated that
adenosine methylation did probably not play a role in the
regulation of the expression of the E2A gene.

The E2A promoter of adenovirus type 2 DNA was also
inserted into the pSVO-CAT construct (Gorman et al.,
1982) and the activity of the unmethylated or the
methylated DNA was tested after transfection into human
HeLa cells. The plasmid construct pSVO-CAT, which
contained the chloramphenicol acetyl transferase (CAT)
gene and a HindIII site immediately in front of it for
experimental insertion of eukaryotic promoters, was used
to test adenovirus promoter activities in the unmethylated and methylated states. We now observed that the E2A
late promoter of adenovirus type 2 DNA also activated the
CAT gene upon transfection into mammalian cells, and this
E2A promoter was inactivated by specific methylations of
three 5'-CCGG-3' sites (Langner et al., 1985). Sur-

prisingly, it was observed that the pSVO-CAT construct, which lacks eukaryotic promoter sequences, was able to express the CAT gene upon transfection into human or hamster cells which harbored the E1 region of adenovirus type 2 or of type 5 DNA (Langner et al., 1985). In contrast, in HeLa or BHK21 cells devoid of adenovirus DNA sequences, the pSVO-CAT construct was not expressed. The adenovirus type 2-transformed hamster cell lines HE5 and HE7, the adenovirus type 5-transformed hamster cell line BHK297-131 or the adenovirus type 5-transformed human cell line 293 were all capable of expressing the pSVO-CAT construct. We adduced evidence that these latter activities were perhaps mediated by prokaryotic promoter-like sequences in the pBR322 section of the construct, and presumably functioned via trans-activation by the E1 region, perhaps by the E1A functions of adenoviruses (Langner et al., 1985). Low levels of expression of the pSVO-CAT construct in HeLa or BHK21 cells devoid of adenovirus sequences were occasionally found and might be due to cellular functions akin to the E1 functions of adenoviruses. The trans-activating effect was less sensitive to DNA methylation. This finding was commensurate with the notion that trans-activation involved prokaryotic promoter-like sequences which, in general, were not affected by methylation of DNA sequences. In cells carrying the left terminal sequences of adenovirus type 2 DNA or of adenovirus type 5 DNA, the expression of the pAd2E2A-CAT construct was enhanced (Langner et al., 1985).

AN INSECT VIRUS PROMOTER IS ALSO SENSITIVE TO SITE-SPECIFIC DNA METHYLATION IN INSECT CELLS

It has been documented by many investigators that Drosophila DNA is devoid of 5-mC (Smith & Thomas, 1981; Urieli-Shoval et al., 1982; Eick et al., 1983). Perhaps, it contains only minute amounts of the modified nucleotide (Achwal et al., 1984). It has also been shown recently that the DNA of the insect cell line Spodoptera frugiperda, that serves as host for the propagation of the insect baculovirus Autographa californica Nuclear Polyhedrosis Virus (AcNPV), does not contain detectable

amounts of methylated nucleotides (T. Müller & W. Doerfler, unpublished). Similarly, methylated nucleotides
cannot be detected in AcNPV DNA (Tjia et al., 1979; Eick
et al., 1983). One could, therefore, reason that 5-mC as
a regulatory signal may be an addition to the arsenal of
regulatory functions which came late in phylogeny.
Although DNA methylation might not play a major role in
insect cells, it was nevertheless conceivable that the
expression machinery in insect cells was sensitive to
site-specific methylations. We investigated this possibility by using a conspicuously strong insect virus promoter in such studies, viz. the p10 gene promoter of
AcNPV DNA (Lübbert & Doerfler 1984a,b).

In lepidopteran insect cells infected with the
baculovirus AcNPV, at least two major late viral gene
products are expressed: the polyhedrin which makes up the
mass of the nuclear inclusion bodies, and a 10,000
molecular weight protein (p10) whose function is unknown.
The structures of the promoters of these genes have been
determined (Hooft van Iddekinge et al., 1983; Kuzio et
al., 1984; Lübbert & Doerfler, 1984a,b). These structures
are similar to those of other eukaryotic promoters,
except that the nucleotide sequences of these promoters
are rich in adenine-thymine base pairs.

We have again used the pSVO-CAT construct (Gorman et
al., 1982) containing the prokaryotic gene chloramphenicol acetyl transferase (CAT) to study the function of the
p10 gene promoter in insect and mammalian cells. Upon
transfection of the pAcp10-CAT construct, which contains
the p10 gene promoter of AcNPV DNA in the HindIII site of
pSVO-CAT, CAT activity was determined. The p10 gene promoter is inactive in human HeLa cells and in uninfected
Spodoptera frugiperda insect cells. The same promoter has
proved active, however, in AcNPV-infected Spodoptera
frugiperda cells and exhibits optimal activity when cells
are transfected 18 h after infection (Knebel et al.,
1985). This finding demonstrates directly that the p10
gene promoter requires additional viral gene products for
its activity in Spodoptera frugiperda cells. The nature
of these products is unknown at present.

The p10 gene promoter sequence contains one (HpaII) 5'-CCGG-3' site 40 bp upstream from the cap site of the gene and two such sites far downstream in the coding sequence of the gene. In view of the fact that Drosophila DNA has been reported to contain no 5-mC, we were interested in determining the effect of site-specific methylation on the insect virus promoter of the p10 gene. Methylation at the 5'-CCGG-3' site led to inactivation of the promoter or to a drastic reduction in its activity (Knebel et al., 1985). These data show that an AcNPV insect virus promoter can be inactivated by site-specific methylation even in insect cells.

The data presented are consistent with the idea that insect cells have the capacity to recognize methylated nucleotides in specific promoter sequences and to respond to this signal in a similar way as vertebrate systems do. This finding was surprising in view of the fact that 5-mC is not a nucleotide modification that abounds in insect cell DNA. We conclude that 5-mC as a regulatory signal, although apparently not extensively used in insect cells, can nevertheless be recognized by their transcriptional machinery. This signal might in fact be used in crucial positions in the insect cell genome.

DNA METHYLATION AS A LONG-TERM INACTIVATING SIGNAL IS SUITABLE ONLY FOR CERTAIN GENES

Since DNA methylation can serve as a long-term signal in the inactivation of genes, it is not likely that this signal should be selected in the transient inactivation of gene functions. It will be useful in this context to operationally subdivide genes into at least three classes:
1. Genes that become permanently inactivated. In this class of genes, DNA methylation can play an important role.
2. Genes that are intermittently active, but inactive for long periods, or genes that can be reactivated, e.g. by hormone treatment. These genes will probably not be inactivated by site-specific promoter methylations,

since it would then be difficult to instantaneously
reactivate them.
3. Active genes. The promoters of these genes are unmethylated or undermethylated.

Of course, this schematic subdivision of gene
classes does not take into account the possibility that
the sites of promoter methylation leading to gene inactivation may have to be highly specific. Thus, the occurrence of 5-mC in a promoter sequence may not **per se** be
associated with the inactive state of a gene. Moreover,
this simple classification presupposes that rapid alterations of levels of DNA methylation are impossible mainly
because active demethylating mechanisms have so far not
been observed. We do in fact not know to what extent
active demethylations could occur.

ACKNOWLEDGMENTS

We are indebted to Petra Böhm for expert editorial
work. Research in the authors' laboratory was supported
by the Deutsche Forschungsgemeinschaft through SFB74-Cl,
by the Ministry of Science and Research of the State of
Northrhine-Westfalia (IV B5 FA 9227) and by a donation of
the Hoechst Comp.

A more extensive version of this paper has been published
in "The Chemistry, Biochemistry and Biology of DNA
Methylation", eds. A. Razin & G. Cantoni, Alan R. Liss,
Inc., New York, 1985.

REFERENCES

Achwal, C. W., Ganguly. P. and Chandra, H. S. (1984) EMBO
     J. 3, 263.
Church, G. M. and Gilbert, W. (1984) Proc. Natl. Acad.
     Sci. USA 81, 1991.
Deuring, R., Klotz, G. and Doerfler, W. (1981) Proc.
     Natl. Acad. Sci. USA 78, 3142.
Deuring, R. and Doerfler, W. (1983) Gene 26, 283.
Doerfler, W. (1981) J. gen. Virol. 57, 1.

Doerfler, W. (1983) Ann. Rev. Biochem. 52, 93.

Doerfler, W. (1984) Adv. Viral. Oncol. 4, 217.

Eick, D., Fritz, H.-J. and Doerfler, W. (1983) Anal. Biochem. 135, 165.

Esche, H. (1982) J. Virol. 41, 1076.

Gorman, C. M., Moffat, L. F. and Howard, B. H. (1982) Mol. Cell. Biol. 2, 1044.

Günthert, U., Schweiger, M., Stupp, M. and Doerfler, W. (1976) Proc. Natl. Acad. Sci. USA 73, 3923.

Hooft van Iddekinge, B. J. L., Smith, G. E. and Summers, M. D. (1983) Virology 131, 561.

Johansson, K., Persson, H., Lewis, A. M., Pettersson, U., Tibbetts, C. and Philipson, L. (1978) J. Virol. 27, 628.

Klimkait, T. and Doerfler, W. (1985) J. Virol. 57, 000.

Knebel, D., Lübbert, H. and Doerfler, W. (1985) EMBO J. 4, 1301.

Kruzcek, I. and Doerfler, W. (1982) EMBO J. 1, 409.

Kruczek, I. and Doerfler, W. (1983) Proc. Natl. Acad. Sci. USA 80, 7586.

Kuhlmann, I. and Doerfler, W. (1982) Virology 118, 169.

Kuhlmann, I., Achten, S., Rudolph, R. and Doerfler, W. (1982) EMBO J. 1, 79.

Kuhlmann, I. and Doerfler, W. (1983) J. Virol. 47, 631.

Kuzio, J., Rohel, D. Z., Curry, C. J., Krebs, A., Carstens, E. B. and Faulkner, P. (1984) Virology 139, 414.

Langner, K.-D., Renz, D., Vardimon, L. and Doerfler, W. (1984) Proc. Natl. Acad. Sci. USA 81, 2950.

Langner, K.-D., Weyer, U. and Doerfler, W. (1985) Proc. Natl. Acad. Sci. USA 82, 000.

Lübbert, H. and Doerfler, W. (1984a) J. Virol. 50, 497.

Lübbert, H. and Doerfler, W. (1984b) J. Virol. 52, 255.

Mann, M. B. and Smith, H. O. (1977) Nucleic Acids Res. 4, 4211.

Marinus, M. G. and Morris, N. R. (1973) J. Bacteriol. 114, 1143.

Razin, A. and Riggs, A. D. (1980) Science 210, 604.

Roberts, R. J., Akusjärvi, G., Aleström, P., Gelinas, R. E., Gingeras, T. R., Sciaky, D. and Pettersson, U. (1986) Developments in Mol. Virol. 8, 000-000.

Smith, S. S. and Thomas, C. A., Jr. (1981) Gene 13, 395.

Sutter, D., Westphal, M. and Doerfler, W. (1978) Cell 14, 569.

Sutter, D. and Doerfler, W. (1979) Cold Spring Harbor Symp. Quant. Biol. 44, 565.

Sutter, D., Doerfler, W. (1980) Proc. Natl. Acad. Sci. USA 77, 253.

Tjia, S. T., Carstens, E. B. and Doerfler, W. (1979) Virology 99, 399.

Urieli-Shoval, S., Gruenbaum, Y., Sedat, J. and Razin, A. (1982) FEBS Lett. 146, 148.

Vardimon, L., Neumann, R., Kuhlmann, I., Sutter, D. and Doerfler, W. (1980) Nucleic Acids Res. 8, 2461.

Vardimon, L. and Doerfler, W. (1981) J. Mol. Biol. 147, 227.

Vardimon, L., Kuhlmann, I., Cedar, H. and Doerfler, W. (1981) Eur. J. Cell. Biol. 25, 13.

Vardimon, L., Kressmann, A., Cedar, H., Maechler, M. and Doerfler, W. (1982a) Proc. Natl. Acad. Sci. USA 79, 1073.

Vardimon, L., Günthert, U. and Doerfler, W. (1982) Mol. Cell. Biol. 2, 1574.

Wienhues, U. and Doerfler, W. (1985) J. Virol. 57, 000.

CARCINOGENESIS AND DNA HYPOMETHYLATION IN METHYL-DEFICIENT ANIMALS

Lionel A. Poirier, Mary J. Wilson and
Narayan Shivapurkar

Nutrition and Metabolism Section, Laboratory
of Comparative Carcinogenesis, National
Cancer Institute, FCRF, Frederick, Maryland

INTRODUCTION

The current increasing interest in the possible role of normal DNA methylation in carcinogenesis has sprung from three major sources: (1) cell culture studies on the role of DNA methylation in cell differentiation; (2) hypomethylation of specific genes in a variety of cancers; and (3) liver cancer causation in methyl-deficient rats. Studies on the role of DNA methylation in mammalian cell differentiation conducted by Christman et al., 1977, and Razin and Riggs, 1980, led to the postulate that undermethylation of the C5 position of cytosine may play a determining role in cancer causation (Holliday, 1979; Riggs and Jones, 1983). Feinberg and Vogelstein (1983b) showed that the genes coding for human growth hormone, α-globin, and γ-globin in human tumors were undermethylated compared to the same genes in the corresponding normal tissues. Subsequent studies have extended these observations to include other tumors and genes (Hoffman, 1984). Finally, dietary deprivation of the methyl donors methionine and choline had been shown to induce liver carcinomas in rats (Copeland and Salmon, 1946). Although these findings were accepted for a period of nearly 10 years, the subsequent demonstration

of aflatoxin contamination in the peanut meal-based diets
used to produce the methionine- and choline-deficiency,
led credence in these findings to be suspended (Newberne,
1965). However, a second system to produce liver tumors
in association with a methyl-deficient state was seen by
the chronic administration of ethionine to rats (Farber,
1963).

LIVER CANCER FORMATION

        Previous studies from our own laboratories (Mikol and
Poirier, 1981) as well as other laboratories (Shinozuka et
al., 1978) indicated that methyl-deficient diets would be
expected to serve as strong promoters of liver cancer formation. In common usage the term "promoter" is used to
describe an agent, the chronic treatment with which results
in enhanced tumor formation in animals previously treated
with a low dose of a complete carcinogen, generally called
an "initiator." We therefore designed a large study to
determine whether methyl-deficient diets would promote
liver cancer formation in rats (Mikol et al., 1983). The
initiator selected was the complete carcinogen diethylnitrosamine administered at single doses of 0, 20, 70, and
200 mg/kg. The animals were given no further treatment for
one week at which time they were placed on one of four amino
acid-defined diets containing (1) both methionine and
choline, (2) neither methionine nor choline, (3) choline
only, or (4) methionine only (Figure 1). All methionine-
deficient diets were supplemented with an equimolar dose of
DL-homocystine. The animals were then maintained on their
respective diets for 18 months. The liver tumor formation
occurring during this study is described in Figure 1. As
indicated in Figure 1, at all initiating doses of diethylnitrosamine, liver tumor formation was enhanced by the
methyl-deficient diets. The enhancement by the diet
deficient in both methionine and choline was always greater
than that observed with the diets singly deficient in
either methionine or choline. Strikingly, as indicated in
Panel 1, a significant incidence of hepatocellular carcinoma was observed in the livers of animals fed the doubly
deficient diet even without an initiating dose of diethylnitrosamine. These results indicated that dietary methyl-
deprivation alone caused liver cancer in rats. Similar
results were obtained by Ghoshal and Farber, 1984. Subsequent studies have shown that dietary methyl deprivation

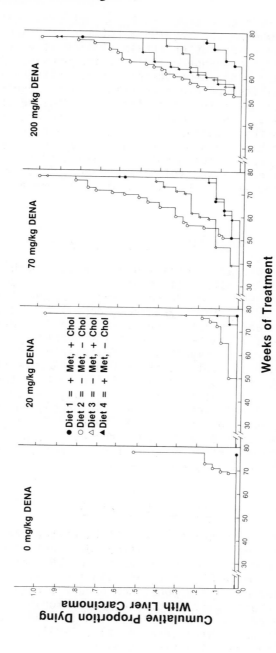

Fig. 1. Formation of hepatocellular carcinomas in rats given a single initial dose of diethylnitrosamine (DENA) and subsequently fed amino acid-defined, methionine- and choline-deficient diets for 18 months.

can induce liver carcinomas in $B_6C_3F_1$ mice but not in
C3H mice (Newberne et al., 1983; Poirier, LA, unpublished
observations). The latter strain of mice is very sensitive, however, to phenobarbitol carcinogenesis. In this
strain phenobarbitol hepatocarcinogenic activity is
markedly inhibited by diets containing high levels of
methionine alone or in combination with choline (Poirier,
et al., 1984). Thus, in addition to hepatocarcinogenesis
by dietary methyl deprivation, diets containing increased
levels of methionine and/or choline have been shown to
inhibit the hepatocarcinogenic activities of several compounds. These include ethionine (Farber, 1963) 2-acetyl-
aminofluorene, and diethylnitrosamine (Rogers and Newberne,
1980).

METHYL INSUFFICIENCY IN VIVO

The chronic administration of the same methyl-
deficient, amino acid defined diets used to produce cancers
in rats also led to decreased ratios of adenosylmethionine
(AdoMet) to adenosylhomocysteine (AdoHcy) (Table 1)
(Shivapurkar and Poirier, 1983). A fifth diet was used in
these studies; it lacked the vitamins necessary for de
novo methyl group biosynthesis: folic acid and vitamin
B_{12}. As shown in Table 1, the ratios of AdoMet to AdoHcy
were found to be proportional to the extent of the severity
of the dietary methyl deprivation. Thus, the administration of methyl-deficient diets to rats resulted in a hypomethylating environment in their livers. Similar findings
were obtained in rats and mice chronically fed a carcinogenic ethionine-containing diet for 1-6 weeks (Poirier et
al., 1982; Hyde and Poirier, 1982).

DNA HYPOMETHYLATION

Figure 2 illustrates the effects of the chronic administration of the amino acid-defined diet deficient in both
methionine and choline on the extent of DNA methylation in
the livers of male F344 rats and C3H mice (Wilson et al.,
1984; Poirier et al., unpublished observations). The
effects of the chronic feeding of an ethionine-containing
diet on the extent of DNA methylation in F344 rats are
also illustrated (Shivapurkar et al., 1984). Chronic
feeding of the methyl-deficient diet to rats for 20 weeks

Table 1. The Effect of 5 Weeks' Administration of Methyl-Deficient Amino Acid-Defined Diets on the Hepatic Levels of S-Adenosylmethionine (SAM) and 5-Adenosylhomocysteine (SAH) in Male Weanling F344 Rats

Diet	Methio-nine	Choline	Dietary Methyl Level (mmoles/kg)	SAM (µg/gm)	SAH (µg/gm)	SAM//SAH
1	+	+	45.7	46.5 ± 1.1	7.5 ± 1.0	6.2 ± 0.8
2	-[a]	-	0	22.5 ± 1.0	14.2 ± 1.8	1.6 ± 0.2
3	-[a]	+	14.3	22.3 ± 0.8	13.2 ± 1.1	1.7 ± 0.1
4	+	-	31.4	27.4 ± 1.2	8.0 ± 0.7	3.4 ± 0.3
5[b]	-[a]	-	0	14.0 ± 1.0	17.7 ± 1.7	0.8 ± 0.1

[a]Replaced with equimolar homocysteine

[b]Same as Diet 2 except that folic acid and vitamin B_{12} were also excluded.

resulted in an 11-14% decrease in the extent of total DNA methylation. In ethionine-fed rats, the hypomethylation occurred as early as 5 weeks after the beginning of treatment. In ethionine-treated rats the extent of DNA methylation was 4% and 8% less than that seen in the corresponding control animals at 5 and 10 weeks respectively (Figure 2). Thus, the long term feeding of the same ethionine-containing or methyl-deficient diets which produced liver tumors in rats also led to DNA hypomethylation in this organ. The C3H mice, which as indicated above did not show neoplastic or preneoplastic changes in their livers during the chronic feeding of the diet deficient in both methionine and

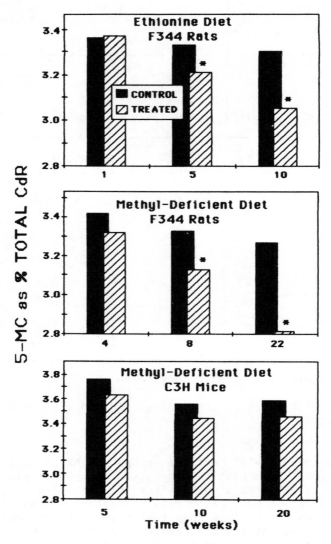

Fig. 2. 5-methylcytosine (5-MC) levels in hepatic DNA of methyl deprived rats and mice and of ethionine-fed rats. *p<0.02 compared to corresponding control.

choline, also had no alterations in the 5-methylcytosine content of their hepatic DNA (Figure 2) (Poirier, et al., unpublished observations). The apparent slight drop noted in the 5-methylcytosine content in the livers of the methyl-deficient mice was not found to be statistically significant (Figure 2). Thus, to the extent investigated in these studies, a good correlation was observed between the diets' ability to induce cancer and their capacity to induce hypomethylated DNA in the livers of rodents.

TRANSFORMATION OF RAT LIVER CELLS IN VITRO

In addition to the studies in vivo, this laboratory has used liver cells in culture to study the tumorigenic effects of a hypomethylating environment. In previous studies we have shown that the incubation of liver cells in complete medium containing ethionine for 12 weeks results in the eventual formation of transformed cells, which upon implantation into syngeneic hosts give rise to tumors (Brown et al., 1983). In the same study, cells grown on a methionine-free, homocysteine-supplemented medium required a much lower dose of ethionine to undergo transformation, and the cells could also be transformed by the AdoMet antagonist S-adenosylethionine (Brown et al., 1983). At the last meeting in this series we speculated that some of the pharmacologically active antagonists of AdoMet used at that time in other laboratories might also prove useful in investigating the mechanism of carcinogenesis of methyl deprivation. The compound selected was 3-deazaadenosine, the mechanism of action of which has been well studied and described by Chiang and Cantoni (1979). Liver cells in culture were treated with one of three different concentrations of 3-deazaadenosine; 0.075, 0.100, 0.150 mM for 4-12 weeks (Wilson, et al., 1985). They were then maintained for an additional 3-12 weeks (Table 2). The cells were then harvested and injected into syngeneic hosts at approximately monthly intervals beginning with week 4 (Table 2). As shown in Table 2, injection site tumors were seen in animals receiving the cells treated with 0.075 and 0.1 mM 3-deazaadenosine. No tumors were seen in animals receiving liver cells that had not been treated with 3-deazaadenosine. No tumors were observed in animals receiving cells treated with 0.150 mM 3-deazaadenosine at a total of 24 weeks in culture, but this effect seems to be the consequence of the cytotoxicity of 3-deazaadenosine

Table 2. Transformation of Rat Liver Cells by Deazaadenosine. Following treatment in culture, the cells were
injected into snygeneic hosts (5 rats/group), maintained
for 1 year.

Weeks of Treatment	Total weeks in Culture	Tumor Yield			
		Control	Deazaadenosine-Treated		
			0.075mM	0.100mM	0.150mM
4-12	≤15	0/14	1/15	3/13	0/12
12	19	0/4	2/4	2/3	0/2
12	24	0/5	3/5	2/5	0/5

at the highest concentration tested. At later time points
tumors have been observed in these animals. Thus,
3-deazaadenosine, which effectively inhibits AdoMet-dependent methylation through its accumulation of AdoHcy and of
3-deazaadenosylhomocysteine transforms rat liver cells in
culture.

The extent of DNA methylation in liver cells treated
with 3-deazaadenosine for 1 and 3 months was also examined
(Table 3). As indicated in Table 3, exposure of the liver
cells in culture to 0.075 mM deazaadenosine for 1-3 months
resulted in a 38-42% decrease in the percentage of deoxycytidine residues modified to 5-methyldeoxycytidine. Yet,
when cells treated with 0.075 mM deazaadenosine for 3
months were allowed to remain in culture for an additional
3 months the extent of DNA methylation returned to normal
levels (Table 3). One should note that although the extent
of the total DNA methylation was apparently normal in the
deazaadenosine-treated cells maintained in normal medium
for an additional 3 months, similarly treated cells were
capable of producing tumors following injection into
syngeneic hosts. It remains to be determined, however,
whether the normal DNA methylation patterns have been
restored in the cells whose total methylcytosine content
has returned to normal.

Table 3. Hypomethylation of DNA from Rat Liver Cells
Following Exposure to 0.075 mM Deazaadenosine

Exposure Time (months)	Total time in culture (months)	Extent of DNA Methylation	
		Control	DAA-Treated
		(100X 5-methylcytosine/total cytosine)	
1	1	3.16 + 0.05	1.97 + 0.02
3	3	2.62 + 0.02	1.53 + 0.03
3	4	2.72 + 0.07	1.92 + 0.06
3	6	2.48 + 0.02	2.47 + 0.02

SUMMARY AND DISCUSSION

The present studies provide evidence that the metabolic and nutritional imbalances regulating the bioavail-
ability of AdoMet may lead to liver tumor formation and to
the transformation of liver cells in culture. To date,
tumor formation also correlates well with the total extent
of DNA methylation in the target tissue or cells. That
such hypomethylation contributes significantly to the
eventual tumor formation remains to be established. However, recent developments in other laboratories lead one
to be optimistic in this regard. For example, the metas-
tatic activity of a series of experimental tumors can be
enhanced by agents inducing hypomethylation of their DNA
(Kerbel et al., 1985). The expression of fes and mos
oncogene activity has been shown to be inhibited by AdoMet-
dependent methylations (Groffen et al., 1983; McGeady et
al., 1983). Feinberg and Vogelstein (1983a) found that
the H-ras oncogene of the human tumors was hypomethylated
in its expressed state. Although specific gene hypomethylation has frequently been described in tumors (Feinberg
and Vogelstein, 1983b), we are unaware of any evidence
indicating such hypomethylation in preneoplastic tissue,
even though the extent of total DNA methylation may be
demonstrably diminished. It would thus seem desirable
to investigate the role of DNA hypomethylation on oncogene

expression in the livers of animals undergoing carcinogenesis through physiological methyl insufficiency.

REFERENCES

Brown, J., Wilson, M. J., and Poirier, L. A. (1983)
Carcinogenesis 4, 173-177.

Chiang, P. K. and Cantoni, G. L. (1979) Biochem. Pharm.
28, 1897.

Christman, J. K., Price, P., Pedrinan, L., and Acs, G.
(1977) Eur. J. Biochem. 81, 53.

Copeland, D. H. and Salmon, W. D. (1946) Am. J. Pathol.
22, 1059.

Farber, E. (1963) Adv. Cancer Res. 7, 383.

Feinberg, A. P. and Vogelstein, B. (1983a) Biochem. Biophys.
Res. Commun. 111, 47.

Feinberg, A. P. and Vogelstein, B. (1983b) Nature 301, 89.

Ghoshal, A. K. and Farber E. (1984) Carcinogenesis 5, 1367.

Groffen, J., Heistercamp, N., Blennerhassett, G., and
Stephenson, J. R. (1983) Virology 126, 213.

Hoffman, R. M. (1984) Biochim. Biophys. Acta 738, 49.

Holliday, R. (1979) Brit. J. Cancer 40, 513.

Hyde, C. L. and Poirier, L. A. (1982) Carcinogenesis 3, 309.

Kerbel, R. S., Frost, P., Liteplo, R. G., and Fidler, R. J.
(1985) Proc. Am. Assoc. Cancer Res. 26, 394.

McGeady, M. L., Jhappan, C., Ascione, R., and VandeWoude,
G. F. (1983) Mol. Cell. Biol. 3, 305.

Mikol, Y. B., Hoover, K. L., Creasia, D., and Poirier,
L. A. (1983) Carcinogenesis 4, 1619.

Mikol, Y. B. and Poirier, L. A. (1981) Cancer Letters 13, 195.

Newberne, P. M. (1965) in Mycotoxins in Foodstuffs (Wogan, G. N., Ed.) pp. 187-208, MIT Press, Cambridge, MA.

Newberne, P. M., Nauss, K. M., and DeCamargo, J. (1983) Cancer Res. 43, 2426s-2634s.

Poirier, L. A., Shivapurkar, N., Hyde, C. L., and Mikol, Y. B. (1982) in Biochemistry of S-Adenosylmethionine and Related Compounds (Usdin, E., Borchardt, R. T. and Creveling, C. R., Eds.) pp. 283-286, MacMillan Press, Ltd., London.

Poirier, L. A., Mikol, Y. B., Hoover, K., and Creasia, D. (1984) Proc. Am. Assoc. Cancer Res. 25, 132.

Razin, A. and Riggs, A. D. (1980) Science 210, 604.

Riggs, A. D. and Jones, P. A. (1983) Adv. Cancer Res. 40, 1.

Rogers, A. E. and Newberne, P.M. (1980) Nutrition and Cancer 2, 104.

Sells, M. A., Kaytal, S. L., Sells, S., Shinozuka, H., and Lombardi, B. (1979) Brit. J. Cancer 40, 274.

Shivapurkar, N. and Poirier, L. A. (1983) Carcinogenesis 4, 1051.

Shivapurkar, N., Wilson, M. J., and Poirier, L. A. (1984) Carcinogenesis 5, 989.

Wilson, M. J., Shivapurkar, N., and Poirier, L. A. (1984) Biochem. J. 218, 987.

Wilson, M. J., Bare, R. M., Kwiecinski, E. D., and Poirier, L. A. (1985) Proc. Am. Assoc. Cancer Res. 26, 506.

THE ROLE OF COENZYMES AND tRNA MODIFICATIONS IN

METABOLIC CONTROL OF GENE EXPRESSION.

H. Kersten
Institut für Physiologische Chemie,
Universität Erlangen-Nürnberg,
Fahrstrasse 17, D-8520 Erlangen

INTRODUCTION

The aim of this article is to discuss mechanims of metabolic control of gene expression involving modified bases and modified nucleosides in tRNA, and to show that tRNA modification serves as a mean to adapt cells to environmental changes, such as starvation or oxidation stress (Kersten, 1984; Buck & Ames, 1984). The metabolic control is triggered by specific alterations of tRNA modifications, caused by (i) changes in the levels or redox-state of coenzymes, or cofactors of the modifying enzymes (e.g. AdoMet, folate, pteridines, iron) or (ii) by the expression of an alternative tRNA gene in which the specific nucleoside to be modified is exchanged. Regulatory mechanisms that involve tRNA modifications are:
(1) Tetrahydrofolate-dependent initiation of the synthesis of proteins,
(2) attenuation of the expression of specific amino acid operons,
(3) suppression of terminator codons,
(4) cotranscription of a tRNA gene with a protein gene encoding a regulatory protein or a specific enzyme,
(5) specification of promotors or of RNA polymerases by (i) a specifically modified tRNA, (ii) a modified base, (iii) a modifying enzyme and or its cofactor.

More than 50 modified nucleosides have been discovered, they are localized in different tRNA species
at defined positions (Kersten, 1982; Björk, 1984;
Sprinzl et al. 1985). A great number are simply methylated nucleosides, the methyl-groups are introduced by
AdoMet-dependent enzymes, except ribosylthymine (T) in
gram-positive bacteria: the methyl-group is derived
from 5,10-methylentretrahydrofolate (see review
Kersten, 1984).

The following tRNA modifications will be discussed: ribosylthymine (T), 7-methylguanosine (m^7G),
2-methylthio-N6-(isopentenyl)adenosine (ms^2i^6A) and
especially queuosine (Q). The corresponding modifying
enzymes developed in facultative anaerobes when oxygen
accumulated in the atmosphere and were conserved
throughout the evolution of organisms. Wybutosine (yW)
occurs in cytoplasmic tRNA of eukaryotes in place of
ms^2i^6A, whereas tRNAs-Phe of mitochondria contain the
isopentenyladenosine modification.

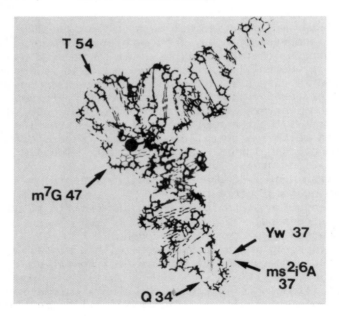

Fig. 1 General three-dimensional structure of tRNA and
positions of the modified nucleosides being discussed

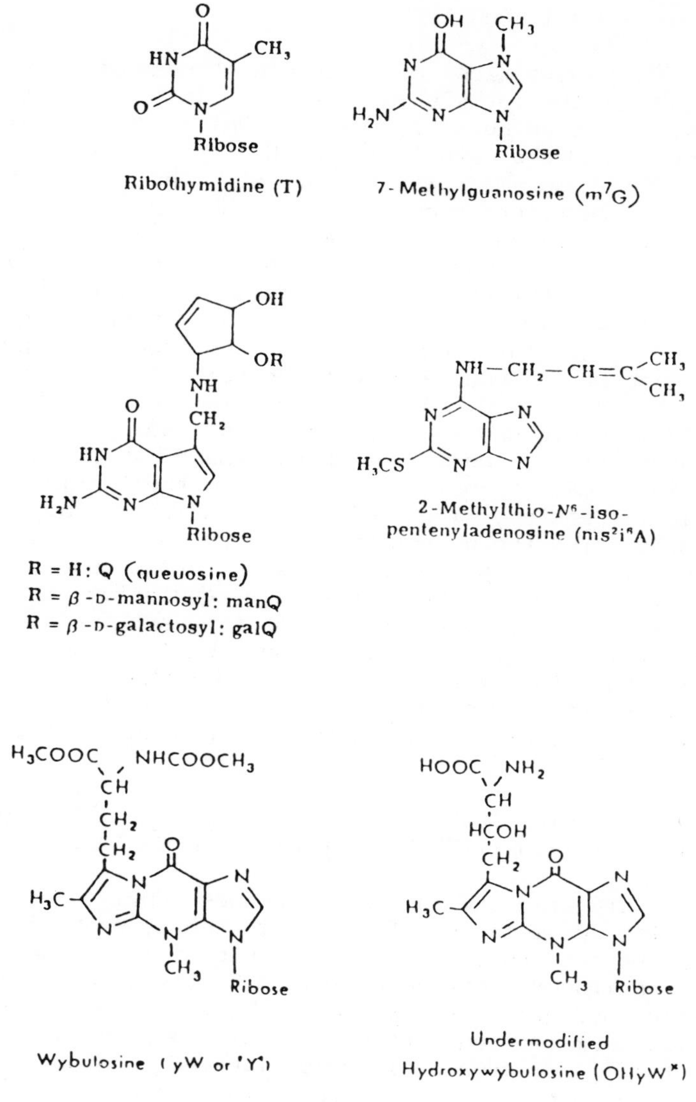

Ribothymidine (T)

7-Methylguanosine (m^7G)

R = H: Q (queuosine)
R = β-D-mannosyl: manQ
R = β-D-galactosyl: galQ

2-Methylthio-N^6-iso-pentenyladenosine (ms^2i^6A)

Wybutosine (yW or 'Y')

Undermodified
Hydroxywybutosine (OHyW*)

Fig. 2 Structures of the modified nucleosides

INTERDEPENDENCE OF METHYLATION AND FORMYLATION OF INI-
TIATOR tRNAs IN EUBACTERIA.

    The initiation of protein synthesis in eubacteria
depends on the formylation of the initiator-methionyl
tRNA. In gram-positive microorganisms the formylation
reaction and the methylation of U54 to T are coupled
via the coenzyme tetrahydrofolate. The methylation of
U54 to T restricts recognition of AUG initiator codons
to prior formylation of tRNA-fMet and thus to metabolic
control. In gram-negative $\underline{E.\ coli}$, U54 in initiator
tRNA is methylated via $\overline{AdoMet}$, in addition G at
position 47 is methylated to m^7G. Interestingly a
second gene for tRNA-fMet has been found, the product
of which has one nucleoside exchange: m^7G is replaced
by an unmodified ´A´. We have observed that the tRNA-
fMet2 is expressed in certain amino acid auxotrophic
strains of $\underline{E.\ coli}$ and have shown that this tRNA
initiates mRNA translation $\underline{in\ vitro}$ without prior formylation (Kersten, 1984). An important regulatory mechanism concerns the corresponding gene, metY: It is localized in one operon with two protein genes, one of
which, nusA, being involved in the regulation of genes,
specifying components of the protein-synthesizing system (Ishii et al., 1984). These results support the
view that formylation and related methylations of the
two initiator tRNAs in $\underline{E.\ coli}$ plays a role in metabolic control of particular genes (Kersten, 1984).

ADAPTATION TO IRON LIMITATION IN $\underline{E.\ COLI}$. IRON-DEPEN-
DENT METHYLTHIOLATION OF ISOPENTENYLADENOSINE.

    A dramatic environmental change during evolution
was the accumulation of oxygen in the atmosphere. Since
then the availability of iron to organisms in an aqueous environment has been limited by the insolubility of
ferric hydroxide (K sp $\gtrsim 10^{-39}$). With the extreme
equilibrium concentration of ferric ions at pH 7 of
about 10^{-18} M, even a diffusion limited transport would
be many orders of magnitude too slow to provide a
sufficient amount of iron to a microbial cell. This
problem has been circumvented by the production of a
great number of siderophore-chelating agents, which
solubilize ferric ions and facilitate their transport

into the bacteria (Raymond and Tufano, 1982).

The modifying enzyme that methylthiolates N6-(iso-pentenyl)adenosine in those tRNAs, cognate for aromatic amino acids, for serine and for leucine, needs iron as a cofactor. Iron limitation in $\underline{E.\ coli}$, causes accumulation of tRNAs with i^6A in place of ms^2i^6A, and these undermodified tRNAs relieve attenuation at the corresponding amino acid operons (Buck & Griffith, 1982). It is proposed that intermediates of this path-way provide the aromatic ring system and serine for the high-affinity iron chelator enterochelin.

The involvement of iron in the pathogenicity of certain bacterial infections has been emphasized (see Raymond & Tufano, 1982 for summarizing references). Iron toxicity in humans in its acute form (infant poi-soning) or in chronic iron overload (as in patients re-quiring periodic blood transfusions) is an important problem. Therapy with iron chelators has been applied but poses some questions with respect to toxicity. Among iron-dependent enzymes in higher organisms from which iron could be disposed, the enzyme that methyl-thiolates i^6A to ms^2i^6A in mitochondrial tRNAs might be affected.

QUEUOSINE-tRNAs AND CELLULAR RESPONSES TO QUEUINE LIMI-TATION.

The deazaguanine-derivative queuosine is a hyper-modified nucleoside, present in tRNAs specific for Asp, Asn, Tyr and His (Nishimura, 1983). It is synthesized by bacteria, but cannot be synthesized by $\underline{Dictyostelium}$ $\underline{discoideum}$ and by mice (Ott & Kersten 1982; Farkas, 1980). Queuine is provided to higher organisms from the nutrition or the intestinal flora. The modification is highly conserved, occurring in facultative anaerobic bacteria and in eukaryotes - except yeast - e.g. in plants, insects, fishes and in mammals and is present in cytoplasmic as well as in mitochondrial tRNAs (Randerath et al., 1984). A precursor of queuine is synthesized in $\underline{E.\ coli}$ from GTP and is inserted into the tRNA by a specific tRNA-transglycosylase. The bio-synthesis of the cyclopenten-moiety occurs at the level of tRNA by an as yet unknown mechanism (Nishimura, 1983). We have found that the accumulation of Q-lacking tRNAs in stationary phase cultures of E. coli can be reversed by iron, indicating that iron is a cofactor of one of the modifying enzymes, that catalyzes the formation of the cyclopentendiol ring.

Queuine-related Changes of Redox Systems in E. coli

To elucidate the function of queuine and the Q-family of tRNAs in facultative anaerobes, mutants of E. coli have been constructed, lacking the transglyco- sylase activity (tgt^-) (Noguchi et al., 1982). We have found, that two tgt^- strains are defective in three anaerobic redox systems: the nitrate reductase (Jänel et al., 1984), the formate dehydrogenase and the trimethylamineoxide reductase. The three anaerobic enzymes need a molybdenum and pteridine containing cofactor for catalytic activity. Whether the synthesis of queuine and the regulation of the molybdenum contain- ing cofactor by pteridines are related is under present investigation. Pteridines and queuine are closely related: (i) they share common biosynthetic pathways, (ii) the E. coli tRNA transglycosylase is inhibited competitively in vitro and also in intact cells by biopterin (Kersten & Jänel, 1984).

When E. coli cells, grown under several restric- tive conditions, enter the stationary phase oxygen be- comes limited and a specific change is observed in the expression of respiratory chains. Cytochrome d, an alternative major oxidase of E. coli with higher affi- nity for oxygen than cytochrome O, appears to be synthe- sized coordinately with cytochrome a_1 and cyto- chrome b_{558} (for review see Ingledew & Poole, 1984). Alterations in cytochromes can be measured in whole cells by low temperature difference spectra. We observe elevated levels in the terminal oxidase cytochrome d_{558} in E. coli, lacking queuosine in tRNA (Kersten & Jänel, 1984).

Queuine or tRNAs of the Q-family are therefore suggested to be involved in adaptation mechanisms of anaer-
obiosis. Oxygen limitation will lead to a decrease of
hydroxylation reactions of aromatic ring systems and
hence to a decrease in the amount of ubiquinone. Recall
that accumulation of tRNA-Phe, with i^6A in place of
ms^2i^6A, compensates for enterochelin deficiency by
increased synthesis of the aromatic ring system. tRNAs
with G in place of Q might - by a similar mechanism -
enhance the hydroxylation of aromatic ring systems and
thereby the synthesis of ubiquinone.

Queuine-related Changes of Redox Systems in Differentiating Cells.

Lower and higher eukaryotes (except yeast) and probably plants cannot synthesize queuine de novo, they
are supplied with queuine by their nutritional environment and insert queuine into tRNA by a tRNA queuine-
transglycosylase. A reduction in the Q-content of specific tRNAs can be caused by limitation of queuine, by
specific inhibition of the transglycosylase reaction
(Farkas et al., 1984), by differences in the turnover
of tRNAs of the Q-family (Ott & Kersten, 1985) and
variations in enzymes involved in the salvage pathway
of queuosine (Gündüz & Katze, 1984).

Two biological systems have been discovered in our
laboratory, suitable to study the responses to queuine
in relation to differentiation: D. discoideum and
virus-transformed Murine eryothroleukemic cells. Both
cell types can be grown and induced to differentiate
(i) in the absence of queuine, (ii) with limiting,
(iii) with sufficient amounts or (iiii) with excess of
queuine.

D. discoideum, when grown in the total absence of
queuine cannot undergo the developmental cycle after a
metabolic stress. The levels of D(-)-lactate are considerably reduced and cytochrome b_{559} accumulates in
queuine-lacking cells. We suggested that cyt b_{559} might
be the coenzyme of an NAD-independent lactate dehydrogenase (iLDH), that oxidizes lactate irreversibly
to pyruvate (Schachner et al., 1984). D-2-hydroxyde-

hydrogenases, E.C.11.99.6 have been found in mitochondria of yeast and occassionaly in mitochondria of rabbit, pig and rat liver. We also find an NAD-independent
enzyme that transfers electrons from lactate to a specific dye in purified mitochondria of D. discoideum.

If vegetative cells are sufficiently supplied with
queuine (1×10^{-7}M) the tRNAs of the Q-family are almost
fully modified. The levels of tRNA-Asp and tRNA-Tyr,
containing Q-derivatives, increase about two-fold (Ott
& Kersten, 1985) and fluctuate during development.
Fluctuations in the levels of tRNAs indicate variations
in the expression of tRNA genes or alterations in their
turnover.

Recently we have observed that Friend virus
transformed Murine erythroleukemic cells, clone $F_4$6,
can be grown in a medium, supplemented with horse serum
and that the adult serum lacks queuine. The addition of
queuine 1×10^{-7}M to the culture medium causes an almost
total shift of Q-lacking to Q-containing tRNAs. The
patterns of proteins on 2-D'O Farrell gels show an
additional 36 K protein in Q-lacking cells and elevated
levels of cytochromes. A substantial increase in the
intensity of the 5 characteristic NAD-dependent LDH isoenzymes on electropherograms is observed in Q-lacking
cells. The characteristic changes of the pattern of
protein synthesis and of redox systems suggest, that
queuine, and alterations in the Q-content of tRNA might
play a role in the switch from respiration to
glycolysis and gluconeogenesis.

With respect to tRNAs that show changes in response to queuine we observe characteristic alterations
in the chromatographic behaviour of tRNA-Phe. Cochro-
matography with mouse tRNA-Phe of known modifcation
pattern, indicates that changes occur in the redox-
state of wybutosine (Fig. 2). The biosynthesis of
wybutosine involves several AdoMet dependent methylation reactions and probably iron-dependent hydroxylation reactions. Wybutosine occurs in cytoplasmic
tRNA-Phe at position 37 as ms^2i^6A in tRNA-Phe of
mitchondria. The modified nucloside occurs in several
forms, differing in the extent of hydroxylation and
acylation. The modification state is dramatically

changed when <u>erythroleukemic cells</u> are induced by
butyrate to differentiate and to synthesize hemoglobin;
this is correlated with the transport of iron into the
cells. These observations led us to assume that queuosine and wybutosine modification are related and play a
role in iron uptake, transport and metabolism in higher
eukaryotes.

Queuine and Derivatives in Chemotherapy?

Q-lacking tRNAs accumulate in tumor cells and
characteristic variations are also found in the wybutosine modification. In tumor cells wybutosine can even
be replaced by m^1G (Kuchino et al., 1982). Since
queuine is a nutrient factor its intracellular concentration may not be sufficient for Q- and related
wybutosine modifications in specific tRNAs. Queuine and
derivatives have been synthesized chemically and are
currently tested for therapeutic effects, especially as
possible competitors of growth factors. The relation of
queuine to cancer has been intensively discussed by
Nishimura, 1983; Elliot et al., 1985; Katze, 1985.

Tissue specificity of tRNA Modification

The lack of queuine is not specific for tumor
cells. It has been observed that leaves of <u>tobacco</u> and
<u>wheat</u> contain tRNA-Tyr, totally lacking queuosine. The
tRNA-Tyr with the anticodon GUA was tested in translation of <u>tobacco mosaic virus</u> RNA in tobacco protoplasts
and found to yield a 17.5 K coat protein and a 126 K
protein and a 183 K protein which is generated by an
efficient readthrough over the UAG termination codon by
tRNA-Tyr$_{GUA}$ (Beier et al., 1984a and Beier et al.,
1984b). Furthermore queuosine modification of the
wobble base in tRNA-His from <u>Drosophila melanogaster</u>
influences decoding properties during the elongation
step of protein synthesis (Meier et al., 1985). These
results support the view that the extent of Q-modifi-
cation in tRNA of eukaryotes is tissue specific and is
probably altered dependent on the metabolic state of
cells and their environment.

CONCLUDING REMARK

Deficiency or alterations in the redox-state of coenzymes and cofactors of tRNA-methylating and tRNA-modifying enzymes might occur during pathogenicity or as a consequence of severe drug treatment in particular cells and tissues. Treatment of patients with coenzymes or cofactors and their derivatives might overcome this deficiency and might be of help to restore metabolic disregulations.

ACKNOWLEDGEMENTS

This work was supported by the Deutsche Forschungs-gemeinschaft (grant Ke 98/17/7) and Fond der Chemischen Industrie.

REFERENCES

Beier, H., Barciszewska, M., Krupp, G., Mitnacht, R. & Gross, H.J. (1984a) EMBO J. 2, 351-356.

Beier, H., Barciszweska, M. & Sickinger, H.-D. (1984b) EMBO J. 5, 1091-1096.

Björk, G.R. (1984) in Processing of RNA (Apirion, D. Ed.) pp 291-330, CRC Press in Inc Florida.

Buck, M. & Ames, B.N. (1984) Cell 36, 523-531.

Buck, M. & Griffith, E. (1982) Nucl. Acids Res. 10, 2609-2624.

Elliott, M.S., Trewyn, R.W. & Katze, J.R. (1985) Cancer Res. 45, 1079-1085.

Farkas, W.R. (1980) J. Biol. Chem. 225, 6832-6835.

Farkas, W.R., Jacobson, K.B. & Katze, J.R. (1984)
Biochem. Biophys. Acta 781, 64-75.

Gefter, M.L. & Russel, R.L. (1969) J. Mol. Biol. 39,
15-147.

Gündüz, U. & Katze, J.R. (1984) J. Biol. Chem. 259,
1110-1113.

Ingledew, W.J. & Poole, R.K. (1984) Microbiological
Reviews 48, 222-271.

Ishii, S., Kuroki, K. & Jamamoto, F. (1984) Proc. Natl.
Acad. Sci., USA 81, 409-413.

Jänel, G., Michelsen, U., Nishimura, S. & Kersten, H.
(1984) EMBO J. 3, 1603-1608.

Katze, J.R. (1985) Proceedings of the Society for
Experimental Biology and Medicine 179, 000-000.

Kersten, H. (1982) in Transmethylations 1982,
(Usdin, E., Borchardt, Th. & Creveling, C.R., Eds.)
pp 357-369, Pittman, London.

Kersten, H. (1984) in Progress in Nucleic Acid Research
and Molecular Biology (Moldave, K. & Cohn, W.E.,
Eds.) 31, pp 59-114, Academic Press, New York,
London.

Kersten, H. & Jänel, G. (1984) in Biochemical and
Clinical Aspects of Pteridines (Pfleiderer, W.,
Wachter, H. & Curtius, H.Ch., Eds.) pp 113-125,
Walter de Gruyter u. Co Berlin, New York.

Kersten, H., Schachner, E., Dess, G., Anders, A.,
Nishimura, S. & Shindo-Okada, N. (1983) in
Biochemical and Clinical Aspects of Pteridines
(Curtius, H.Ch., Pfleiderer, W. & Wachter, H., Eds.)
pp 367-382, Walter de Gruyter u. Co Berlin, New York.

Kuchino, Y., Borek, E., Grunberger, D., Mushinski, J.F.
    & Nishimura, S. (1982) Nucl. Acids Res. 10,
    6421-6432.

Meier, F., Suter, B., Grosjean, H., Keith, G. &
    Kubli, E. (1985) Embo J. 4, 823-827.

Nishimura, S. (1983) in Progress in Nucleic Acid
    Research and Molecular Biology (Cohn, W.E., Ed.) 28,
    49-74, Academic Press, New York, London.

Noguchi, S., Nishimura, Y., Hirota, Y. & Nishimura, S.
    (1982) J. Biol. Chem. 257, 6544-6550.

Ott, G., Kersten, H. & Nishimura, S. (1982) FEBS Lett.
    146, 311-314.

Ott, G. & Kersten, H. (1985) Biol. Chem. Hoppe Seyl.,
    366, 69-76.

Randerath, E., Agrawal, H.P. & Randerath, K. (1984)
    Cancer Res. 44, 1167-1171.

Raymond, K.N. & Tufano, P. (1982) in The Biological
    Chemistry of Iron (Dunford, H.B., Dolphin, P.,
    Raymond, K.N. & Sieker, L., Eds.) pp 85-105,
    D. Reidel Publishing Company, London, Boston.

Sprinzl, M., Moll, J., Meissner, F. & Hartmann, Th.
    (1985) Nucl. Acids Res. 13, rl-r49.

Schachner, E., Aschhoff, H.-J. & Kersten, H. (1984)
    Eur. J. Biochem. 139, 481-487.

RELATIONSHIP BETWEEN METHYLATION AND MATURATION OF RIBOSO-

SOMAL RNA IN PROKARYOTIC AND EUKARYOTIC CELLS

Jean-Hervé ALIX

Institut de Biologie Physico-Chimique

13 rue P. et M. Curie, 75005 PARIS, FRANCE

A. GENERAL CHARACTERISTICS OF RIBOSOMAL RNA METHYLATION

All ribosomal RNAs (except the 5 S rRNA present in the large subunit of ribosomes) contain a relatively large number of methylated nucleosides (about 1 % of the total number) (Attardi and Amaldi, 1970 ; Hall, 1971), but the distribution of methyl groups in prokaryotic and eukaryotic ribosomal RNAs is strikingly different (see Table 1 of Maden, 1976 and Table 1 of Björk, 1983). *E.coli* 16 S and 23 S rRNAs contain a small number of 2'-O methylated ribose residues (Xm) (Nichols and Lane, 1967, 1968) and most (> 80 %) of methyl groups occurs as methylated bases (Fellner and Sanger, 1968 ; Van Charldorp et al., 1981), whereas more than 90 % of the methyl groups found in eukaryotic 18 S and 28 S rRNAs are present in 2'-O methylated ribose residues (Singh and Lane, 1964 ; Hashimoto et al., 1975 ; Maden and Salim, 1974 ; Cecchini and Miassod, 1979 ; Connaughton et al., 1984). The 5.8 S rRNA, hydrogen-bonded to the 28 S rRNA and present in the large subunit of eukaryotic (but not of prokaryotic) ribosomes, contains two 2'-O methylated ribose residues (Nazar et al., 1975a, b ; MacKay and Doolittle, 1981 ; Schnare and Gray, 1982). Whereas phosphodiester bonds adjacent to methylated bases in RNA display normal sensitivity to ribonucleases and alkaline pH, those which bear a 2'-O methylated ribose on the 3' side are resistant to these agents since formation of a 2'-3' cyclic phosphate intermediate is impossible.

175

Determination of ribosomal RNA primary structures has shown that methyl groups are not distributed at random, but are grouped in specific regions of these molecules. For example, twelve of the thirteen methyl groups of *E.coli* 16 S rRNA are located in the 3' half of the molecule (Fellner et al., 1972 ; Carbon et al., 1978). Similarly the 2'-O methylated ribose residues and the methylated bases of eukaryotic 18 S rRNA are concentrated towards respectively the 5' and 3' terminal regions of the molecule. In eukaryotic 28 S rRNA methyl groups are rare in the 5' terminal region, more frequent in the central part and abundant in the 3' terminal region of the molecule (Maden, 1980).

A remarkable feature of the post-transcriptional methylation of ribosomal RNA is its evolutionary stability. The striking similarity of the methylation patterns observed in a wide range of cell types from prokaryotic organisms (Sogin et al., 1972 ; Hsuchen and Dubin, 1980) as well as from eukaryotic organisms such as yeast, drosophila, toad, chicken, plants, mouse, hamster, rat and man (Khan et al., 1978 ; Klagsbrun, 1973 ; Khan and Maden, 1976 ; Maden and Tartof, 1974 ; Klootwijk and Planta, 1973 ; Cecchini and Miassod, 1979 ; Maden and Reeder, 1979 ; Brand and Gerbi, 1979 ; Gray, 1979 ; Miassod and Cecchini, 1979 ; Woese et al. 1975 ; Choi et al., 1982) reveals a high degree of evolutionary conservation. rRNA sequences containing methylated bases are even more highly conserved than those containing methylated ribose residues. The best illustration is the extremely conserved methylated sequence Gm_2Am_2AC universally present (Van Knippenberg et al., 1984) near the 3' end of the small ribosomal subunit RNA of all prokaryotic and eukaryotic organisms (only two exceptions have been found in organellar ribosomes , Klootwijk et al., 1975 ; Steege et al., 1982 ; Van Buul et al., 1984), and this may be related to the direct involvement of this region of RNA in initiation of protein synthesis and in subunit interaction.

The high degree of conservation of rRNA methylation specificity throughout evolution and the nearly completion of ribose methylation of eukaryotic rRNA at the stage of the primary pre-rRNA (see part B) support the view that this modification of the polynucleotide chain is of fundamental importance for correct assembly of pre-ribonucleoparticles or/ and for correct processing of 45 S precursor RNA to the mature 28 S and 18 S RNA species. I shall examine here the role of methylation for pre-rRNA processing in *E.coli* and in eukaryotic cells, in relation to the basic differences of the methylation pathway in both systems.

B. RIBOSOMAL RNA PROCESSING IN *E.coli* AND IN EUKARYOTIC CELLS

Conversion of the 30 S precursor RNA of prokaryotic cells and of the 45 S precursor RNA of eukaryotic cells into the mature species involves excision of transcribed spacer sequences (and for some eukaryotic precursor rRNAs excision of introns and subsequent splicing) and modifications of ribose and purine and pyrimidine residues.

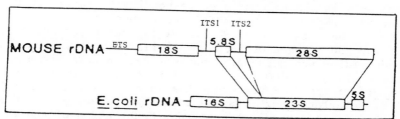

Fig. 1 : *Organization of rRNA genes in prokaryotes (E.coli) and eukaryotes (mouse). Note 1) the presence of the 5 S rRNA gene in the bacterial 16 S - 23 S rRNA operon, but its absence from the eukaryotic 18 S - 28 S rRNA operon ; 2) the presence inside the E.coli 23 S rRNA (5' end) of a region homologous in sequence to the eukaryotic 5.8 S rRNA (see Walker and Pace, 1983) ; and 3) The following sequence in the initial 45 S rRNA transcript (from the 5' end) : an external transcribed spacer (ETS), 18 S rRNA, an internal transcribed spacer (ITS1), 5.8 S rRNA, a second internal transcribed spacer (ITS2) and 28 S rRNA.*

The organization of the mature rRNA sequences in the precursor species and the sequence of cleavage processes are similar in prokaryotic and eukaryotic cells with the exception that 5 S rRNA is present in the prokaryotic 30 S but not in the eukaryotic 45 S precursor species. The initial transcript is immediately associated with a group of proteins, and all further processing occurs within the framework of this ribonucleoprotein particle. However, the sequence of the cleavages at different sites of pre-rRNA may not be the same in all organisms. Even in a single species, simultaneous operation of alternate pathways may be operating (Bowman et al., 1981). Organization and transcription of eukaryotic rRNA genes, maturation of pre-RNA and preribosomes in eukaryotes and maturation of bacterial RNA have been reviewed in detail respectively by Mandal (1984), Hadjiolov and Nikolaev (1976), Apirion and Gegenheimer (1981) and Apirion (1983).

Post-transcriptional modifications of rRNA precursors
other than cleavage processes differ in two important aspects in prokaryotic and eukaryotic organisms :
a) In eukaryotic organisms, methylation of pre-rRNA takes place in the nucleolus, the site of its synthesis, during or shortly after pre-rRNA transcription ; it is almost
entirely completed before cleavage of this molecule into
intermediate precursor species occurs. Methyl groups are
added only in the sequences corresponding to mature 28 S
rRNA, 18 S rRNA and 5.8 S rRNA, the transcribed spacer segments in the primary pre-rRNA remaining unmethylated. The
distribution of pseudouridine is similar. The numbers of
pseudouridine and methylated nucleotides in rRNA are almost equal, about 100 each. A different situation is found
in $E.coli$: the 30 S precursor RNA is only partially methylated. Methylation of 16 S and 23 S rRNA sequences in 30 S
pre-rRNA follows distinct patterns. Methylation of the 23 S
rRNA segment appears to be already complete in the 30 S pre-
rRNA (Dahlberg et al., 1975) but methylation of the 16 S
rRNA is not completed until the final stages of its maturation and of 30 S subunit assembly (Hayes et al., 1971 ;
Sogin et al., 1972).
b) as already mentioned in part A, all except six or seven of the approximately one hundred methyl groups introduced into eukaryotic 45 pre-rRNA are present as ribose 2'-0
methyl groups whereas methylation of bacterial ribosomal
RNA is confined almost entirely to purine and pyrimidine
bases. The small number of modified bases in eukaryotic ribosomal RNAs occur mainly in the 17 S - 18 S species and are
almost all introduced at late stages in the rRNA maturation
process probably at sites which are exposed in the 40 S ribosomal subunits, after transport to the cytoplasm. This is
the case for the N^6-dimethyladenine in the ubiquitous
Gm_2Am_2AC sequence (see part A) (Brand et al., 1977 ; Alberty
et al., 1978 ; Hagenbüchle et al., 1978 ; Samols et al.,
1979). There are two examples of stepwise modification in
two successive cellular compartments = a) 5.8 S rRNA : one
2'-0 methylation occurs in the nucleus and the other in the
cytoplasm (Nazar et al., 1980) ; b) The hypermodified uridine residue, 1-methyl-3(α-amino-α-carboxy-propyl)-pseudo-
uridine, in which both the methyl and the aminocarboxypro-
pyle substituents are derived, like all the methyl groups,
from methionine (Saponara and Enger, 1974 ; Maden et al.,
1975 ; Brand et al., 1978) : the pseudouridylation and the
methylation processes take place on the 45 S or 37 S pre-
rRNA in the nucleus, whereas the aminocarboxypropyl group is

introduced in the cytoplasm at a very late stage in 18 S
rRNA maturation.

C. METHYLATION AND MATURATION OF RIBOSOMAL RNA IN *E.coli*

A series of observations show that a role of methylation for pre-rRNA maturation in *E.coli* is an unlikely possibility. First, an *E.coli* mutant lacking the single m^1G
residue normally present in 23 S rRNA is not impaired in
ribosome formation and function (Björk and Isaksson, 1970).
Second, a kasugamycin-resistant *E.coli* mutant (KsgA) which
lacks the four methyl groups present in the $m_2^6Am_2^6ACCUG$ sequence of 16 S rRNA contains 16 S rRNA of normal (mature)
chain length (Helser et al., 1971). Third, incubation of a
methionine minus strain of *E.coli* in a medium containing
ethionine in place of methionine can be used as a method
to block all cellular post-synthetic methylations : this
is because ethionine is not accepted by prokaryotic L-me-
thionine-S-adenosyltransferase whose product, S-adenosyl-
L-methionine, is used for methylation reactions (Alix,
1982). Analysis of 16 S rRNA synthesized in these conditions shows that it lacks the methyl groups present in normal 16 S rRNA. But it possesses the same 3'-OH and 5'-phos-
phate terminal sequences as the latter. 23 S rRNA and 5 S
rRNA formed in ethionine-treated cells also contain normal
terminal sequences. Therefore, in *E.coli*, methylation is
not necessary for the maturation of pre-rRNA to products
with normal chain lengths (Chelbi-Alix et al., 1981). If the
rates of maturation of methylated and unmethylated rRNAs
are the same (this has not yet been shown) it can be concluded that methylation plays no role in this process.

D. METHYLATION AND MATURATION OF RIBOSOMAL RNA IN EUKARYOTIC CELLS

The relationship between the methylation and maturation
of rRNA precursors is apparently different in *E.coli* and eukaryotic organisms. Numerous studies have been carried out
either with isolated nucleoli (Liau and Hurlbert, 1975 ;
Liau et al., 1976) or with intact cells in which all possible methods to inhibit methylation have been used.

1) The deficiency in 28 S rRNA maturation and assembly of
60 S ribosomal subunits observed at non-permissive temperature (39°C) in a temperature -sensitive mutant of BHK cells
has been related to the observed undermethylation of 28 S
cytoplasmic rRNA and its 45 S and 32 S precursors (Ouellette

et al., 1976), although this conclusion has been challenged by others (Toniolo and Basilico, 1976 ; Levin and Clark, 1979).

2) Methionine deprivation of HeLa cells in culture (Vaughan et al., 1967) and methionine limitation of a me-thionine-requiring strain of *Saccharomyces cerevisiae* (Wej-ksnora and Haber, 1974) cause the accumulation of rRNA pre-cursors and lead to the conclusion that methylation of ribo-somal RNA or other methionine-dependent events plays a role in the processing of precursor rRNA.

3) Exposure of Novikoff ascites hepatoma cells to poly (I).poly(C) impairs the methylation of ribosomal precursor RNA, which in turn is responsible for the destruction of ri-bosomes, preferentially the small subunits, during the matu-ration processes (Liau et al., 1975).

4) Histidine starvation of Ehrlich ascites cells provo-kes a decrease in the methylation of both 45 S pre-rRNA and mature rRNAs and a slowdown of ribosome formation. This sug-gests that correct methylation, although not a pre-requisite for maturation, is involved at some step of ribosome matura-tion, affecting for example, the rate of pre-rRNA processing (Grummt, 1977).

5) Infection of baby hamster kidney cells by foot-and-mouth disease virus causes extensive inhibition of the methy-lation of host nuclear rRNA precursors, which is directly res-ponsible, according to the authors, for the loss of formation of nascent ribosomes (Ascione and Van de Woude, 1969).

6) In eukaryotic cells treated with ethionine, the syn-thesis of S-adenosylethionine, an inhibitor of methylation, and the reduction in the concentration of ATP and thus of S-adenosylmethionine leads to undermethylation of nuclear and cytoplasmic rRNA (Alix, 1982), at 2'-hydroxyribose sites, but not at base sites in hepatic pre-rRNA (Wen and Tsukada, 1983). This effect is apparently the cause of the inhibition of pro-cessing of nuclear pre-rRNA to cytoplasmic rRNA observed in these cells. However, processing is not entirely blocked since earliest cleavage step (45 S→32 S RNA) is observed to take place to a limited extent (Swann et al., 1975 ; Wolf and Schlessinger, 1977). In *S. cerevisiae* treated with ethionine, rRNA processing is also altered, but rRNA methylation is not extensively affected (Singer et al., 1978).

7) The treatment of Chinese hamster ovary cells with cycloleucine, a competitive inhibitor of methionine, leads to the same conclusion as the treatment of other mammalian

cells with ethionine, i.e., that the maturation pathway of
the undermethylated pre-rRNA is severely affected at several
stages, particularly the last stage (appearance of 28 S
rRNA in the cytoplasm) (Caboche and Bachellerie, 1977).Im-
pairment by cycloleucine of the transport of newly synthesized tRNAs into the cytoplasm (Amalric et al., 1977) and of
processing of mitochondrial RNA (Dubin et al., 1982) and of
avian retrovirus RNA (Stoltzfus and Dane, 1982) has also
been shown, resulting most likely from interference with methylation.

8) Other methods generally used to inhibit cellular methylations act at the level of either S-adenosylmethionine,
the methyl group donor (inhibition of its synthesis ; synthesis of S-adenosylmethionine analogs which competitively inhibit the methyltransferases) or S-adenosylhomocysteine, the
product and inhibitor of most methyltransferases (increase
of its cellular level ; synthesis of S-adenosylhomocysteine
analogs). As a potent inhibitor of transmethylation reactions,
S-adenosylhomocysteine must be efficiently catabolized, for
normal cellular function, to adenosine and L-homocysteine.
The equilibrium constant of this reaction which is catalyzed
by S-adenosylhomocysteine hydrolase strongly favors *the synthesis* of S-adenosylhomocysteine, and therefore, physiologically, degradation of S-adenosylhomocysteine occurs only because of the efficient metabolic removal of the reaction products. It is therefore possible to increase the S-adenosylhomocysteine level and inhibit transmethylations by treatment of cells with adenosine or/and homocysteine (or homocysteine thiolactone, its lipophilic analog), or by drugs inhibiting adenosine deaminase (Glazer, 1980).

For example, culture of human myeloma cells in the presence of adenosine causes inhibition of 18 S rRNA accumulation
(Bynum and Volkin, 1975). Most adenosine analogs used (e.g.
cordycepin, xylosyladenine), are inhibitors of transmethylation, but this is not always the case since *neither* toyocamy-
cin nor sangivamycin, two closely related pyrrolopyrimidine
nucleoside analogs, causes a reduction in the methylation of
the 45 S rRNA precursor (Cohen and Glazer, 1985b) although
the former inhibits RNA processing whereas the latter does
not (Cohen and Glazer, 1985a). Therefore, all the effects of
a drug must be known before drawing conclusions.

9) A contradictory result has been recently obtained with
a cyclopentenyl analog of adenosine, neplanocin A (Keller
and Borchardt, 1984 ; Borchardt et al., 1984) which, while

inhibiting RNA methylation, neither inhibits RNA synthesis, nor causes accumulation of rRNA precursors (Glazer and Knode, 1984).

With the exception of the last observation, all the results listed tend to the following conclusions :

1) Inhibition of methylation of the nucleolar 45 S RNA affects its processing to mature cytoplasmic products 18 S and 28 S RNA, but not its synthesis.

2) The initial maturation step (45 S rRNA→32 S rRNA) is less affected than the subsequent steps by the absence of methylation.

3) When they are not processed, rRNA molecules are degraded.

4) Ribose methylation and not base methylation of nucleolar pre-rRNA appears to be important for its processing.

5) Methylation is not a prerequisite for rRNA maturation but controls its efficiency at some step(s), probably in the cytoplasm or during the nucleocytoplasmic transport.

E. DISCUSSION AND CONCLUSIONS

Evidence has been presented that most of the methods which inhibit RNA methylation in eukaryotic cells also severely inhibit rRNA processing, which however is blocked neither completely nor at a definite stage : several elementary stages of the maturation pathway are affected. On the other hand, non-dependence of rRNA maturation on methylation has been demonstrated in the case of a prokaryote, *E.coli*. This apparent discrepancy may be related to the differences between the processes of RNA methylation in prokaryotic and eukaryotic cells : the former occurs essentially at base sites, late in the ribosome assembly process, and in the cytosol, whereas the latter occurs mainly at ribose sites, very early during primary transcription, and in the nucleus. Ribose methylation would thus play an important role. This could be in protecting eukaryotic rRNA precursors against enzymatic degradation. The basis for this currently accepted hypothesis is the early advent (co-transcriptional) of methylation and the fact that inhibition of methylation leads to extensive degradation of rRNA precursor species. One also can note that phenobarbital stimulates the activity of nucleolar RNA methyltransferases, which in turn increases the stability of 45 S pre-rRNA (Smith et al., 1976).

Alternatively ribose methylation would play a role either in the recognition of the cleavage sites by the processing enzymes, or in the determination of conformation of RNA in the cleavage sites or in the binding sites of specific proteins. Because of the small amounts of 28 S and 18 S rRNA still formed when methylation is inhibited, the first possibility is less likely. Therefore, ribose methylation appears to be non essential but important in controlling the rate or the efficiency of processing, which suggests that it has a role in conformation determination. Physical studies have shown that 2'-O alkylation enhances ordered structure in single-stranded RNA (Rottman et al., 1974). 2'-O methylation of 5.8 S RNA (on the U at position 14) influences its conformation and plays a role in the 5.8 S - 28 S rRNA interaction (Nazar et al., 1983).

The noticeable feature that the initial nuclear maturation step (45 S→32 S rRNA) is less affected by the absence of methylation than the subsequent cytoplasmic steps may be related to the likely existence of different cellular pools of S-adenosylmethionine in eukaryotes (Judes and Jacob, 1972 ; Farooqui et al., 1983).

In the case of tRNAs where, as in prokaryotic rRNA, base modification is predominant, studies of the time course of methylation during tRNA maturation did not reveal any interdependence of the two processes. Formation of the various methylated residues, although it is not clear if this is an ordered (Munns and Sims, 1975) or random (Davis and Nierlich, 1974) process, is likely to occur late in tRNA maturation (Sakano et al., 1974 ; Harada et al., 1984).

REFERENCES

- Alberty, H., Raba, M. and Gross, J.H. (1978) Nucleic Acids Research 5, 425-434.
- Alix, J.H. (1982) Microbiological Reviews 46, 281-295.
- Amalric, F., Bachellerie, J.P. and Caboche, M. (1977) Nucleic Acids Research 4, 4357-4370.
- Apirion, D., and Gegenheimer, P. (1981) FEBS Letters 125, 1-9.
- Apirion, D. (1983) Prog. Nucleic Ac. Res. Mol. Biol. 30, 1-40.
- Ascione, R. and Vande Woude, G.F. (1969) J. Virology 4, 727-737.
- Attardi, G. and Amaldi, F. (1970) Ann. Rev. Biochem. 39, 183-226.
- Björk, G.R. and Isaksson, L.A. (1970) J. Mol. Biol. 51, 83-100.

- Björk, G.R. (1983) in Processing of RNA. D. Apirion ed., CRC Press.
- Borchardt, R.T., Keller, B.T. and Patel-Thombre, U. (1984) J. Biol. Chem. 259, 4353-4358.
- Bowman, L.H., Rabin, B. and Schlessinger, D. (1981) Nucleic Acids Research 9, 4951-4966.
- Brand, R.C., Klootwijk, J., Van Steenbergen, T.J.M., De Kok, A.J. and Planta, R.J. (1977) Eur. J. Biochem. 75, 311-318.
- Brand, R.C., Klootwijk, J., Planta, R.J. and Maden, B.E.H. (1978) Biochem. J. 169, 71-77.
- Brand, R.C. and Gerbi, S.A. (1979) Nucleic Acids Research 7, 1497-1511.
- Bynum, W. and Volkin, E. (1975) J. Cell. Physiol. 88, 197-206.
- Caboche, M. and Bachellerie, J.P. (1977) Eur. J. Biochem. 74, 19-29.
- Carbon, P., Ehresmann, C., Ehresmann, B. and Ebel, J.P. (1978) FEBS Letters 94, 152-156.
- Cecchini, J.P. and Miassod, R. (1979) Eur. J. Biochem. 98, 203-214.
- Chelbi-Alix, M.K., Expert-Bezançon, A., Hayes, F., Alix, J.H. and Branlant, C. (1981) Eur. J. Biochem. 115, 627-634.
- Choi, Y.C., Reddy, R. and Busch, H. (1982) In : Biochemistry of S-adenosylmethionine and related compounds, Usdin, E., Borchardt, R.T. and Creveling, C.R., eds., Mac Millan Press, Ldt, pp. 313-320.
- Cohen, M.B. and Glazer, R.I. (1985a) Molecular Pharmacology 27, 308-313.
- Cohen, M.B. and Glazer, R.I. (1985b) Molecular Pharmacology 27, 349-355.
- Connaughton, J.F., Rairkar, A., Lockard, R.E. and Kumar, A. (1984) Nucleic Acids Research 12, 4731-4745.
- Dahlberg, J.E., Nikolaev, N. and Schlessinger, D. (1975) Processing of RNA, Brookhaven Symposia in Biology 26,194-200.
- Davis, A.R. and Nierlich, D.P. (1974) Biochem. Biophys. Acta 374, 23-37.
- Dubin, D.T., Green, C.M. and Prince, D.L. (1982) In : Biochemistry of S-adenosylmethionine and related compounds, Usdin, E., Borchardt, R.T. and Creveling, C.R. eds., Mac Millan Press Ldt, pp. 289-296.
- Farooqui, J.Z., Lee, H.W., Kim, S. and Paik, W.K. (1983) Biochim. Biophys. Acta 757, 342-351.
- Fellner, P. and Sanger, F. (1968) Nature 219, 236-238.

- Fellner, P., Ehresmann, C., Stiegler, P. and Ebel, J.P. (1972) Biochimie 54, 853-967.
- Glazer, R.I. (1980) Cancer Chemother. Pharmacol. 4, 227-235.
- Glazer, R.I. and Knode, M.C. (1984) J. Biol. Chem. 259, 12964-12969.
- Gray, M.W. (1979) Can. J. Biochem. 57, 914-926.
- Grummt, I. (1977) Eur. J. Biochem. 79, 133-141.
- Hadjiolov, A.A., and Nikolaev, N. (1976) Prog. Biophys. Molec. Biol. 31, 95-144.
- Hagenbüchle, O., Santer, M., Steitz, J.A. and Mans, R.J. (1978) Cell 13, 551-563.
- Hall, R.H. (1971) The Modified Nucleosides in Nucleic Acids, Columbia University Press, New York.
- Harada, F., Matsubara, M. and Kato, N. (1984) Nucleic Acids Research 12, 9263-9269.
- Hashimoto, S., Sakai, M. and Muramatsu, M. (1975) Biochemistry 14, 1956-1964.
- Hayes, F., Hayes, D.H., Fellner, P. and Ehresmann, C. (1971) Nature New. Biol. 232, 54-55.
- Helser, T.L., Davies, J.E. and Dahlberg, J.E. (1971) Nature New Biol. 233, 12-14.
- Hsuchen, C.C. and Dubin, D.T. (1980) J. Bact. 144, 991-998.
- Judes, C. and Jacob, M. (1972) FEBS Letters 27, 289-292.
- Keller, B.T. and Borchardt, R.T. (1984) Biochem. Biophys. Res. Commun 120, 131-137.
- Khan, M.S.N. and Maden, B.E.H. (1976) J. Mol. Biol. 101, 235-254.
- Khan, M.S.N., Salim, M. and Maden, B.E.H. (1978) Biochem. J. 169, 531-542.
- Klagsbrun, M. (1973) J. Biol. Chem. 248, 2612-2620.
- Klootwijk, J., Klein, I. and Grivell, L.A. (1975) J. Mol. Biol. 97, 337-350.
- Klootwijk, J. and Planta, R.J. (1973) Mol. Biol. Rep. 1, 187-191.
- Levin, E.G. and Clark, J.L. (1979) J. Cell. Physiol. 101, 361-368.
- Liau, M.C., Smith, D.W. and Hurlbert, R.B. (1975) Cancer Research 35, 2340-2349.
- Liau, M.C. and Hurlbert, R.B. (1975) Biochemistry 14, 127-134.
- Liau, M.C., Hunt, M.E. and Hurlbert, R.B. (1976) Biochemistry 15, 3158-3164.
- MacKay, R.M. and Doolittle, W.F. (1981) Nucleic Acids Research 9, 3321-3334.

- Maden, B.E.H. and Salim, M. (1974) J. Mol. Biol. 88, 133-164.
- Maden, B.E.H. and Tartof, K. (1974) J. Mol. Biol. 90, 51-64.
- Maden, B.E.H., Forbes, J., de Jonge, P. and Klootwijk, J. (1975) FEBS Letters 59, 60-63.
- Maden, B.E.H. (1976) Trends Biochem. Sci. 1, 196-199.
- Maden, B.E.H. and Reeder, R.H. (1979) Nucleic Acids Research 6, 817-830.
- Maden, B.E.H. (1980) Nature 288, 293-296.
- Mandal, R.K. (1984) Prog. Nucleic Ac. Res. Mol. Biol. 31, 115-160.
- Miassod, R. and Cecchini, J.P. (1979) Biochim. Biophys. Acta 562, 292-301.
- Munns, T.W. and Sims, H.F. (1975) J. Biol. Chem. 250, 2143-2149.
- Nazar, R.N., Sitz, T.O. and Busch, H. (1975a) J. Biol. Chem. 250, 8591-8597.
- Nazar, R.N., Sitz, T.O. and Busch, H. (1975b) FEBS Letters 59, 83-87.
- Nazar, R.N., Sitz, T.O. and Somers, K.D. (1980) J. Mol. Biol. 142, 117-121.
- Nazar, R.N., Lo, A.C., Wildeman, A.G. and Sitz, T.O. (1983) Nucleic Acids Research 11, 5989-6001.
- Nichols, J.L. and Lane, B.G. (1967) J. Mol. Biol. 30, 477-489.
- Nichols, J.L. and Lane, B.G. (1968) Can. J. Biochem. 46, 109-115.
- Ouellette, A.J., Bandman, E. and Kumar, A. (1976) Nature 262, 619-621.
- Rottman, F., Friderici, K., Comstock, P. and Khan, M.K. (1974) Biochemistry 13, 2762-2771.
- Sakano, H., Shimura, Y. and Ozeki, H. (1974) FEBS Letters 48, 117-121.
- Samols, D.R., Hagenbüchle, O. and Gage, L.P. (1979) Nucleic Acids Research 7, 1109-1119.
- Saponara, A.G. and Enger, M.D. (1974) Biochim. Biophys. Acta 349, 61-77.
- Schnare, M.N. and Gray, M.W. (1982) Nucleic Acids Research 10, 2085-2092.
- Singer, R.A., Johnston, G.C. and Bedard, D. (1978) Proc. Natl. Acad. Sci. USA 75, 6083-6087.
- Singh, H. and Lane, B.G. (1964) Can. J. Biochem. 42, 1011-1021.
- Smith, S.J., Liu, D.K., Leonard, T.B., Duceman, B.W. and Vesell, E.S. (1976) Molecular Pharmacology 12, 820-831.

- Sogin, M.L., Pechman, K.J., Zablen, L., Lewis, B.J. and Woese, C.R. (1972) J. Bact. 112, 13-16.
- Steege, D.A., Graves, M.C. and Spremulli, L.L. (1982) J. Biol. Chem. 257, 10430-10439.
- Stoltzfus, C.M. and Dane, R.W. (1982) In : Biochemistry of S-adenosylmethionine and related compounds, Usdin, E., Borchardt, R.T. and Creveling, C.R. eds. Mac Millan Press Ldt pp. 345-353.
- Swann, P.F., Peacock, A.C. and Bunting, S. (1975) Biochem. J. 150, 335-344.
- Toniolo, D. and Basilico, C. (1976) Biochim. Biophys. Acta 425, 409-418.
- Van Buul, C.P.J.J., Hamersma, M., Visser, W. and Van Knippenberg, P.H. (1984) Nucleic Acids Research 12, 9205-9208.
- Van Charldorp, R., Heus, H.A. and Van Knippenberg, P.H. (1981) Nucleic Acids Research 9, 2717-2725.
- Van Knippenberg, P.H., Van Kimmenade, J.M.A. and Heus, H.A. (1984) Nucleic Acids Research 12, 2595-2604.
- Vaughan, M.H., Soeiro, R., Warner, J.R. and Darnell, J.E. (1967) Proc. Natl. Acad. Sci. USA 58, 1527-1534.
- Walker, T.A. and Pace, N.R. (1983) Cell 33, 320-322.
- Wejksnora, P.J. and Haber, J.E. (1974) J. Bact.120, 1344-1355.
- Wen, L.T. and Tsukada, K. (1983) Biochim. Biophys. Acta 741, 153-157.
- Woese, C.R., Fox, G.E., Zablen, L., Uchida, T., Bonen, L., Pechman, K., Lewis, B.J. and Stahl, D. (1975) Nature 254, 83-86.
- Wolf, S.F. and Schlessinger, D. (1977) Biochemistry 16, 2783-2791.

DISTRIBUTION OF m^{6}A IN mRNA AND ITS POSSIBLE BIOLOGICAL ROLE.

F. Rottman, P. Narayan, R. Goodwin, S. Camper,
Y. Yao, S. Horowitz, R. Albers, D. Ayers,
P. Maroney and T. Nilsen

Department of Molecular Biology and Microbiology
Case Western Reserve University
School of Medicine, Cleveland, Ohio 44106

INTRODUCTION

Methylation of cellular and viral mRNA is a common post-transcriptional event whose function is not well understood. Although a role for 5' terminal methylated cap structures in translation and mRNA stability has been demonstrated (Both et al., 1975), the function of internal methylation of specific adenine residues, to form N^6-methyladenosine (m^{6}A), is not clear. It has been suggested that m^{6}A serves some nuclear role in precursor processing and/or transport (Camper et al., 1984) although m^{6}A is not universally found in eukaryotic messages (Perry and Scherrer, 1975; Surrey and Nemer, 1976). The postulated nuclear role for m^{6}A correlates positively with its presence in viral RNAs which spend a portion of their replicative cycle within the nucleus. Internal m^{6}As are found in both cellular and viral mRNAs within the consensus sequence, $\overset{G}{A}$m^{6}AC, (Dimock and Stoltzfus, 1979; Wei et al., 1976) and it has been suggested that these residues may be involved in mRNA precursor splicing (Aloni et al., 1979; Canaani et al., 1979; Chen-Kiang et al; 1979).

Any model for m^{6}A function would benefit from a more detailed description of the distribution of this modification within cellular and viral mRNAs. We have approached this problem by developing methods for the

189

determination of m^6A in individual mRNA species and
defining the location of these residues within the mRNA.
For cellular mRNA we have focused mainly on the abundant
pituitary message coding for prolactin. For viral mRNAs
we chose influenza, which had previously been shown to
contain internal m^6A residues. In an attempt to determine
the role of internal m^6A we have used a methylation
inhibitor to alter, in vivo, the m^6A levels in cellular
and viral mRNAs.

RESULTS

Effect of S-tubercidinylhomocysteine (STH) on cellular mRNA Methylation.

One approach to studying the possible function of
 m^6A residues is to observe the metabolism of mRNAs
which do not possess a full complement of m^6A . We
have earlier described the use of the methylation inhibitor STH to partially block mRNA methylation, thereby
producing undermethylated mRNA species for study in vivo
(Camper et al., 1984). Concentrations of 500 µM STH
lead to undermethylated mRNA species which still have
 m^7G within the terminal cap structure, but contain reduced amounts of internal m^6A and the 2'-O- methyl-
nucleoside residues (Nm) immediately adjacent to the m^7G
moiety of the cap ($m^7GpppN'm$). As a result of STH
treatment one also generates "cap 0" structures (m^7GpppN')
which contain no 2'-O-methylnucleosides and also up to a
90% reduction in internal m^6A residues. The physiological
fate of undermethylated mRNAs generated in this manner
can be studied to provide some clue regarding the function
of mRNA methylation. Using STH-treated HeLa cells, it
was shown that once undermethylated mRNA reached the
cytoplasm it behaved normally, i.e. the cytoplasmic stability of undermethylated and methylated mRNA was indis-
tinguishable, and both species were found on polysomes.
In contrast, the rate of appearance of undermethylated
mRNAs entering the cytoplasm was significantly delayed,
possibly reflecting a nuclear processing or transport
event which relied on methylation (Camper et al., 1984).
This result, which utilized total poly A^+ RNA populations,
suggested some role for m^6A residues in mRNA maturation
and underlined the necessity of obtaining information on
the distribution of m^6A within individual mRNA species.

Distribution of m^{6}A in m RNA

Determination of m^{6}A in unlabeled steady state mRNA populations.

A major difficulty in determining m^{6}A in individual mRNA species is related to the low levels of m^{6}A normally found in mRNA and the problems encountered in obtaining homogeneous mRNA species from total poly A$^+$ mixtures. From [^{3}H]-methyl-methionine labeling of steady state mRNA populations we had earlier estimated that, on average, a typical eukaryotic cellular mRNA contains 1-3 m^{6}A residues. Thus the amount of radioactivity expected in a single cellular mRNA of average abundance is extremely low and generally precludes any direct analysis of in vivo labeled material by conventional analytical methods. In an attempt to circumvent this problem, we have developed a method for m^{6}A determination which relies upon prior purification of an unlabeled mRNA species by hybridization, followed by in vitro [^{32}P] labeling of nucleotides from the protected fragment (Horowitz et al., 1984). Briefly, this procedure involves hybridization of unlabeled mRNA with a cloned single strand M13 cDNA sequence corresponding to either full length message or a selected restriction enzyme generated sub-fragment. Following hybridization, the unprotected RNA species are digested by nuclease and the protected fragment resolved by gel electrophoresis. The RNA recovered from the gel is degraded to mononucleotides and labeled by polynucleotide kinase with γ-[^{32}P]-ATP. The phosphorylated m^{6}A derived from the protected fragment is enriched by binding to m^{6}A-specific antibody and subsequently resolved on TLC. Elution and counting of the [^{32}P]-labeled m^{6}A and comparison with unmodified nucleotide spots permits detection of m^{6}A within an mRNA molecule or sub-fragment. The advantages of this method include its sensitivity, the ability to utilize unlabeled steady state mRNAs and the possibility of locating m^{6}A residues within regions of an individual mRNA molecule. The major disadvantage of the method is that due to the number of manipulations in the procedure, m^{6}A recovery is not quantitative. Nonetheless the method is reliable for determining relative amounts of m^{6}A within fragments of a given mRNA or in relative comparisons between several mRNA species.

This in vitro labeling method was ideally suited for determining m^{6}A in bovine prolactin (bPRL) mRNA, because of the high steady state levels of this message in the pituitary and the difficulty of in vivo labeling due to low transcriptional rates. Furthermore, by using specific M13 restriction fragments corresponding to regions within bPRL mRNA, it has been possible to locate the m^{6}A residues to a 127 nucleotide region in the 3' untranslated portion of the message which contains 3 potential consensus sites (AAC) of m^{6}A methylation (Horowitz et al. 1984). We have not at this time determined which of these 3 potential sites are methylated. Because the method is not entirely quantitative, we cannot determine the absolute levels of m^{6}A in prolactin mRNA and it is entirely possible that methylation at any single site is less than stoichiometric.

Theoretically this method should be applicable to any mRNA which accumulates to reasonable steady state levels and for which appropriate cDNA clones are available. To determine the relative levels of m^{6}A in other selected cellular mRNAs, M13 clones containing complimentary sequences to rat albumin and mouse dihydrofolate reductase (DHFR) mRNAs were used to protect corresponding mRNAs from rat liver and a methotrexate-resistant CHO cell line, respectively. The cDNA clone for rat albumin was nearly full length whereas the cDNA for mouse DHFR corresponded to a 750 nucleotide region found mainly in the portion of the message coding for the DHFR protein. The m^{6}A levels in albumin mRNA were extremely low and barely detectable by the antibody-TLC method, whereas the levels of m^{6}A in the mouse DHFR message were substantially greater, relative to either prolactin mRNA or total CHO cell A+ RNA. Although the in vitro labeling approach does not allow us to determine precise levels of m^{6}A within a specific mRNA, it does enable us to identify for future study those cellular messages which are highly enriched in m^{6}A, such as DHFR mRNA, and to focus on the role of m^{6}A in the metabolism of these mRNAs.

Effect of STH on synthesis of influenza virus-specific proteins.

We have taken a similar approach to the study of mRNA methylation events and its potential role in the expression of flu-specific mRNAs. The synthesis of flu

specific proteins provides a convenient method for monitoring the terminal events in the overall expression
of information contained in the virion. Furthermore, it
had previously been shown (Krug et al. 1976) that the
immediate transcription products of the viral genome
contained substantial levels of m^{6}A. Because STH was
known to markedly affect the methylation pattern of mRNA
in HeLa cells, this inhibitor was added to flu-infected
cultures prior to infection to determine its overall
effect on the kinds of proteins synthesized in uninfected
and flu-infected cultures. Flu-specific proteins, corresponding to the translation of the 8 individual flu
mRNAs, can be readily detected on SDS polyacrylamide
gels. Increasing concentrations of STH were added and
labeled cellular and flu-specific proteins detected by
radioautography (Figure 1). Under conditions (500 µM
STH) in which approximately 90% of cellular m^{6}A is
suppressed along with some inhibition of cap-containing
2'-0-methylnucleosides, the synthesis of flu specific
proteins was reduced to nearly nondetectable levels.
In contrast, the presence of 500 µM STH had no discern-
able affect on the synthesis of cellular proteins (Figure
1). In light of no direct translational effect of STH,
these results imply a major effect on the metabolism of
flu mRNA.

Characterization of m^{6}A and methylation patterns in flu-specific mRNAs.

Many of the difficulties encountered in characterizing m^{6}A in specific mRNAs and studying their functional
role can be minimized by use of a viral system such as
flu in which only a few mRNAs are produced in large
amounts. The extremely active transcription of flu-specific mRNAs allows one to use in vivo labeling with ^{3}[H]-
methyl-methionine to obtain sufficient material for detailed analyses. It should then be possible to determine the complete methylation profile of an mRNA species,
including cap components and internal m^{6}A, utilizing an
HPLC separation system we have specifically devised for
this purpose (Albers et al., 1981). This HPLC analytical
system provides a complete profile of methylated constituents found in eukaryotic mRNAs, including resolution of
all cap structures, 2'-0-methylnucleosides from the second N"m in cap 2 and most importantly, internal m^{6}A.

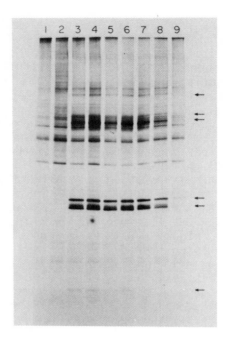

Figure 1. Effect of STH on flu specific proteins

Monolayers of HeLa cells were infected with influenza virus (WSN strain) in Dulbecco's modified Ea-
gle's medium containing 1% BSA. Cells were treated with
various concentrations of STH after the virus was adsorbed for 2 hr at 37°C. At 7 hr postinfection, cells
were labeled for 60 min with ^{35}S-methionine (100 μCi/ml)
in methionine free media. Cell extracts were prepared
by lysis in 2% SDS and labeled proteins analyzed by
electrophoresis on SDS-17.5% polyacrylamide gel. The
gel was dried and autoradiographed Lane 1. Mock infected
control; 2 - mock infected control treated with 500 μM
STH; 3 and 4 - virus infected cells; 5-9 virus infected
cells treated with 0.5, 5, 50, 250 and 500 μM STH respectively. Arrows indicate position of representative
virus-specific proteins.

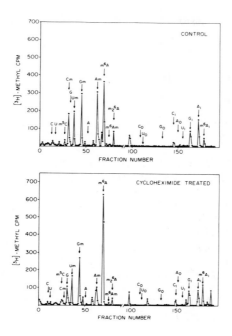

Figure 2. HPLC separation of methyl-labeled mRNA from influenza virus infected cell.

Cytoplasmic poly A⁺ RNA from flu infected control and cycloheximide treated cells were digested and chromatographed with standards on HPLC essentially as described previously (Camper et al., 1984). Arrows indicate the peak of absorbance of the standard in each individual run.

In addition it provides an accurate determination of m⁶A levels per 5'-terminal cap.

Influenza viral RNAs seem to be a particularly appropriate subject for such studies in light of the fact that earlier unfractionated flu mRNAs were reported to contain approximately 3 m⁶A residues per molecule (Krug

Table 1. m^{6}A Content in Flu RNA

	Control	Cycloheximide	Cordycepin	Cycloheximide and Cordycepin	Control NS1
m^{6}A (CPM)	502	1123	982	742	45
CAP (CPM)	231	242	179	288	59
m^{6}A/CAP	2.2	4.6	5.5	2.6	0.77

Infection of MDBK cells with influenza (WSN strain) was performed as described previosly (Krug et al., 1976). After 2 hr and 10 min the cells were transferred to methionine free media for 35 min at which time the media was replaced with methionine free media containing L-[methyl-^{3}H] methionine (1mCi/ml, 50 Ci/mM) and $\pm$ cycloheximide (100 μg/ml). After 3 hr the cells were harvested as previously described (Nilsen et al., 1982) and cytoplasmic poly A$^+$ RNA prepared. NS1 mRNA was selected by hybridization to NS1 cDNA (Nilsen and Maroney, unpublished experiments). RNA was analyzed by HPLC as described in the legend to Figure 2.

et al., 1976). Furthermore, flu is the only non-oncogenic RNA virus that replicates in the nucleus and 2 of its 8 capped primary transcripts, NS_1 and M_1, can give rise to the spliced products, NS_2 and M_2. A typical HPLC separation of [^{3}H]-methyl labeled constituents from flu-specific mRNA is shown in Figure 2. The relative level of m^{6}A per 5' terminal cap is shown in Table 1. The data indicate the presence of 3 m^{6}A residues per cap structure, or 3 residues per RNA molecule in total, unfractionated flu mRNA. This is essentially in agreement with levels of m^{6}A reported earlier (Krug et al., 1976). These m^{6}As do not appear, however, to be equally distributed among each of the flu RNAs. NS_1 and M_1, the two mRNAs which can be spliced, contain less than 1 (Table 1) and no detectable m^{6}A, (data not shown) respectively. Although NS and M by size are the two smallest flu RNA species, on a total mass basis they account for approximately 30% of the flu RNAs. Thus they are significantly underrepresented in m^{6}A content relative to the total flu RNA population. The m^{6}A levels in each of the remaining individual flu RNAs remain to be determined.

Cycloheximide and cordycepin are two inhibitors which have been used in earlier studies characterizing methylnucleotides in flu mRNAs (Krug et al., 1976). In order to determine the effect of these inhibitors on methylation patterns they were included during infection and methylated constituents resolved by HPLC. There was a marked elevation in the relative levels of m⁶A compared to cap constituents, as shown in Figure 2. and Table 1.

Discussion

Use of the methylation inhibitor STH has been shown in HeLa cells to result in the delayed appearance of undermethylated mRNAs into the cytoplasm. Under conditions employed in these studies internal methylation at m⁶A is inhibited to nearly 90% and the delayed cytoplasmic appearance would lead one to suspect an interference in some nuclear processing or transport event. However, one cannot rule out the possiblity that STH indirectly affects a processing step or transport via some essential non-nucleic acid component which requires methylation.

The correspondence of consensus methylation sites (ᴳᴬm⁶AC) with consensus lariat acceptor sites (ᴬ̲AY) used in intron removal during splicing, has led to the hypothesis that m⁶A residues may play some determinative role in intron excision (Zeitlin and Efstratiadis, 1984). It would seem more likely, however, that such methylation events might function in a negative sense by preventing lariat formation at potentially aberrant splice sites rather than specifying the location of normal splicing events. These and other questions regarding m⁶A residues await studies on specific cellular and viral mRNA precursors both in vivo and in vitro.

The location of m⁶A residues within a single mRNA molecule can be determined by in vitro labeling of nucleotides derived from hybrid-protected mRNA fragments. Using this approach it was shown that the m⁶A found in bovine PRL mRNA is clustered in the 3' untranslated portion of the molecule. The precise location of m⁶A

could not be determined by this method but could be
limited to 3 methylation sites contained in a 3' terminal
fragment of 127 nucleotides out of a total of 27 possible
consensus methylation sites in the entire prolactin mRNA
molecule. A major advantage of this in vitro labeling
method for detecting m^6A is that it does not depend on
prior labeling of mRNAs with [^{3}H]-methyl-methionine. In
studies on several other cellular mRNAs including rat
albumin and mouse DHFR, it was shown that mRNA m^6A
content varies widely between different mRNAs. A cellular mRNA with a high m^6A content such as DHFR, should
serve as a useful candidate for further studies on the
role of m^6A in post-transcriptional events.

The dramatic effect of the methylation inhibitor,
STH, on flu-infected cells suggests a highly differential
mode of action on cellular and flu-specific expression.
The end point of viral expression, flu-specific proteins,
was used to monitor the overall effect of the methylation
inhibitor. Whereas host protein synthesis apparently
remained unaffected, synthesis of flu proteins was dramatically inhibited at higher concentrations of STH.
However, because STH is also known to result in the
appearance of "cap 0" structures by blocking 2'-O-methyl-
ation, the inhibition of flu expression by STH might
conceivably reflect disruption of the earlier step in
replication in which a cap structure derived from host
mRNA is used as a primer for flu-mRNA synthesis. If
this is true, it would suggest that 2'-O-methylnucleo-
sides are required on the host-derived RNA to serve as a
primer in the synthesis of flu RNAs. Of particular
interest will be the effect of STH induced undermethylation at m^6A positions on those flu RNAs containing high
levels of this modification.

The influence of cycloheximide and cordycepin on
the relative number of m^6A residues per molecule indicates that these inhibitors have a significant affect
on RNA methylation by some mechanism which is not obvious. These results would suggest that the use of such
inhibitors in such processing studies should be approached with some caution.

The flu virus offers a particularly attractive model

system for studying the role of m^{6}A modification. The expression of large amounts of flu RNAs in infected cells permits efficient _in_ _vivo_ labeling with [^{3}H]-methyl-methionine and subsequent analysis by HPLC. This analytical procedure provides detailed information on each of the methylated constituents found in mRNA. Another advantage of the flu system is that viral mRNAs contain, on average, a high level of m^{6}As. In light of the fact that both M$_1$ and NS$_1$ undergo splicing, these RNAs were selected as initial targets for methylation analysis. As shown in these studies, m^{6}A's are not distributed evenly among all 8 flu RNAs and it was somewhat surprising to note the low levels of this modification in NS and M. By inference the remaining flu RNAs must contain relatively high levels of m^{6}A and these will be the object of further study.

References:

Albers, R.J., Coffin, B. and Rottman, F.M. (1981) Anal. Biochem. 113, 118-123.

Aloni, Y., Dhar, R. and Khoury, G. (1979) J. Virol. 32, 52-60.

Both, G.W., Furichi, Y., Muthukrishman, S. and Shatkin, A.J. (1975) Cell 6, 185-195.

Camper, S.A., Albers, R.J. Coward, J.K. and Rottman, F.M. (1984) Mol. Cell. Biol. 4, 538-543.

Canaani, D., Kahana, C., Lavi, S. and Groner, Y. (1979) Nucleic Acids Res. 6, 2879-2899.

Chem-Kaing, A., Nevins, J.R. and Darnell, J.R. (1979) J. Mol. Biol. 135, 733-752.

Dimock, K. and Stoltzfus, C.M. (1979) J. Biol. Chem. 254, 5591-5594.

Horowitz, S., Horowitz, A., Nilsen, T.W., Munns, T.W. and Rottman, F.M. (1984) Proc. Natl. Acad. Sci USA 81, 5667-5671.

Krug, R.M., Morgan, M.A. and Shatkin, A.J. (1976) J. Virol. 20, 45-53.

Nilsen, T.W., Maroney, P.A. and Baglioni, C. (1982) J. Virol. 42, 1039-1045.

Peary, R.P. and Scherrer, K. (1975) FEBS Lett. 57, 73-78.

Surrey, S. and Nemer, M. (1976) Cell 9, 589-595.

Wei, C.M., Giershowitz, A. and Moss, B. (1976) Biochemistry 15, 397-401.

Zeitlin, S. and Efstratiadis, A. (1984) Cell 39, 589-602.

C. Regulation of S-Adenosylmethionine, S-Adenosylhomocysteine, and Methylthioadenosine Metabolism

REGULATION OF S-ADENOSYLMETHIONINE SYNTHESIS IN HUMAN LYMPHOCYTES

Nicholas M. Kredich, Malak Kotb, Deborah

Campano German and Craig A. Bloch

Howard Hughes Medical Institute Laboratories,

Duke University Medical Center, Durham, NC

27710

INTRODUCTION

The biochemistry of S-adenosylmethionine (AdoMet) provides several possible strategies for drug design. One focuses on the ability of S-adenosylhomocysteine (AdoHcy) and its analogues to inhibit transmethylation reactions; and involves the design of agents that inhibit transmethylases directly, or inhibit AdoHcy hydrolase causing AdoHcy accumulation, or react intracellularly with homocysteine to form inhibitory analogues of AdoHcy.

Another general approach is to perturb AdoMet metabolism either by inhibiting its synthesis, or by using analogues of ATP or methionine that AdoMet synthetase (ATP:L-methionine S-adenosyltransferase) can convert into toxic analogues of AdoMet. Cycloleucine is a well-known inhibitor of AdoMet synthetase, which lowers AdoMet levels in vivo (Chou et al., 1977); and both selenomethionine and ethionine have been useful as methionine analogues in studies of AdoMet metabolism. In addition, several ATP analogues, which can be provided to cells as nucleosides for in vivo conversion to triphosphates, have been found to serve as substrates for AdoMet synthetase giving the corresponding analogues of

203

AdoMet as products (Kredich, 1980; Garrett and Kredich, 1981). The latter are known to be inhibitory for some transmethylases and to serve as methyl donors for others (Borchardt et al., 1976). In those instances where a methyl group is transferred, an analogue of AdoHcy is produced, which itself can be inhibitory either directly or by inhibiting AdoHcy hydrolase or by both mechanisms. Cordycepin (3'-deoxyadenosine) and xylosyladenine are two well-documented examples of nucleosides that are converted in vivo to AdoHcy analogues by de-methylation of AdoMet analogues rather than by reversal of the AdoHcy hydrolase reaction (Kredich, 1980; Garrett and Kredich, 1981).

Thus, manipulation and exploitation of AdoMet synthetase appears to have considerable potential for chemotherapeutic interference with AdoMet metabolism. It is obvious, however, that realization of this potential requires a better understanding of human AdoMet metabolism – in particular AdoMet synthetase and those factors regulating its activity.

MULTIPLE FORMS OF ADOMET SYNTHETASE

Given the diverse involvement of AdoMet in trans-methylation and its role in polyamine metabolism, it is reasonable to assume that AdoMet synthesis should be subject to a global system of regulation. In considering this topic in humans one must distinguish between hepatic and non-hepatic tissues, for in the former the AdoMet requirement for creatine synthesis alone is several times greater than that of all other tissues combined (Mudd and Poole, 1975). Studies from a number of laboratories indicate that mammalian tissues contain several forms of AdoMet synthetase with differing physical and kinetic properties. In rats and humans three hepatic enzymes are found with K_m values for methionine that are "low", "intermediate" or "high" (Liau, et al., 1979b). These have also been designated MAT II, MAT I, and MAT III (Sullivan and Hoffman, 1983) or γ, α and β (Okada et al., 1981). Non-hepatic, normal tissues appear to have only the low K_m form, which is probably identical to its counterpart in liver, but malignant tissues have an intermediate K_m enzyme, which unlike that of liver can be

converted to a low Km species by two cycles of
DEAE-cellulose chromatherapy (Liau et al., 1979a,b).
Reactivity of rat liver intermediate Km enzyme with
antibody to highly purified high Km enzyme (Abe et al.,
1982) indicates these two enzymes are closely related.
Both appear to be unique to liver, and one possible
explanation for their presence is to subserve that
organ's special function as the body's major utilizer of
AdoMet in creatine syntheis. The low Km AdoMet
synthetase might then be considered to be the
"housekeeping" enzyme of non-hepatic tissues and perhaps
of liver as well.

With this multiplicity of AdoMet synthetases, it is
clear that detailed knowledge of several or all is
important for a rational approach to drug design. In
most instances the non-hepatic enzyme would be the target
of chemotherapy, and agents that interact with this
species and not the liver-specific enzymes might have the
advantage of less hepatic toxicity. Furthermore,
differences between the enzymes of normal and malignant
tissues might be exploited to provide additional
specificity (Sufrin and Lombardini, 1982).

Regulation of the hepatic-specific enzymes might be
keyed to creatine demand, but perhaps more specifically
to methionine availability owing to the important
regulatory role of AdoMet in homocysteine metabolism.
Through its ability to inhibit methylene tetrahydrofolate
reductase (Kutzbach and Stokstad, 1971) and to stimulate
cystathionine synthetase (Finkelstein et al., 1975),
AdoMet is believed to be a major factor in determining
whether homocysteine is remethylated to methionine or
irreversibly committed to transsulfuration (Finkelstein,
1979). It seems appropriate then that the major hepatic
enzyme has a Km value for methionine that is so high (c.
1 mM) that its reaction rate is essentially first order
at any physiologic concentration of this amino acid.
Such a property would allow AdoMet synthesis, and
presumably AdoMet levels in the liver to be relatively
sensitive to methionine availability.

Fluctuations in methionine concentration over a
physiologic range (10-30 µM in human plasma) are less
likely to influence AdoMet levels in non-hepatic tissues,

which contain an enzyme with a low Km for methionine.
AdoMet is known to inhibit this enzyme with Ki values
[2–60 µM (Sullivan and Hoffman, 1983; Oden and
Clark,1983)] that are in the range of AdoMet
concentrations reported in non–hepatic tissues (Chou et
al., 1977; Oden and Clark, 1983). This suggests that
AdoMet synthesis in non–hepatic tissues is controlled, at
least in part, by feedback inhibition. The purpose of
this communication is to describe studies performed in
our laboratory that indicate additional factors may be
involved in the regulation of AdoMet synthesis.

TRANSMETHYLATION AND ADENOSINE DEAMINASE DEFICIENCY

Our original interest in AdoMet metabolism resulted
from studies on heritable adenosine deaminase (ADA)
deficiency, a condition causing severe combined
immunodeficiency disease with marked to near–total
depletion of circulating and tissue lymphocytes. A
number of theories have been proposed to explain the lack
of lymphocytes in ADA deficiency, most of which are based
on the toxic effects of the ADA substrates adenosine and
2'–deoxyadenosine noted in cell culture models (Kredich
and Hershfield, 1983). One such effect is inhibition of
transmethylation reactions by AdoHcy, which can
accumulate either from reversal of the AdoHcy hydrolase
reaction by adenosine (Kredich and Martin, 1977) or by
inactivation of this enzyme by 2'–deoxyadenosine
(Hershfield, 1979). In attempting to determine whether
this mechanism is responsible for the immune defect in
ADA deficient patients, we reasoned that lymphocytes
might be particularly sensitive to AdoHcy if they
differed from other types of cells in some special aspect
of AdoMet metabolism. To evaluate this possibility we
directed our efforts toward measuring AdoMet
concentrations and turnover rates in cultured human
lymphocytes.

AdoMet Metabolism in Human Lymphocytes

Cultured WI–L2 human lymphoblasts readily incorporate
exogenous ^{35}S–methionine into intracellular free
methionine and AdoMet. By measuring rates of radio–

isotope equilibration we found pool turnover rates of
0.8/min and 0.076/min for methionine and AdoMet (German,
et al., 1983). With an intracellular AdoMet
concentration of 59 μM this amounts to utilization of
4.5 μM AdoMet/min in a culture growing with a doubling
time of about 20 h. Measurements of extracellular
homocysteine accumulation in WI-L2 cultures gave values
that were 79% those of AdoMet utilization, while
transsulfuration to cysteine and remethylation of
homocysteine to methionine accounted for an additional 5%
and <0.5%. Thus, transmethylation reactions utilize at
least 84% of the AdoMet synthesized in cultured WI-L2
cells, with the remainder used for polyamine synthesis or
lost to detection by our techniques. Comparison of total
AdoMet turnover with the amount of methionine removed
from the culture medium indicates as much as 23% of
methionine consumption is used for AdoMet synthesis
(German et al., 1983).

From the data of Mudd and Poole (1975) one can
estimate that labile methyl group turnover, exclusive of
that required for creatine synthesis, is approximately 3
mmol/day. Assuming a 28 liter cell volume for a 70 Kg
individual, this is equivalent to an average total body
turnover rate of 0.074 nmol/min/ml cell volume (0.074
μM/min), which is less than 2% of that found for
cultured WI-L2 cells. This comparison is prejudiced,
however, by the fact that cultured WI-L2 cells are
rapidly dividing, and most cells in the body are not.
Therefore, we turned our attention to a cultured cell
system that may be more representative of lymphoid cells
in an intact human.

Human peripheral blood mononuclear cells, composed of
approximately 80% lymphocytes, were isolated by
Ficoll-Hypaque density gradients and studied in culture
with the same techniques used for WI-L2 cells (German, et
al., 1983). AdoMet pool turnover in unstimulated,
non-dividing cells varied between 0.029/min and 0.06/min,
which is about one-half the rate found for WI-L2. Owing
to much smaller AdoMet pool sizes, absolute turnover
rates (0.12-0.40 μM/min) were less than 10% of those
found with WI-L2, but still 2-5 times the total body
average for non-creatine related AdoMet consumption.
Although these data are by no means conclusive they do

suggest that non–dividing lymphocytes have AdoMet
requirements that are greater than those of many other
tissues. Of interest also is that AdoMet levels are very
low in resting peripheral blood lymphocytes, at least
when compared to those reported for other tissues (Chou
et al., 1977). This finding may be relevant to the
lymphocyte defect in ADA deficiency, since cells with
high turnover rates and low levels of AdoMet should be
more sensitive to AdoHcy accumulation owing to the fact
that inhibition of transmethylases by AdoHcy is usually
competitive with AdoMet.

Within 24–48 h after PHA–stimulation of peripheral
blood mononuclear cells, absolute rates of AdoMet
turnover increase to approximately 1.5 µM/min, which is
about one–third the rate found in WI–L2 cells. More
rapid turnover is accompanied by a 5 to 10–fold expansion
of AdoMet pool size, and little or no change in the pool
fractional turnover rate. These findings are not
surprising considering the fact that virtually all
metabolic activities are increased by stimulating resting
cells to grow and divide. Of interest, however, is the
time course of this effect on AdoMet metabolism. In most
experiments AdoMet turnover and intracellular
concentration increased 30% or more within 2–3 h after
lectin stimulation and by as much as four–fold after 7 h
(German, et al., 1983).

Synthesis of additional AdoMet synthetase is one
possible cause of the increase in AdoMet turnover in
PHA–stimulated cells, and undoubtedly plays an important
role after 24–48 h. However, since significant effects
on total new protein synthesis are not observed until
12–16 after lectin–stimulation, other factors affecting
the rate of AdoMet synthesis must be considered as well.
A kinetic explanation is suggested by the known sensitivity of the low Km enzyme to inhibition by AdoMet.
Conceivably, increased utilization of AdoMet in processes
associated with early events of lectin stimulation could
lower steady state levels of AdoMet and thus stimulate
AdoMet synthesis by "pulling" on the pathway from
downstream. However, such a mechanism is contrary to our
findings that AdoMet levels actually rise as turnover
increases. If product inhibition by AdoMet is
significant at the concentrations found in these cells,

the observed increases in AdoMet pool size would actually
tend to decrease absolute turnover rates. In light of
these considerations we purified human lymphocyte AdoMet
synthetase in order to characterize factors that might be
involved in the regulation of its activity.

LYMPHOCYTE ADOMET SYNTHETASE

Chronic lymphocytic leukemia lymphocytes were used as
an enzyme source because they are readily available as a
by-product of therapeutic leukophoresis. Our purification
scheme gave 2 mg of protein from 880 g of frozen cells,
which represented a 2700-fold purification and a 17%
overall recovery of enzyme activity. Judging from native
and denaturing polyacrylamide gel electropherograms the
final product was about 95% pure (Kotb and Kredich, 1985).

The molecular weight of purified native enzyme, as
determined by equilibrium sedimentation, is 185,000.
SDS-polyacrylamide gel electrophoresis gives three
separate bands: two termed α and α' with molecular
weights of 53,000 and 51,000; and a smaller peptide
designated β with a molecular weight of 38,000. Limited
peptide mapping indicates that α and α' are virtually
identical and probably differ by post-translational
modification. These data are consistant with native
structures of $\alpha\alpha'\beta_2$, $\alpha_2\beta_2$ and $\alpha'_2\beta_2$. The significance
of this subunit composition is unknown, but it is
tempting to speculate whether one of these peptides, or
the conversion of α to α' (or α' to α) plays a role in
the regulation of catalytic activity.

Initial velocity kinetic studies of human lymphocyte
AdoMet synthetase indicate a steady state, sequential
mechanism with ordered addition of ATP before methionine
(Kotb and Kredich, 1985). At the near optimum pH of 7.4
in 0.05 M potassium TES, 0.05 M KCl, 10 mM free Mg^{++}
(in excess of MgATP) and 10 mM DTT, the K_m values for ATP
and methionine are 32 μM and 3.8 μM, and the K_{ia} for
ATP is 100 μM. MgATP is probably the actual substrate
for the reaction, but free Mg^{2+} is also required as
an essential activator with a half-maximal effect at 1.0
mM. KCl is not necessary for full activity but was
included in our kinetic studies to provide a more
physiologic environment. As expected AdoMet,

orthophosphate (Pi) and pyrophosphate (PPi) are produced
in equimolar amounts.

   Inhibition of the enzyme by AdoMet is uncompetitive
with ATP, and noncompetitive with respect to methionine,
indicating that this product is released first. Ordered
release of all three products in a Bi Ter steady state,
sequential mechanism requires that the second product
give uncompetitive inhibition with respect to both
substrates, and the final product released should give
competitive inhibition with respect to the first
substrate bound (Cleland, 1963). Since both Pi and PPi
show noncompetitive inhibition with respect to ATP and
methionine, we conclude that these two products are
released randomly after AdoMet. When tested singly,
inhibition constants for the three products vary between
18–32 μM for AdoMet, 2–6 mM for Pi and 0.25–0.8 mM for
PPi depending on whether slope or intercept effects are
measured and on whether ATP or methionine is varied
(Table 1) (Kotb and Kredich, 1985).

Table 1. Kinetic Properties of Human Lymphocyte AdoMet
          Synthetase

Compound	Constant	Value	Type of Inhibition*
ATP	Km	32 μM	–
	Kia	100 μM	–
Methionine	Km	3.8 μM	–
AdoMet	Kii vs ATP	18 μM	UC
	Kii and Kis vs methionine	32 μM	NC
Pi	Kii,app vs ATP	2 mM	NC, parabolic
	Kis,app vs ATP	6 mM	NC, parabolic
	Kii and Kis vs methionine	6 mM	NC
PPi	Kii vs ATP	0.8 mM	NC
	Kis vs ATP	0.25 mM	NC
	Kii and Kis vs methionine	0.8 mM	NC

*Inhibition is uncompetitive (UC) or noncompetitive (NC).
For parabolic inhibition, Kii,app and Kis,app are values
that double the intercept or slope of double reciprocal
plots (Kotb and Kredich, 1983; unpublished).

Regulation by Phosphate and Pyrophosphate

Recently, we have carried out a more detailed analysis of product inhibition, which has forced us to postulate an additional binding site for Pi. Of a number of kinetic models tested the simplest that is consistant with our data involves binding of Pi to the PPi site giving rise to two additional enzyme forms designated E-Pi-Pi* and E-Pi*, where Pi* represents Pi bound to the PPi site (Fig. 1). The complete rate equation for this steady state mechanism is lengthy with 65 denominator terms and 5 numerator terms in the forward direction. By systematically measuring the kinetic effects of each product, first individually and then in various combinations, we have obtained values for the coefficients contained in 33 of these terms and have eliminated the others as too small to be of significance at reactant concentrations likely to occur in cells (Kotb, M. and Kredich, N.M., unpublished). Using these parameters we can accurately describe the kinetic behavior of purified human lymphocyte AdoMet synthetase over a wide range of substrate and product concentrations.

Our model shows a considerable amount of synergism in product inhibition, particularly with combinations including PPi. At 1 mM ATP and 20 µM methionine, the single addition of 2 mM Pi or 0.2 mM PPi decreases activity from 81% of Vm to 72% or 68%; in combination they lower activity to 36% of Vm (Table 2). Inhibition by AdoMet is relatively insensitive to Pi alone, but

Table 2. Product Inhibition of Human Lymphocyte AdoMet Synthetase

Pi	PPi	AdoMet (µM)				
		0	5	10	30	60
(mM)				(% Vm)		
0	0	81	68	59	38	25
2	0	72	61	53	36	24
0	0.2	68	47	36	19	11
2	0.2	36	25	19	12	6

ATP and methionine were present at 1 mM and 20 µM.

Ordered Segment

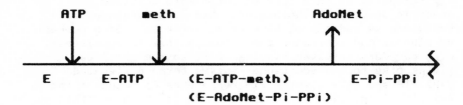

Random Segment

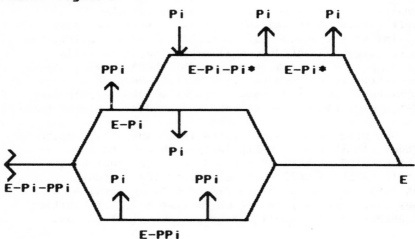

Fig. 1. Reaction mechanism for human lymphocyte AdoMet synthetase. Addition of ATP and methionine is ordered, steady state, and AdoMet is the first product released. Pi and PPi are released randomly, and Pi can bind to an additional site, which may be identical to the PPi site. Pi bound to this other site is designated Pi*.

increases significantly with PPi alone and to an even greater extent with a combination of Pi and PPi. The data given in Table 2 show that equivalent velocities (in this case 31% of Vm) can be achieved at 5 µM AdoMet when 2 mM Pi and 0.2 mM PPi are present, and at 60 µM AdoMet in the absence of these two products. Thus, Pi and PPi have the effect of sensitizing AdoMet synthetase to inhibition by AdoMet.

SUMMARY

The kinetic properties of human lymphocyte AdoMet synthetase raise the possibility that the enzyme is regulated in vivo by product inhibition involving not only AdoMet but Pi and PPi as well. Combinations of Pi and PPi at physiologic concentrations are inhibitory themselves and markedly enhance inhibition by AdoMet. These product interactions could provide the cell with a mechanism, i.e. a lowering of Pi and/or PPi levels, by which both the steady state concentration and turnover rate of AdoMet could be increased simultaneously without the need for synthesis of additional enzyme. Whether this is the explanation for the early changes in AdoMet metabolism in lectin-stimulated peripheral blood lymphocytes is yet to be determined.

Availability of pure non-hepatic, human AdoMet synthetase should facilitate a number of other investigations involving questions of substrate specificity, sensitivity to drugs and the relationships between enzymes from normal and malignant tissues. The enzyme we have studied was derived from leukemic cells, and it would be interesting to compare its subunit structure and kinetic properties with those of normal lymphocytes and of other tissues. Kinetic data already available on partially purified human erythrocyte AdoMet synthetase are significantly different from ours (Oden and Clarke, 1983), but it is not known whether this is due to differences between lymphocytes and erythrocytes or between malignant and normal tissues.

REFERENCES

Abe, T., Okada, G., Teraoka, H. and Tsukada, K. (1982) J. Biochem. 91, 1081-1084.

Borchardt, R.T., Wu, Y.S., Huber, J.A. and Wycpalek, A.F. (1976) J. Med. Chem. 18, 300-304.

Chou, T.-C., Coulter, A.W., Lombardini, J.B., Sufrin, J.R. and Talalay, P. (1977) in The Biochemistry of Adenosyl-methionine (Salvatore, F., Borek, E., Zappia, V., Williams-Ashman, H.G. and Schlenk, F., Eds.) pp 18-36, Columbia University Press, New York.

Cleland, W.W. (1963) Biochim. Biophys. Acta 67, 173-187.

Finkelstein, J.D. (1979) in Transmethylation (Usdin, E., Borchardt, R. and Creveling, C.R., Eds.) pp 49-58, Elsevier/North Holland, New York.

Finkelstein, J.D., Kyle, W.E., Martin, J.J. and Pick, A.-M. (1975) Biochem. Biophys. Res. Commun. 66, 81-87.

Garrett, C. and Kredich, N.M. (1981) J. Biol. Chem. 256, 12705-12709.

German, D.C., Bloch, C.A. and Kredich, N.M. (1983) J. Biol. Chem. 258, 10997-11003.

Hershfield, M.S. (1979) J. Biol. Chem. 254, 22-25.

Kotb, M. and Kredich, N.M. (1985) J. Biol. Chem. 260, 3923-3930.

Kredich, N.M. (1980) J. Biol. Chem. 255, 7380-7385.

Kredich, N.M. and Hershfield, M.S. (1983) in The Metabolic Basis of Inherited Disease (Stanbury, J.B., Wyngaarden, J.B., Fredrickson, D.S., Goldstein, J.L. and Brown, M.S., Eds.) pp 1157-1183, McGraw-Hill, New York.

Kredich, N.M. and Martin, D.W. Jr. (1977) Cell 12, 931-938.

Kutzbach, C. and Stokstad, E.L.R. (1971) Biochim. Biophys. Acta 250, 459-477.

Liau, M.C., Chang, C.F. and Becker, F. (1979a) Cancer Res. 39, 2113-2119.

Liau, M.C., Chang, C.F., Belanger, L. and Grenier, A. (1979b) Cancer Res. 39, 162-169.

Mudd, H.S. and Poole, J.R. (1975) Metabolism 24, 721-735.

Oden, K.L. and Clarke, S. (1983) Biochemistry 22, 2978-2986.

Okada, G., Teraoka, H. and Tsukada, K. (1981) Biochemistry 20, 934-940.

Sullivan, D.M. and Hoffman, J.L. (1983) Biochemistry 22, 1636-1641.

CANCER, METHIONINE, AND TRANSMETHYLATION

Robert M. Hoffman and Peter H. Stern

Department of Pediatrics, M-009F
University of California, San Diego
La Jolla CA 92093

ABSTRACT

The nature of cancer is outlined and it is concluded that many changes in the cellular program are required for clinical cancer to occur in humans. These large program changes are not as compatible with mutation theories as they are with altered methionine metabolism and imbalanced transmethylation including DNA hypomethylation which are prevalent in all surveys of human cancer. Transmethylation is affected by many and diverse carcinogens further supporting our hypothesis. Applications of altered methionine metabolism/transmethylation for cancer prevention and treatment are discussed.

Nature of Cancer

Cancer is due to many cellular changes. Cells must first undergo changes in their growth regulation and the way they interact with their neighbors. Cells which originally responded to growth factors synthesized elsewhere in the body often become independent of them, possibly due to the newly acquired ability of oncogenically transformed cells to synthesize their own growth factors. Cells which originally responded to neighboring cells often lose this ability and proliferate and migrate independently of them. As the newly formed tumor progresses, cells within the tumor acquire more and more new properties. Cells may acquire the ability to detach from their tissue of origin, lyse structural proteins such as collagen enabling them to enter blood vessels, and migrate great distances in the body, implant in tissues different from their origin and

215

grow in their newly found milieu. Often this process may take many years in human beings, ten, twenty or even more.

Is Cancer Due to Mutations?

Some of the current literature indicates that cancer may be due to a limited number of mutations in oncogenes, possibly only one or two (Land, et al, 1983). However, these very limited alterations do not explain the data of cells undergoing many changes in order to become clinically observable, metastasizing cancers. One must consider therefore that cancer involves many and profound changes in the cellular program and the cell's ability to regulate itself. One need not postulate that all or even the majority of these changes involve point mutations. Indeed, in surveys of human cancers, (Table 1), oncogenes as potent as those of the ras family are rarely found to be activated by mutation or gene amplification (Feinberg et al., 1983; Fujita et al., 1984; Fujita et al., 1985) even though transcriptional and immunohistochemical studies have indicated abnormally high ras gene activity frequently occuring in human cancers (Slamon et al., 1984; Thor et al., 1984; Hand et al., 1984). What changes can occur in the cell such that the oncogenic program alterations result?

TABLE 1

Comparison of incidence of abnormally elevated ras[H] oncogene activity and genetic alteration with incidence of altered methionine metabolism and transmethylation in human cancer

% human cancers with elevated ras[H] oncogene activity:	64% (Slamon et al., 1984) 49% (Thor et al., 1984) 56% (Hand et al., 1984)
% human cancers with mutated or amplified ras[H]:	6.3% (Fujita et al., 1985) 0% (Feinberg et al., 1983
% human cancer tissues or cell types with under-methylated DNA:	95% (Diala et al., 1983) 55% (Gama-Sosa et al., 1983) 80% (Feinberg et al., 1983) 100% (Goelz et al., 1985)
% human cancer cell types methionine-dependent:	60% (Mecham et al.,1983)
% human cancer cell types with defective methionine metabolism or overall transmethylation:	100% (Stern et al., 1984) 100% (Stern & Hoffman, 1984)

Altered Methionine Metabolism/Transmethylation and Cancer

Possible solutions to the origin of large program changes in cancer come from studies of altered methionine metabolism and transmethylation in cancer cells (Hoffman, 1984; Hoffman, 1985). The alteration is often expressed as an inability of the cancer cells to grow when methionine (Met) is replaced by homocysteine (Hcy) in the culture medium, a condition that allows essentially optimal growth of normal cells. This metabolic defect is termed methionine dependence, and in our laboratory we have found it to occur in the majority of cell lines tested from diverse types of human cancers. (Mecham et al. 1983). It must be emphasized that all normal cell strains tested, as well as normal animals, are methionine independent and grow well when methionine is replaced by homocysteine, vitamin B_{12} and folic acid in the cell culture medium or diet (Hoffman

1984; 1985).

Methionine dependence has been shown not to be due to reduced levels of methionine synthesis in cancer cells (Hoffman and Erbe, 1976), but seems to be determined by the intracellular ratio of S-adenosylmethionine (AdoMet) to S-adenosylhomocysteine (AdoHcy) when cells are growing in methionine-free, homocysteine-containing (Met$^-$Hcy$^+$) medium. When the AdoMet/AdoHcy ratios are low, often going well below 1, the cells are almost always methionine dependent (see Table 2; Coalson et al., 1982; Stern et al., 1983; Stern et al., 1984).

TABLE 2

Altered methionine metabolism/transmethylation in human cancer*+

Free Met	Free $\frac{Met}{Hcy}$	Adomet	$\frac{AdoMet}{AdoHcy}$	Rate of *** Transmeth.
Methionine-dependent human cancer cells				
Carcinomas (Average for 6 cancers)				
8,826	0.029	13,158	0.941	5.48
Sarcomas (Average for 4 cancers)				
8,159	0.081	5,472	0.63	3.84
Neurologic Cancers (Average for 2 cancers)				
9,769	0.080	3,693	0.40	7.94
Average for 12 total cancers				
8,761	0.055	9,018	0.748	5.34
Methionine-independent human cancer cells				
Carcinomas (Average for 3 cancers)				
7,473	0.196	22,804	7.42	8.75
Sarcomas (Average for 2 cancers)				
17,187	0.228	102,918	13.26	7.93
Melanoma				
10,018	0.051	4,536	0.65	4.86
Average for 6 total cancers				
11,135	0.183	46,646	8.24	7.83
Normal Diploid Human Fibroblasts	(Average for 4 strains)			
203,900	0.97	22,798	8.96	1.19

* All data are from Stern et al., 1984 and Stern and Hoffman, 1984 and are expressed in cpm.
+ All cells incubated in Met$^-$Hcy$^+$ media with [^{35}S]Hcy except for rate of transmethylation experiments where cells were in Met$^+$Hcy$^-$ media with [^{35}S]Met.

TABLE 2 (continued)

*** cpm AdoHcy formed per mg protein in 2.5 hours in the presence of AdoHcy hydrolase inhibitor periodate-oxidized 3-deazaadenosine divided by the value for that of a normal diploid human fibroblast strain RO the value for which is given as 1.00 for relative comparison.

– – –

However, further experimentation indicated that altered ratios of AdoMet to AdoHcy may reflect more fundamental changes in cancer cells. Data from both methionine-dependent and methionine-independent human tumor cell lines in our laboratory indicated that when both types of cancer cells are incubated in Met^-Hcy^+ media the steady-state levels of free methionine are very low despite apparent normal amounts of methionine synthesis (see Table 2; Stern, et al., 1984). The levels of free methionine are approximately equal in methionine-dependent and methionine-independent cancer cell lines and are over 20 times lower than the free-methionine levels in normal, methionine-independent diploid human fibroblasts incubated in Met^-Hcy^+ media. (see Table 2 and Stern, et al., 1983; Stern, et al., 1984). Thus the data indicate that both methionine-dependent and methionine-independent cancer cells are altered in methionine metabolism. The data raise the possibility that the free-methionine pools are low in the cancer cells because their overall rate of transmethylation is elevated and when in Met^-Hcy^+ medium, the cancer cells can not replenish their levels of free methionine sufficiently, even though approximately normal rates of methionine synthesis are occurring (Stern, et al., 1984).

Measurements of the overall rate of transmethylation in human normal and cancer cells were then made in our laboratory by blocking AdoHcy hydrolase with periodate-oxidized 3-deazaadenosine, and measuring the rate of accumulation of AdoHcy as a function of time. Each molecule of AdoHcy accumulated represents one transmethylation event. In a study of 18 different cell lines derived from diverse human cancers compared to four strains of normal human diploid fibroblasts, using the above measurement, we found that all 18 tumor-cell lines had an elevated rate of transmethylation compared to the rate of normal diploid fibroblasts (Table 2 and Stern and Hoffman, 1984). We hypothesized that methionine dependence usually resulted when cancer cells could not compensate for the elevated rates of transmethylation occurring and generate a normal AdoMet/AdoHcy ratio when incubated in Met⁻Hcy⁺ media. Cancer cells that could compensate for elevated transmethylation rates, and generate a normal ratio of AdoMet to AdoHcy despite low steady-state levels of free methionine could become at least partially methionine independent and grow to varying degrees in Met⁻Hcy⁺ media.

That cancer cells have excess rates of overall transmethylation indicates that certain substances within the cancer cells must be overmethylated. However, experiments from our laboratory and others have indicated that there are substances in human cancer cells that are undermethylated such as DNA and certain residues of tRNA (Hoffman, 1984; Hoffman, 1985; Diala and Hoffman, 1982; Diala, et al., 1983; Gama-Sosa et al., 1983; Feinberg and Vogelstein, 1983a, 1983b; Cheah et al., 1984). Therefore one gets the idea that in cancer cells there is an imbalance of methylation, which results in the overmethylation of some substances and the undermethylation of others.

Our hypothesis at this point was that the set of cellular transmethylases is altered in a quantitative and qualitative way in the cancer cells. To test this hypothesis we passed [^{3}H]leucine-labeled extracts of human cancer cells and normal cells over an AdoHcy-agarose affinity column. Since AdoHcy is bound to and inhibits all known cellular transmethylases, it was thought that the majority, if not all the proteins binding the AdoHcy-agarose column and specifically eluted by Adomet are cellular transmethylases. Initial results indicated that the cancer cell types with the highest rates of transmethylation had approximately twice the amount of protein bound to the column and specifically eluted by AdoMet than the normal cell strains. Two-dimensional electrophoretic analysis of these affinity-purified proteins suggested qualitative and quantitative differences between the normal and cancer cells, thereby supporting our hypothesis.

What are some of the ramifications with regard to cancer for imbalanced transmethylation occurring in cells? A number of types of experiments indicate that DNA methylation plays an important role in gene regulation in mammalian cells. A large number of studies using methyl-specific DNA restriction enzymes have shown a correlation between undermethylation of genes and their level of activity in the majority of genes investigated.

(Riggs and Jones, 1983; Hoffman, 1984; Razin et al., 1984; Hoffman, 1985)

Experiments that have gone beyond a mere correlation show that a number of DNA sequences which have been methylated in vitro are found to have their activity inhibited when assayed by insertion into specific cells by various means (Keshet et al., 1985). Further evidence for the ability of DNA methylation to have an important effect on the program of gene expression comes from experiments with sperm DNA where it is found that point sites of undermethylation occur within constitutively expressed genes but not within tissue-specific genes or inactive genes. These sites of undermethylation in sperm DNA correspond to the location of regions of altered chromatin structure in somatic tissue which result in hypersensitivity to specific nucleases. These undermethylated regions are postulated to play a role in the activation of the paternal genome during embryogenesis, an important regulation of cell programming (Groudine and Conkin, 1985). Thus it can be seen that when DNA methylation is disrupted, great changes in cellular programming may take place, possibly enabling cancer to result and progress.

With regard to changes in DNA methylation in cancer, it should be noted that human cancer cells in vitro (Diala and Hoffman, 1982; Diala et al., 1983; Cheah et al., 1984) and in vivo (Gama-Sosa et al., 1983; Feinberg and Vogelstein, 1983a, 1983b; Goelz et al., 1985) have been found to have highly hypomethylated DNA (Table 1). Even pre-cancerous cell types such as benign polyps of the human colon have been found to have DNA that is hypomethylated demonstrating that defective DNA methylation may be an early event in oncogenesis. (Goelz et al., 1985). Indeed, many carcinogens can affect DNA methylation either indirectly, such as the ethionine which affects methionine metabolism and transmethylation (Shivapurkar, et al., 1985) or directly such as 5-azacytidine, which can induce the oncogenic transformation of cells in culture (Benedict et al, 1977; Taylor and Jones, 1982) as well as in vivo (Riggs, et al., 1984). Many other carcinogens have a large inhibitory effect on methylation of DNA (Wilson and Jones, 1983; Boehm and Drahovsky, 1983). Thus, consistent with our hypothesis that altering methionine metabolism and transmethylation may have a causative effect in oncogenic transformation are the results that methionine metabolism and transmethylation are frequently found to be defective in cancer, and substances which alter these pathways are carcinogenic. Therefore, it is possible that large changes in DNA methylation induce the activation of sets of genes which may include oncogenes and thereby alter cells such that they become malignant. Perhaps oncogenes are more frequently activated by demethylation than by mutation or amplification. In this light Table 1 indicates that the ras^H oncogene is frequently abnormally highly active in human cancers but only very rarely mutated or amplified. On the other hand, Table 1 indicates that altered DNA methylation, altered overall transmethylation and altered methionine metabolism are very frequent occurrences in the human cancer cells and tissues surveyed. The actual relationship between altered oncogene activity and altered methionine metabolism/transmethylation needs to be investigated.

Imbalance in methylation is also found in other molecules of cancer cells, for example in tRNA. A unique characteristic of of tRNA is that normally many of the bases are modified, frequently by methylation. In cancer cells, the methylation of tRNA has been found to be imbalanced with certain residues being undermethylated and others being overmethylated (Hoffman, 1985). The altered methylation of tRNAs in cancer may have important functional consequences as well. The phenylalanine tRNA of mammalian tissues contains the hypermodified guanine derivative "Y"-base (Wye) adjacent to the 3'- end of the anticodon and two O-methylated bases in the 5'- portion of the anticodon loop. These positions are hypomodified in a variety of tumor cells including a mouse neuroblastoma. It has been shown that the tumor-specific hypomodified phenylalanine tRNA is generally utilized preferentially in the synthesis of rabbit globins in a reticulocyte cell-free protein- synthesizing system. It is postulated that the bulky "Y" base or other modifications of normal tRNA may modulate protein synthesis and that tumor cells may achieve a growth advantage if specific tRNAs are hypomodified (Smith et al., 1985). Thus the alteration of tRNA function by imbalanced methylation may be another means of changing the cellular program such that cancer may result and progress.

Applications of Altered Methionine Metabolism /Transmethylation in cancer

A corollary to the fact that methionine metabolism and transmethylation are altered in cancer cells is that prevention of their alteration may be important in the prevention of cancer. Indeed, it has been known for close to forty years that when animals are given a diet low in methionine and related molecules, the animals incur spontaneous cancers that they would not normally get and become much more susceptible to certain carcinogens (Hoffman, 1984; 1985). It has been shown that when animals are on this diet low in methyl groups their level of DNA methylation decreases (Wilson, et al., 1984). Therefore, a methyl-rich diet may prevent decreases in DNA methylation, possibly even those decreases occurring due to the presence of carcinogens, as well as decreases in the methylation of other molecules such as tRNA. A methyl-rich diet may be important in preventing the cellular program changes that would lead to cancer.

Another corollary is that alterations of transmethylation and methionine metabolism in cancer can possibly be exploited for treatment. Taking advantage of the fact that methionine-dependent cancer cells arrest in the late-S/G_2 phase of the cell cycle when incubated in Met$^-$Hcy$^+$ medium (Hoffman and Jacobsen, 1980), we have found that in mixed cultures of human methionine- dependent cancer cells and normal diploid methionine-independent fibroblasts, the inclusion of adriamycin in Met$^-$Hcy$^+$ medium and then the repletion with Met$^+$Hcy$^-$ medium and vincristine allows the complete killing of the cancer cells while allowing the neighboring normal cells to survive and subsequently proliferate (Stern and Hoffman, unpublished results). It is thought that the adriamycin in Met$^-$Hcy$^+$ medium helps to kill methionine –dependent cancer cells which are being synchronized in late-S/G_2 and then the vincristine in Met$^+$Hcy$^-$ medium kills the cancer cells as they synchronously leave late-S/G_2 for mitosis where they are most susceptible to anti-mitotic drugs such an vincristine. It is important to attempt this type of methionine –dependent chemotherapy in animals, for example in nude mice carrying methionine-dependent human tumors. Success in this phase would certainly warrant such experimental chemotherapy in humans.

ACKNOWLEDGEMENTS
The reasearch was supported by grant CA27564 and research career development award CA00804 from the National Cancer Institute; grants 1348 and 1496 grom the Council for Tobacco Research - USA, Inc.; The George A. Jacobs Memorial Fund for Cancer Research; and the Dr. Louis Sklarow Memorial Fund, all to Robert M. Hoffman.

REFERENCES

Benedict, W., Banerjee, A., Gardner, A., & Jones, P. (1977) Canc. Res. 37, 2202-2208.

Boehm, T. & Drahovsky, D. (1983) J. Natl. Canc. Inst. 71, 429-433.

Cheah, M.S.C., Wallace, C.D., & Hoffman, R.M. (1984) J. Natl. Canc. Inst. 73, 1057-1065.

Coalson, D.W., Mecham, J.O., Stern, P.H., & Hoffman, R.M. (1982) Proc. Natl. Acad. Sci. USA 79, 4248-4251.

Diala, E.S., Cheah, M.S.C., Rowitch, D. & Hoffman, R.M. (1983) J. Natl. Canc. Inst. 71, 755-764.

Diala, E.S. & Hoffman, R.M. (1982) Biochem. Biophys. Res. Commun. 107, 19-26.

Feinberg, A.P., Vogelstein, B., Droller, M.J., Baylin, S.B., & Nelkin, B.D. (1983) Science 220, 1175-1177.

Feinberg, A.P., & Vogelstein, B. (1983a) Nature 301, 89-92.

Feinberg, A.P., & Vogelstein, B. (1983b) Biochem. Biophys. Res. Commun. 111, 47-54.

Fujita, J., Srivastava, S.K., Kraus, M.H., Rhim, J.S., Tronick, S.R., & Aaronson, S.A. (1985) Proc. Natl. Acad. Sci. USA 82, 3849-3853.

Fujita, J., Yoshida, O., Yuasa, Y., Rhim, J.S., Hatanaka, M. & Aaronson, S.A. (1984) Nature 309, 464-466.

Gama-Sosa, M.A., Slagel, V.A., Trewyn, R.W., Oxenhandler, R., Kuo, K.C., Gehrke, C.W. & Ehrlich, M. (1983) Nucl. Acids Res. 11, 6883-6894.

Goelz, S.E., Vogelstein, B., Hamilton, S.R. & Feinberg, A.P. (1985) Science 228, 187-190.

Groudine, M. & Conkin, K.F. (1985) Science 228, 1061-1068.

Hand, P.H., Thor, A., Wunderlich D., Muraro, R., Caruso, A., & Schlom, J. (1984) Proc. Natl. Acad. Sci. 81, 5227-5231.

Hoffman, R.M. (1984) Biochim. Biophys. Acta 738, 49-87.

Hoffman, R.M. (1985) Anticanc. Res. 5, 1-30.

Hoffman, R.M. & Jacobsen, S.J. (1980) Proc. Natl. Acad. Sci. USA 77, 7306-7310.

Hoffman, R.M. & Erbe, R.W. (1976) Proc. Natl. Acad. Sci. USA 73, 1523-1527.

Keshet, I., Yisraeli, J. & Cedar, H. (1985) Proc. Natl. Acad. Sci. USA 82, 2560-2564.

Land H., Parada, L. & Weinberg, R. (1983) Nature 304, 596-602.

Razin, A., Cedar H. & Riggs, A.D., Eds. (1984) in DNA Methylation, Biochem. & Biol. Significance, Springer, New York.

Riggs, A.D., Singer-Sam, J., Keith, D. & Carr, B.I. (1984) ICSU Short Rep. I, 32-35.

Riggs, A.D. and Jones, P.A. (1983) Adv. Canc. Res. 40, 1-30.

Shivapurkar, N. & Poirier, L.A. (1985) Biochem. Pharmacol. 34, 373-375.

Slamon, D.J., deKernion, J.B., Verma, I.M. and Cline, M.J. (1984) Science 224, 256-262.

Smith, D.W.E., McNamara, A.L., Mushinski, J.F. and Hatfield, D.L. (1985), J. Biol. Chem. 260, 147-151.

Stern, P.H. and Hoffman, R.M. (1984) In Vitro Rapid Commun. in Cell Biol. 20, 663-670.

Stern, P.H. Wallace, C.D. and Hoffman, R.M. (1984) J. Cell. Physiol. 119, 29-34.

Stern, P.H., Mecham, J.O., Wallace, C.D. and Hoffman, R.M. (1983) J. Cell. Physiol. 117, 9-14.

Taylor, S. and Jones, P. (1982) J. Cell. Physiol. 111, 187-194.

Thor, A., Hand, P.H., Wunderlich, D., Caruso, A., Muraro, R. and Schlom, J. (1984) Nature 311, 562-565.

Wilson, M., Shivapurkar, N. and Poirier, L.A. (1984) Biochem. J. 218, 987-990.

Wilson, V.L. and Jones, P.A. (1983) Cell 32, 239-246.

THE CENTRALITY OF S-ADENOSYLHOMOCYSTEINASE IN THE REGULATION OF THE BIOLOGICAL UTILIZATION OF S-ADENOSYLMETHIONINE

Giulio L. Cantoni, Laboratory of General and Comparative Biochemistry, National Institute of Mental Health, Bethesda, MD 20205

S-Adenosylhomocysteine (AdoHcy), first isolated as one of the products of transmethylation reactions from S-adenosylmethionine (AdoMet) (Cantoni & Scarano, 1954) has been shown to be a competitive inhibitor of all methyltransferases. This was first shown by Gibson et al. (1961) for phosphatidylethanolamine methyltransferase and later extended to other methyltransferases (Borchardt, 1977). Of special interest is the fact that AdoHcy is a competitive inhibitor of most of the reactions in which AdoMet participates, both those where it serves as a methyl or an alkyl donor, and those where it functions as an allosteric effector.

With few exceptions, all cells metabolize AdoHcy through a single pathway catalyzed by S-adenosylhomocysteine hydrolase (AdoHcyase), an enzyme first described in rat liver by de la Haba and Cantoni several years ago. We established that the reaction catalyzed by AdoHcyase is reversible and that in fact the equilibrium is predominantly in the direction of synthesis. Physiologically however the reaction proceeds in the direction of hydrolysis because of the widespread distribution of enzymes that further metabolize the products of the hydrolysis of AdoHcy, namely, adenosine deaminase or adenosine kinase and cystathionine synthase, 5-methyl-tetrahydrofolate-homocysteine or dimethylthetin-homocysteinase methyltransferases (de la Haba & Cantoni, 1959). AdoHcyase was not further studied for almost 20 years, but in the last few years the biological role of AdoHcy and the significance of AdoHcyase in its metabolism has been the focus of interest in my laboratory as well as in various other laboratories.

227

In this paper, I propose to review the principal developments of recent studies that permit the formulation of a coherent picture of the role of AdoHcyase and of AdoHcy in the control of AdoMet utilization.

The realization that AdoHcy is a competitive inhibitor of most of the reactions in which AdoMet participates led directly to two lines of research. In the first place, the relative ease with which analogs of AdoHcy can be chemically synthesized suggested that it might be useful to search for synthetic analogs of AdoHcy capable of exerting, both in vitro and in vivo, inhibitory effects specific for one or a limited number of methyltranspherases (Coward et al., 1974; Robert-Gero et al., 1980; Borchardt, 1977). Such compounds could have important therapeutic significance; e.g. in the control of the metabolism of norepinephrine, serotonin or other neurohormones. In pursuit of this objective, a very large number of AdoHcy analogs has been synthesized and tested in vitro for inhibitory activity against a limited number of methyltranspherases. While these studies have so far failed to produce a therapeutically useful drug, they have been very valuable for they have revealed that it is possible to synthesize congeners of AdoHcy that, in vitro, have a spectrum of inhibitory activity significantly different from that of AdoHcy. Furthermore, these studies served to provide an insight into the interaction between substrate, inhibitor, and enzyme thereby defining some of features of the active centers of various methyltranspherases. The reason why it has not been possible to extend productively to studies in vivo the relatively high degree of specificity demonstrated by these analogs in vitro is that AdoHcy and most of its synthetic analogs do not enter cells easily, if at all (Walker & Duerre, 1975). A related approach has come from the discovery that a number of naturally occurring compounds which exhibit specific antibiotic, antifungal and/or cytostatic activities, such as tubercidin (Chang & Coward, 1975), neplanosin A (Borchardt et al., 1984), aristeromycin (Guranowski et al., 1981), eritadenine (Votruba & Holy, 1982), cordycepin (Kredich, 1980) and sinefungin (Fuller & Nagarajan, 1978) are analogs of adenosine (or AdoHcy) and in some cases inhibitors of AdoHcyase or of methyltranspherases. The relationship between the biological activity of these compounds and their interaction with AdoHcyase is being investigated very actively in several laboratories. De Clercq and Cools have recently reported that there is an excellent correlation between inhibition of AdoHcyase and antiviral activity for a series of these analogs (De Clercq & Cools, 1985).

I took a rather different approach that has been based on the following considerations: Metabolic regulation is exerted primarily at branchpoints, where a metabolite is partitioned between two or more pathways (Atkinson, 1977). AdoMet is a branchpoint metabolite since it can function as a substrate for numerous methyltranspherases, and for AdoMet decarboxylase. The regulation of the relative fluxes of AdoMet through the transmethylation and the transalkylation pathways should be determined by the relative affinity of AdoHcy for the various methyltranspherases and the decarboxylase. While AdoHcy is not a branchpoint metabolite, the two products of its enzymatic hydrolysis can be partitioned between multiple metabolic pathways and are therefore branchpoint metabolites. Furthermore, as already mentioned, the reaction catalyzed by AdoHcyase is readily reversible and the fact that the equilbrium is far in the direction of synthesis strongly suggests that the modulation of the activity of AdoHcyase could form the basis for regulation of the relative fluxes of AdoMet between different pathways by changing the intracellular levels of AdoHcy.

The working hypothesis that we decided to explore experimentally proposes that changes in AdoMet/AdoHcy ratios would affect in different ways various AdoMet-utilizing enzymes, and that the different sensitivity of these enzymes to the inhibitory effects of AdoHcy would form the basis for establishing a physiological hierarchy for the utilization of AdoMet. It became of interest therefore to investigate in detail the characteristics and properties of AdoHcyase with two objectives in mind: in the first place, we began a search for compounds capable of inhibiting AdoHcyase in vivo and of changing the pattern of biological methylation. With regard to the second objective, we had hoped to gain an insight into the mechanisms that regulate the activity of the enzyme under physiological conditions.

I believe that the first objective has been attained, at least partially, through studies in my own lab, and here I wish to acknowledge contributions of P. Chiang, H. Richards, A. Guranowski, J. Seegal, Young Kim, R. Aksamit, P. Backlund, A. Bozzi, G. de la Haba, A. Merta and C. Unson, and in the laboratories of Abeles and of Ueland. The second objective still eludes us, but along the way considerable progress has been made and we have learned that AdoHcyase is an enzyme of unexpected complexity capable of binding several different ligands.

The reaction catalyzed by the enzyme involves the hydrolysis of a thiol ester, or, in the synthetic direction, the replacement of the adenosine 5'OH group with a thiol. The realization that there is no obvious chemical mechanism of catalysis for this reaction stimulated Palmer and Abeles to study the mechanism of AdoHcyase and led to the very important discovery that the enzyme contains tightly bound NAD^+ which participates in the reaction by undergoing an oxidation reduction cycle without dissociation from the enzyme (Palmer & Abeles, 1976). The enzyme derived from different tissues has been purified to homogeneity and crystallized from beef and rat liver and from Alkaligenes faecalis; at all stages during purification procedures the enzyme is active without the need for exogenous NAD.

The enzyme as isolated in pure form from different mammalian sources and from slime molds is a tetramer composed of subunits with m.w. ranging from 43,000–48,000. The purified enzyme contains four moles of NAD/mole of enzyme. AdoHcyase isolated from lupin seeds is a dimer, m.w. 90.000 (Guranowski & Pawelkiewicz, 1977) whereas the enzyme obtained from Alkaligenes faecalis (Shimizu et al., 1984) is composed of six subunits each with a slightly higher molecular mass.

The enzyme subunits of the mammalian enzyme seem to be very similar as judged by the fact that a) only one molecular species can be recognized on 2D gel electrophoresis; b) only one kind of amino acid is found at the carboxyl terminus and all the amino end groups are blocked, and c) the number of peptides that are produced upon fragmentation of the enzyme by chemical or enzymatic procedures agrees, more or less, with what might be expected from amino acid analysis (Gomi et al., 1985). On the other hand, there is evidence that the four subunits are not functionally equivalent and that only two of the four subunits participate in catalysis. This was first shown by Abeles et al. (1982) who demonstrated that when radiolabeled adenosine is added to the enzyme, radioactivity corresponding to only 2.0 moles of substrate/moles of enzyme tetramer remains associated with the protein after gel filtration. These investigators showed furthermore that only two of the four NAD participate in the reaction by being reduced to NADH, whereas two remain unchanged in the oxidized state. As I will discuss later in more detail by an entirely different approach, we have recently obtained evidence that the enzyme is fully active when only two NAD's/tetramer are bound to the enzyme (de la Haba et al., unpublished data). These data lead to the inescapable conclusion that the four subunits of the mammalian enzyme are not functionally equivalent.

Further work will be required to determine if the difference between the two pairs of subunits is due to the expression of half the sites reactivity of the enzyme with respect to adenosine, or AdoHcy or whether the difference between the subunits indicates that the enzyme has an $\alpha_2\beta_2$ subunit structure.

Additional complexity was revealed by the work of Ueland and his collaborators, who as early as 1977 had reported the presence in mouse liver of a cAMP binding protein not related to the classical protein kinases (Ueland & Doskeland, 1977). This protein had a molecular weight and subunit structure similar to or identical with that of liver AdoHcyase. Shortly thereafter, Hershfield & Kredich (1978) identified the cAMP binding protein as AdoHcyase. This observation was confirmed by Saebo and Ueland (1978) for the binding protein from mouse liver. The significance of the cAMP binding to the activity of AdoHcyase, however, remained unclear since both Ueland and Saebo (1979) and others (Guranowski et al, unpublished) had found that addition of cAMP had no effect on the catalytic activity of AdoHcyase. A clue to the significance of the cAMP binding was to be found in the observation of Ueland and Doeskeland (1978) and Ueland and Saebo (1979) that the capacity of the

native protein to bind cAMP can be markedly increased by
incubation at 37° with ATP, Mg^{++} and KCl. Under these same
conditions, as first reported by Ueland and Saebo (1979)
the activity of AdoHcyase is gradually lost, and the
enzyme, is converted from an active to an inactive form.
The inactivated enzyme binds cAMP whereas the native enzyme
does not. Recently in my lab with de la Haba, Bozzi and
Unson (see abstract of this meeting) we have extended these
observations. We find that during incubation with ATP,
Mg^{++}, and KCl, when the active enzyme is converted to an
inactive enzyme, 4 moles of NAD are released from the
enzyme (m.w. 190,000) and can be recovered in the protein
free fraction after gel filtration. The inactivated enzyme
can be almost fully reactivated by incubation with NAD.
Whether the reversible inactivation of the enzyme by ATP,
Mg^{++} and KCl is relevant to the physiological regulation
of the activity of the enzyme is not yet clear.

Considerable information on the properties and characteristics of the active center of the enzyme has accumulated as the result of the work of Fujioka and others
(Takata & Fujioka, 1984; Takata & Fujioka, 1983; Patel-
Thombre & Borchardt, 1985). The availability of the enzyme
from rat liver and from Alkaligenes faecalis in crystalline
form should permit X-ray diffraction studies and definition
of the three dimensional structure of the enzyme and the
binding sites for the different ligands.

As noted above, different methyltranspherases exhibit
different sensitivity towards the inhibition by various
congeners of AdoHcy. Earlier studies in my laboratory had
shown that the substrate specificity of AdoHcyase for
purines was rather broad and this observation suggested
that a systematic survey of adenosine analogs for their
capacity to serve as substrates for the enzyme in vitro
might lead to the identification of a number of alternate
substrates capable of entering the cells through the
adenosine channel and of generating intracellularly
congeners of AdoHcy.

The most interesting outcome of these studies was the discovery that replacement of the adenine moiety of adenosine with 3-deazaadenine yields a series of adenosine analogs namely, 3-deazaadenosine (3-DZA), 3-deazarabinosyladenosine and 3-deazaaristeromycin (3-DZAari) with novel and interesting characteristics (Chiang et al., 1977; Montgomery et al., 1982). 3-Deazaadenine analogs of adenosine are neither substrates for, nor inhibitors of, adenosine deaminase or adenosine kinase. As far as it is known, 3-DZA and 3-DZAari interact with a high degree of specificity only with AdoHcyase.

3-DZA is both a substrate and a competitive inhibitor of AdoHcyase; it has a K_m similar to that of adenosine and a slightly higher V_{max} (Richards et al., 1978). In vitro S-3-deazaadenosyl-L-homocysteine (3-DZAHcy) is a potent competitive inhibitor of AdoMet in methyl and alkyl-transfer reactions (Cantoni et al., 1979; Gordon et al., 1983). 3-DZAari, the carbocyclic analog of 3-deaza-adenosine, is another interesting compound. Unlike 3-DZA, 3-DZAari in most cells is not a substrate but is a very potent inhibitor of AdoHcyase. Comparison of the biochemical and biological consequences of the administration of 3-DZA and 3-DZAari emphasizes a critical difference between compounds that are only inhibitors (Kim et al., 1982). The increase in the AdoHcy concentration that follows administration of the 3-DZAari is related to, and limited by, the rate of AdoMet utilization, and by the degree of inhibition of AdoHcyase. In liver, for example, where as much as 10 mmoles/day of AdoMet are utilized for the synthesis of creatine, the rate of accumulation of AdoHcy if AdoHcyase is inhibited will be very much greater than in other tissues where the AdoMet serves principally as a donor of methyl groups for macromolecular or posttranscriptional modifications that consume only micromoles of AdoMet. It is important to keep in mind that in vertebrates AdoHcy is the sole source of homocysteine, and that homocysteine is needed not only for synthesis of cystathionine and cysteine but also as a substrate for 5-methyltetrahydrofolate (MTHF)-homocysteine methyltransferase a reaction that is essential for the recycling of tetrahydrofolate (THFA). In the absence of homocysteine, THFA will be trapped as MTHF. We have shown that the cytostatic effects of 3-DZAari are due

to the failure to produce Hcy from AdoHcy and cells treated
with cytostatic doses of 3-DZAari can be rescued by administration of very small amounts of Hcy (Kim et al., 1982). On
the other hand, it is possible to overcome the limitations
in the availability of homocysteine and to take advantage
of the fact that the equilibrium of AdoHcyase favors synthesis of AdoHcy or its congeners. One can supply homocysteine thiolactone and adenosine or a utilizable analog,
and thereby generate in vivo very high levels of AdoHcy,
3-DZAHcy or other PuHcy congeners.

I believe that the experiments just reviewed validate
the hypothesis that modulation of the activity of AdoHcyase
is of importance in the regulation of the biological
utilization of AdoMet. Further support comes from experiments that show that the biochemical or biological effects
of adenosine or its analogs can be potentiated by the
simultaneous administration of homocysteine thiolactone.
I must point out, however, that the working hypothesis
just outlined predicted that modulation in the activity of
AdoHcyase should be demonstrable in vivo under a variety
of physiological conditions and this has not yet been
achieved.

It is conceivable that the reversible removal of NAD
plays a role in the regulation of the enzyme activity,
and/or that the two NAD's that are not reduced during the
enzyme catalysis are involved in regulation as suggested
by Abeles et al. (1980). Further work will be needed to
clarify the picture.

Even though it has not yet been demonstrated that
changes in AdoMet/PuHcy ratios can occur physiologically,
it has become well established that modulation of AdoMet/
AdoHcy ratios can be utilized to probe for the involvement
of methylation reactions in a variety of physiological
systems since changes in AdoMet/AdoHcy ratios brought about
by pharmacological manipulations can be associated with
striking biological effects. These include inhibition of
macrophage chemotaxis (Aksamit et al., 1982; Aksamit et
al., 1983), of histamine release from lung mast cells
(Benyon et al., 1984) or insulin release from pancreatic
isles (Best et al., 1984), of aldosterone stimulated Na^+

transport (Weismann et al., 1985), or of thrombin induced release of van Willebrand factor (De Groot et al., 1984), and inhibition of growth of RNA and DNA viruses (Bader et al., 1978; Stoltzfus & Montgomery, 1981; Montgomery et al., 1982; De Clercq & Montgomery, 1983) as well as stimulation of the differentiation of myoblasts (Scarpa et al., 1984), of erythroleukemic cells in tissue culture (Dean, Schechter, Wu, Backlund, Aksamit and Cantoni, in preparation), and of 3T3 fibroblasts into adipocytes (Chiang, 1981).

It has not yet been possible to identify which specific transmethylation or transalkylation reaction is correlated with any one of these biological responses because alterations in AdoMet/AdoHcy ratios have pleiotropic effects. It should be borne in mind, however that the administration of different analogs of adenosine capable of affecting AdoMet/AdoHcy ratios can result in discrete and specific physiological effects. 3-DZA, for instance, inhibits chemotaxis of RAW 264 macrophages while neither adenosine nor anyone among several other AdoHcyase inhibitors does. 3-DZA in the presence of homocysteine stimulates myoblast differentiation under conditions where 3-DZAari or adenosine, have no effect. Neplanosin A, 3-DZA and 3-DZAari have rather specific antiviral effects where other analogs are much less active. It should therefor be possible to examine critically these different systems in order to identify which specific biochemical change correlates with a given physiological effect. If pursued vigorously this approach should, in due course, permit a definition of the specific role of AdoMet in different physiological processes.

ACKNOWLEDGMENTS:

I am grateful to Dr. de la Haba for many stimulating discussions and to Drs. P. Backlund and R. Aksamit for critical reading of the manuscript.

ABBREVIATIONS:

AdoHcy, S-adenosylhomocysteine; AdoMet, S-adenosyl-methionine; MTHF, methyltetrahydrofolate; THFA, tetrahydro-folic acid; Hcy, homocysteine; 3-DZA, 3-deazaadenosine; 3-DZAHcy, S-3-deazaadenosylhomocysteine; PuHcy, purinyl-homocysteine.

REFERENCES:

Abeles, R. H., Tashjuan, A. H. and Fish, S. (1980) Biochem. Biophys. Res. Commun. 95, 612-617.

Abeles, R. H., Fish, S. and Lapinskas, B. (1982) Biochemistry 21, 5557-5562.

Aksamit, R. R., Falk, W. and Cantoni, G. L. (1982) J. Biol. Chem. 257, 621-625.

Aksamit, R. R., Backlund, P. S. Jr. and Cantoni, G. L. (1983) J. Biol. Chem. 258, 20-23.

Aswad, D. W. and Koshland, D. E. Jr. (1975) J. Mol. Biol. 97, 207-223.

Atkinson, D. E. (1977) in Cellular Energy Metabolism and Its Regulation. Academic Press, New York.

Bader, J. P., Brown, N. R., Chiang, P. K. and Cantoni, G. L. (1978) Virology 89, 494-505.

Benyon, R. C., Church, M. K. and Holgate S. T. (1984) Biochem. Pharmacol. 33, 2881-2886.

Best, L., Lebrun, P., Saceda, M., Garcia-Morales, P., Hubinont, C., Juvent, M., Herchuelz, A., Malaisse-Lagae F., Valverde, I. and Malaisse, W. J. (1984) Biochem. Pharmacol. 33, 2033-2039.

Borchardt, R. T. (1977) in The Biochemistry of Adenosyl-methionine (Salvatore, F., et al., eds.) pp. 151-171, Columbia University Press, New York.

Borchardt, R. T., Keller, B. T. and Patel-Thombre, U. (1984) J. Biol. Chem. 259, 4353-4358.

Cantoni, G. L. and Scarano, E. (1954) J. Am. Chem. Soc. 76, 4744.

Cantoni, G. L., Richards, H. H. and Chiang, P. K. (1979) in Transmethylation (Usdin, E., et al. eds.) pp. 155-164, Elsevier, New York.

Chang, C. -D. and Coward, J. K. (1975) Mol. Pharmacol. 11, 701-707.

Chiang, P. K., Richards, H. H. and Cantoni, G. L. (1977) Mol. Pharmacol. 13, 939-947.

Chiang, P. K. (1981) Science 211, 1164-1166.

Coward, J. K., Bussolotti, D. L. and Chang, C. -D. (1974) J. Med. Chem. 93, 1286-

De Clercq, E. and Montgomery, J. A. (1983) Antiviral Res. 3, 17-24.

De Clercq, E. and Cools, M. (1985). Biochem. Biophys. Res. Commun. 129, 306-311.

De Groot, P. G., Gonsalves, M. D., Loesberg, C., van Buul-Wortelboer, M. F., van Aken, W. G., van Mourik, J. A. (1984) J. Biol. Chem. 259, 13329-13333.

de la Haba, G. and Cantoni, G. L. (1959) J. Biol. Chem. 234, 603–608.

Fuller, A. N. and Nagarajan, A. (1978) Biochem. Pharmacol. 27, 1981–1983.

Gibson, K. D., Wilson, J. D. and Udenfriend, S. (1961) J. Biol. Chem. 236, 673–679.

Gomi, T., Ishiguro, Y. and Fujioka, M. (1985) J. Biol. Chem. 260, 2789–2793.

Gordon, R. K., Brown, N. D. and Chiang, P. K. (1983) Biochem. Biophys. Res. Commun. 114, 505–510.

Guranowski, A. and Pawelkiewicz, J. (1977) Eur. J. Biochem. 80, 517–523.

Guranowski, A., Montgomery, J. A., Cantoni, G. L. and Chiang, P. K. (1981) Biochemistry 20, 110–115.

Hershfield, M. S. and Kredick, N. M. (1978) Science 202, 757–760.

Kim, I. -K., Aksamit, R. R. and Cantoni, G. L. (1982) J. Biol. Chem. 257, 14726–14729.

Kredich, N. M. (1980) J. Biol. Chem. 255, 7380–7385.

Montgomery, J. A., Clayton, S. J., Thomas, H. J., Shannon, W. M., Arnett, G., Bodner, A. J., Kim, I. -K., Cantoni, G. L. and Chiang, P. K. (1982) J. Med. Chem. 25, 626–629.

Palmer, J. L. and Abeles, R. H. (1976) J. Biol. Chem. 251, 5817–5819.

Patel-Thombre, U. and Borchardt, R. T. (1985) Biochemistry 24, 1130–1136.

Platzer, E. G. (1972) Transactions of the New York Academy of Science, Series II 34, 200–207.

Richards, H. H., Chiang, P. K. and Cantoni, G. L. (1978) J. Biol. Chem. 253, 4476–4480.

Robert-Gero, M., Pierre, A., Vedel, M., Enouf, J., Lawrence, F., Raies, A. and Lederer, E. (1980) in Enzyme Inhibitors (Brodbeck, U., ed) pp. 61–74, Verlag Chemie, Weinheim.

Saebo, J. and Ueland, P. M. (1978) FEBS Lett. 96, 125–128.

Scarpa, S., Strom, R. Bozzi, A., Aksamit, R. R., Backlund, Jr, P. S., Chen, J. and Cantoni, G. L. (1984) Proc. Natl. Acad. Sci. USA 81, 3064–3068.

Shimizu, S., Shiozaki, S., Ohshiro, T. and Yamada, H. (1984) Eur. J. Biochem. 141, 385–392.

Stoltzfus, C M. and Montgomery, J. A. (1981) J. Virol. 38, 173–183.

Takata, Y. and Fujioka, M. (1983) J. Biol. Chem. 258, 7374–7378.

Takata, Y. and Fujioka, M. (1984) Biochemistry 23, 4357–
    4362.
Ueland, P. M. and Døskeland, S. O. (1977) J. Biol. Chem.
    252, 677–686.
Ueland, P. M. and Døskeland, S. O. (1978) Arch. Biochem.
    Biophys. 185, 195–203.
Ueland, P. M. and Saebo, J. (1979) Biochemistry, 18, 4130–
    4135.

S-ADENOSYLHOMOCYSTEINE HYDROLASE

Peter K. Chiang and George A. Miura

Division of Biochemistry
Walter Reed Army Institute of Research
Washington, DC 20307-5100
U.S.A.

S-Adenosylhomocysteine hydrolase (AdoHcyase; EC 3.3.1.1) catalyzes the overall reaction first described by de la Haba and Cantoni (1957):

$$AdoHcy + H_2O \rightleftharpoons Ado + Hcy$$

The equilibrium of the reaction favors synthesis with a K_{eq} of about 10^{-6} M. While the enzyme was being crystallized by Richards et al. (1978), Palmer and Abeles (1979) demonstrated that it contains NAD and proposed a catalytic mechanism based on the oxidation and reduction of the enzyme-bound NAD. Richards et al. (1978) first showed that the enzyme exists as a tetramer, but in contrast, the plant AdoHcyase is dimeric (Guranowski and Pawełkiewicz, 1977) while the bacterial enzyme is hexameric (Shimizu et al., 1984). In general, the native molecular weight of the mammalian enzyme is between 180,000 and 200,000.

Discrete steps in the mechanism of action of AdoHcyase have been elucidated by Palmer and Abeles (1979), and are depicted in Scheme 1. The enzymatic synthesis of AdoHcy starts with the oxidation of the 3'-OH of adenosine (Ado) by an enzyme-bound NAD (1). Ado is converted to 3'-keto Ado and NAD to NADH. A base at the active site removes the 4' proton from the 3'-keto Ado to form an α-carbanion (2). After the abstraction of H_2O, 3'-keto-4',5'dehydro Ado is formed (3). The latter then reacts with Hcy to form 3'-keto AdoHcy α-carbanion (4),

239

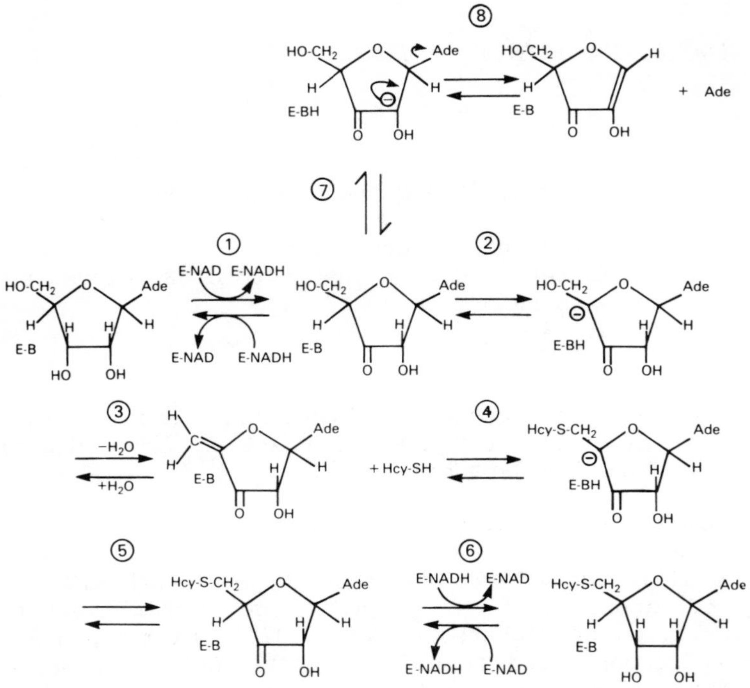

SCHEME 1

which accepts a proton at the 4' position to form 3'-keto
AdoHcy (5). AdoHcy is formed after the reduction of 3'-
keto AdoHcy by enzyme-bound NADH (6). The hydrolysis of
AdoHcy to Ado and Hcy is the reversal of steps (6) to
(1).
     Interest has been focused on steps (7) and (8),
particularly with respect to the possibility of the
release of adenine during the irreversible inactivation
of the enzyme by nucleoside analogs. The transient 3'-
keto Ado, if not converted immediately to other
intermediates, is highly unstable and leads to
spontaneous trans-elimination of adenine. Lately,
conflicting results have been reported by several
laboratories on the release of adenine from nucleosides
upon incubation with AdoHcyase isolated from different

Table I

Comparison of the Observation of Adenine Release from Adenosine

AdoHcyase source	Nucleoside	Adenine released
Plant[1]	Ado	observed
Bovine liver[2]	Ado	observed
	Ara-A	observed
Bovine liver[3]	2'-deoxy-Ado	observed
L1210 cells[4]	2-F-Ado	not observed
	Ara-A	not observed
	Ado	not observed
Human placenta[5]	Ara-A	observed
Hamster liver[6]	Ara-A	not observed
	Ado	not observed

[1] Jakubowski and Guranowski (1981).
[2] Chiang et al. (1981).
[3] Abeles et al. (1982).
[4] White et al. (1982).
[5] Hershfield et al. (1982).
[6] Kim et al. (1985).

sources. The results are summarized in Table I. In spite of the conflicting results from various laboratories, the oxidation-reduction of enzyme-bound NAD is most likely the mechanism of action, and may indicate very efficient catalytic cycles without releasing adenine from Ado under normal conditions. Why there are discrepancies regarding the release of adenine is not apparent at present.

Before presenting a detailed discussion on the interaction of various nucleoside analogs with AdoHcyase, in particular with respect to the inhibition of the enzyme activity, it is opportune for us to propose here that there are three main categories of inhibitors for the enzyme: (1) competitive inhibitors; (2) irreversible and the pseudo-irreversible inactivators; and (3) mixed

Table II

K$_i$ Values for the Competitive Inhibition of AdoHcyase

Nucleoside	K$_i$ (M)	Source
3-Deaza-(±)aristeromycin	1×10^{-9}	hamster liver[1]
(±)Aristeromycin	5×10^{-9}	bovine liver[2]
3-Deaza-Ado	4×10^{-6}	bovine liver[2]
	7×10^{-7}	hamster liver[1]
3-Deaza-(±)aristeromycinyl-Hcy	3×10^{-6}	hamster liver[1]
Adenine	1×10^{-6}	rat liver[3]
	9×10^{-6}	hamster liver[1]
3-Deaza-adenine	2×10^{-5}	hamster liver[1]
AdoHcy	5×10^{-5}	bovine liver[2]
3-Deaza-AdoHcy	6×10^{-5}	hamster liver[1]
8-Aza-Ado	2×10^{-4}	bovine liver[2]
N^6-Methyl-Ado	2×10^{-4}	bovine liver[2]
Formycin A	3×10^{-4}	bovine liver[2]
2-Aza-3-deaza-Ado	3×10^{-4}	bovine liver[2]
1-Deaza-(±)aristeromycin	5×10^{-4}	rabbit liver[4]
Inosine	1×10^{-3}	bovine liver[2]
Ado-N^1-oxide	2×10^{-3}	bovine liver[2]
Pyrazomycin	10×10^{-3}	bovine liver[2]

[1]Kim et al. (1983).
[2]Guranowski et al. (1981).
[3]Briske-Anderson and Duerre (1982).
[4]Ohno et al. (1984).

type inhibitors which consist of nucleosides that can inhibit competitively and/or irreversibly.

The K$_i$ values for the competitive inhibition of AdoHcyase are listed in Table II. In contrast to their ineffectiveness as substrates (Guranowski et al., 1981; Montgomery et al., 1982), the carbocyclic analogs are among the best competitive inhibitors found. The conjugation of 3-deaza-adenine to the cyclopentyl ring to yield 3-deaza-(±)aristeromycin (Montgomery et al., 1982) is an example of rational design, based on the known potency of 3-deaza-adenosine (Chiang et al., 1977). On the other hand, the efforts of Ohno et al. (1984) were not so fortunate. Their 1-deaza-(±)aristeromycin-Hcy has a disappointing K_i of about 0.5 mM, but this is not unexpected since we found that 1-deaza-Ado has no inhibitory effect on the activity of AdoHcyase (P. K. Chiang, unpublished observation). This shows the importance of the nitrogen at position 1 of the purine ring for activity, while the deletion of the nitrogen at position 3 (3-deaza nucleosides) enhances the competitive inhibition of a nucleoside tremendously. Although bulky substituents at position 6 are not well tolerated, the 6-amino is required for activity. Substitution at the 8-position results in decreased inhibition. The 9-nitrogen is required for activity; this is evidenced by the inability of 9-deaza-Ado to inhibit AdoHcyase in any manner (P. K. Chiang, unpublished observation), and also that formycin B (8-aza-9-deaza-Ado) is a mediocre inhibitor. There is an absolute requirement for the 7-nitrogen, because tubercidin (7-deaza-Ado) or tubercidinylhomocysteine are without any effect on the activity of AdoHcyase (Guranowski et al., 1981).

Table III shows the inactivation constants, K_I values, calculated for the irreversible inactivation of enzyme activity by nucleoside analogs. The inactivation experiments were conducted by first incubating AdoHcyase with a particular nucleoside in a buffer lacking the normal substrates (Ado and Hcy). At the designated time, an aliquot of the preincubation mixture is assayed for enzyme activity remaining (Chiang et al., 1981; Kim et al., 1985). The most potent inactivator is neplanocin A, with a K_I of 2 nM, which is about the same as that calculated (8 nM) by Borchardt et al. (1984) using the Ackermann-Potter plot. Next, with K_I values differing by 3 orders of magnitude are S-iso-butyl-Ado (SIBA), S-isobutyl-3-deaza-Ado (3-deaza-SIBA), and 5'-cyano-Ado. In comparison, both Ara-A (9-β-D-arabinofuranosyl-adenine) and 5'-azido-Ado are moderate inactivators. 3-Deaza-Ara-A is less potent than the parent compound, Ara-A. While 2'-deoxy-Ado and 2-Cl-Ado can inactivate reasonably well, it is perplexing to find that 2-Cl,2'-deoxy-Ado is completely inactive. The substitution of a halogen (Cl or F) to the 2 position of Ara-A results in weaker inactivators. The ability of 2',3'-dideoxy-Ado to inactivate AdoHcyase implies that the 2',3'-OH groups are not required for inactivation. In sharp contrast to the

potency of 5'-cyano-Ado, 5'-Cl-5'-deoxyadenosine is the
least effective inactivator.

Table III
Inactivation Constants, K_I*, of Nucleoside Analogs

Nucleoside	K_I (μM)	Source
Neplanocin A	0.002	hamster liver[1]
S-Isobutyl-Ado (SIBA)	0.5	hamster liver[1]
S-Isobutyl-3-deaza-Ado (3-deaza-SIBA)	4	hamster liver[1]
5'-Cyano-Ado	5	hamster liver[2]
Ara-A	19	L1210 cells[3]
	11	hamster liver[2]
5'-Azido-Ado	14	hamster liver[2]
3-Deaza-Ara-A	41	hamster liver[2]
2'-Deoxy-Ado	62	hamster liver[2]
5'-Amino-Ado	65	hamster liver[2]
2-Cl-Ado	66	hamster liver[2]
Nucleocidin	71	hamster liver[2]
2-Cl-Ara-A	143	hamster liver[2]
2-Aza-Ado	181	hamster liver[2]
2-F-Ara-A	122	L1210 cells[3]
	188	hamster liver[2]
2',3'-Dideoxy-Ado	260	hamster liver[2]
2-Cl-3-Deaza-Ado	378	hamster lvier[2]
5'-Cl-5'-Deoxy-Ado	597	hamster lvier[2]

*The inactivation constant, K_I, was calculated according
to the following equation:

$$\frac{1}{K_{app}} = \frac{K_I}{k_2[I]} + \frac{1}{k_2}$$

where K_{app} is the pseudo-first order rate constant, and
k_2 is the rate constant of inactivation.

[1]G. A. Miura (unpublished observation).
[2]Kim et al. (1983).
[3]White et al. (1982).

Table IV
Comparison of The Competitive K_i and Inactivating K_I
Values of Mixed Type Inhibitors for AdoHcyase

Nucleoside	Source	Competitive K_i (M)	Inactivating K_I
Neplanocin A	HeLa cells[1]	2×10^{-9}	4×10^{-10}
	HL-60 cells[1]	2×10^{-9}	1×10^{-9}
	red blood cell[1]	3×10^{-9}	2×10^{-9}
Ara-A	hamster liver[2]	18×10^{-6}	2×10^{-6}
3-Deaza-Ara-A	hamster liver[2]	86×10^{-6}	41×10^{-6}

[1] G. A. Miura (unpublished observation).
[2] Kim et al. (1985).

In addition to 2-Cl,2'-deoxy-Ado, the following compounds are also devoid of any time-dependent inactivating activity against AdoHcyase isolated from hamster or bovine liver: 3-deaza-guanosine, guanine, diazepam, N,N-dimethyl-Ado, sangivanmycin, erthythro-9-(2-hydroxyl-3-nonyl)-adenine (EHNA), S-isobutyl-tubercidin, S-isobutyl-(ethoxymethyl)adenine, and methylthioacyclo-Ado. Neither 3-deaza-Ado nor 3-deaza-(±)aristeromycin will inactivate AdoHcyase irreversibly.

Table IV shows neplanocin A, Ara-A and 3-deaza-Ara-A can inhibit competitively and also inactivate AdoHcyase irreversibly. While objections can be raised on measuring both the competitive inhibition and the irreversible inactivation of the enzyme by the same nucleosides, the K_i and the K_I values are almost identical as clearly shown here. It is also a fact that most other nucleosides cannot exhibit this kinetic anomaly. These mixed inhibitors may well be pseudo-irreversible inhibitors; i.e. if given enough time and the right conditions, the enzyme activity might be recovered. Pseudo-irreversible inactivation of AdoHcyase has been described by Patel-Thombre and Borchardt (1985). Although not entirely similar in terms of kinetics, a parallel anomaly exists in that 3-deaza-Ado and 3-deaza-(±)aristeromycin can competitively inhibit the enzyme and function as substrates at the same time.

There are several similarities between the competitive inhibitors and the irreversible inactivators:

(1) There is an absolute requirement for a nitrogen at position 7. (2) Bulky substitutions at the N-6 position are not well tolerated. (3) The purine moiety is required for recognition. (4) The absence of a nitrogen at the 9-position decreases activity. (5) Modification of the ribose to a carbocyclic pentose enhances activity. On the other hand, there are some subtle differences: (1) A deletion of the nitrogen at the 3-position decreases the potencies of the inactivators, while it enhances the inhibition of the competitive inhibitors, e.g. Ara-A vs. 3-deaza-Ara-A. (2) Substitutions at the 5' position do not seem to hinder the irreversible inactivators, but they decrease the potencies of competitive inhibitors. (3) Substituting at the 2-position with a Cl restricts 2-Cl-Ado to an inactivator only (see also Shimizu et al., 1984).

The mechanism for the inactivation of the enzyme by nucleosides was first proposed by Hershfield (1979) to be a suicide type involving catalysis of the inactivators. Since then, revisions have been forwarded by various laboratories, and also by Hershfield et al. (1982). Although the results obtained by Abeles et al. (1982) using 2'-deoxy-Ado are convincing, the release of adenine from nucleosides, as mentioned earlier, could not be clearly demonstrated in all cases (Kim et al., 1985; White et al., 1982). Furthermore, nucleosides lacking 3'- or 5'-OH groups (2',3'-dideoxy-Ado; 5' substituted; dialdehyde analogs) a priori should not be able to undergo a catalytic conversion or the so-called "K_{cat}" mechanism to reactive intermediates according to the scheme put forth by Abeles. It also has been demonstrated by Gomi and Fujioka (1984) that nucleosides (adenine and 3'-deoxy-Ado) bind to AdoHcyase mainly through hydrophobic interactions. A reduction of the enzyme-bound NAD could not be shown in the inactivation by cAMP (Hohman et al., 1984) or by aliphatic adenine analogs (Schanche et al., 1984) of AdoHcyase, purified from Dictyostelium discoideum and mouse liver, respectively. However, it is entirely possible that para-catalytic self-inactivation of AdoHcyase could occur with respect to some of the nucleosides that have the 3'- and 5'-OH groups. In such a case, transiently reactive intermediates are generated during the oxidation of the enzyme-bound NAD, and serve to modify groups at the active site without being released from the enzyme.

Mechanisms aside, it is our opinion that the

competitive inhibitors are the nucleosides of choice to achieve the desired inhibition of the enzyme activity in vivo and in cells. This is based on the observation that, although both S-iso-butyl-Ado (SIBA) and S-iso-butyl-3-deaza-Ado (3-deaza-SIBA) have inactivating K_I values which are about the same as the competitive K_i's of 3-deaza-Ado (about 1 µM; Tables II and III), there is no change in the level of AdoHcy when the HeLa cells are incubated with 3-deaza-SIBA (Fig. 2). Moreover, it has been demonstrated by Kim et al. (1985) that, in spite of the similar rates of inactivation of AdoHcyase in the rat hepatocytes, the cellular levels of AdoHcy and AdoMet were much higher in the cells treated with 3-deaza-Ara-A (a mixed type) than in those treated with 2-Cl-Ado, a strictly irreversible inactivator. In collaboration with E. De Clerq, we found that nucleosides having the capacity to inhibit the enzyme competitively are better antiviral agents than the irreversible inactivators.

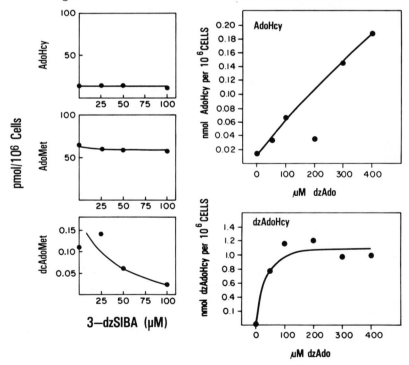

Fig. 2.   Levels of metabolites in HeLa cells treated with 3-deaza-SIBA (left), and 3-deaza-Ado (right).

Table V

Effectiveness of Nucleosides to Form S-Nucleosidyl-homocysteine Analogs (NucHcy) and S-Nucleosidylcysteine Analogs (NucCys) Catalyzed by Bovine Liver AdoHcyase

| | Relative Velocity | |
Nucleoside	NucHcy	NucCys[b]
Ado	100[a]	100
3-Deaza-Ado	165[a]	33
2-Aza-3-deaza-Ado	113[a]	?
Purine riboside (nebularine)	34[a]	40
Formycin A	18[a]	12
N^6-Methyl-Ado	16[a]	12
8-Aza-Ado	9[a]	0
Ado N^1-oxide	5[a]	6
Pyrazomycin	5[a]	0
8-Amino-Ado	4[a]	0
Inosine	1.5[a]	0
(±)Aristeromycin	0.1[a]	0
2-Amino-Ado	+[b]	70
N^6-Hydroxy-Ado	+[b]	70
2-Hydroxy-Ado	+[b]	0
2-Cl-Ado	+[b]	0
3-Deaza-(±)aristeromycin	+[b]	0

[a]Guranowski et al. (1981).
[b]Guranowski and Jakubowski (1983).

One of the unique features of AdoHcyase is its ability to use a variety of nucleosides as substrates. For this reason, it is probably more appropriate that the enzyme be renamed nucleosidylhomocysteine hydrolase. Table V compares the ability of various nucleosides that can function as alternative substrates. 3-Deaza-Ado is the best nucleoside substrate, irrespective of enzyme source or cell type used. In contrast, 3-deaza-(±)-aristeromycin is at best a poor substrate, thus indicating the importance of the ribose for substrate ability but not for inhibition. Based on indirect evidence, 2-F-Ado may also be a substrate for AdoHcyase of mouse lymphocytes (Zimmerman et al., 1980). Guranowski and Jakubowski (1983) reported that cysteine is also a substrate and can form S-nucleosidylcysteine when incubated with various nucleosides (Table V) using bovine AdoHcyase. However, we have not been able to indentify the formation of S-adenosylcysteine in cells incubated with radioactive cysteine or cystathione as precursors, using a new high performance liquid chromatography method (Miura et al., 1984). For now, S-nucleosidylcysteine remains an enzymatic oddity.

An interesting kinetic property reported by Kim et al. (1983) was that the enzyme activity of AdoHcyase from hamster liver can be affected bimodally by nucleosides or adenine. At high concentrations, they of course inhibit the enzyme competitively, but at very low concentrations, they can actually stimulate the enzyme activity by 10-30%. It has been demonstrated that bovine AdoHcyase exhibits half-site reactivity (Chiang et al., 1981), i.e. one mole of AdoHcyase (per tetramer) binds two moles of Ado. It has recently been confirmed that two moles of Ado dialdehyde are bound per mole of bovine AdoHcyase (Patel-Thombre and Borchardt, 1985). Considering all available evidence, AdoHcyase is most likely a regulatory enzyme. Indeed, it has been suggested by Abeles et al. (1982) that AdoHcyase consists of two pairs of non-identical subunits, and only two of the four enzyme-bound NAD molecules participate in the catalytic cycle. We postulate that the other two subunits are probably regulatory subunits, which bind nucleosides to modulate the activity of the enzyme via conformational changes. Nonidentical catalytic sites have also been postulated by Guranowski and Jakubowski (1983), based on the observation that the enzymatic reactions with Hcy and cysteine are not mutually exclusive.

A murine lymphoid cell line partially deficient in AdoHcyase activity has been cloned by Kamatani et al. (1983); the mutant clone (Sahn 12) has 11-13% of wild-type activity. Attempts by us (R. P. Siraganian and P. K. Chiang) to clone rat basophilic leukemia cells resist-ant to 3-deaza-Ado resulted in cells with enzyme activity either twice or half that of the wild-type enzyme activity. Taken together, cells extremely deficient in AdoHcyase activity are probably lethal mutants.

AdoHcyase is obviously a fascinating enzyme with kinetic anomalies. More interesting phenomena have yet to unfold, especially from the cell mutants with altered AdoHcyase activities. Furthermore, the biological effects of the enzyme inhibitors/inactivators (Chiang,

1985) may prove to be even more exciting.

REFERENCES

Abeles, R. H., Fish, S. and Lapinskas, B.   (1982)
  Biochemistry 21, 5557-5562.
Borchardt, R. T., Keller, B. T.and Patel-Thrombre, U.
  (1984) J. Biol. Chem. 259, 4353-4358.
Briske-Anderson, M. and Duerre, J. A.   (1982) Canad. J.
  Biochem. 60, 118-123.
Chiang, P. K. (1985) Methods Pharmacol. 6, 127-145.
Chiang, P. K., Richards, H. H. and Cantoni, G. L.
  (1977) Mol. Pharmacol. 13, 939-947.
Chiang, P. K., Guranowski, A. and Segall, J. E.   (1981)
  Arch. Biochem. Biophys. 207, 175-184.
de la Haba, G and Cantoni, G. L.   J. Biol. Chem. 234,
  603-608 (1959).
Gomi, T. and Fujioka, M.   (1984) Biochim. Biophys. Acta
  785, 177-180.
Guranowski, A. and Jakubowski H.   (1983) Biochim.
  Biophys. Acta 742, 250-256.
Guranowski, A. and Pawełkiewcz, J.   (1977) Eur. J.
  Biochem. 80, 517-523.
Guranowski, A., Montgomery, J. A., Cantoni, G. L. and
  Chiang, P. K. (1981) Biochemistry 20, 110-115.
Hershfield, M. S. (1979) J. Biol. Chem. 254, 22-25.
Hershfield, M. S., Small, W. C., Premakumar, R.,
  Bagnara, A. S. and Fetter, J. E.   (1982) in
  Biochemistry of S-Adenosylmethionine and Related
  Compounds (Usdin, E., Borchardt, R. T. and Creveling,
  C. R., Eds.) pp.657-665, Macmillan, London.
Hohman, R. J., Guitton, M. C. and Véron, M.   (1984)
  Arch. Biochem. Biophys. 233, 785-795.
Jakubowski, H. and Guranowski, A.   (1978) Biochem.
  Biophys. Res. Commun. 84, 1060-1068.
Kamatani, N., Willis, E. H. and Carson, D. A.   (1983)
  Biochem. Biophys. Acta 762, 205-214.
Kim, I.-K., Zhang, C.-Y., Chiang, P. K. and Cantoni, G.
  L. (1983) Arch. Biochem. Biophys. 226, 65-72.
Kim, I.-K., Zhang, C.-Y., Cantoni, G. L., Montgomery, J.
  A. and Chiang, P. K.   (1985) Biochem. Biophys. Acta
  829, 150-155.
Miura, G. A., Santangelo, J. R., Gordon, R. K. and
  Chiang, P. K. (1984) Anal. Biochem. 141, 161-167.
Montgomery, J. A., Clayton, S. J., Thomas, J. J.,
  Shannon, W. M., Arnett, S. G., Bodner, A. J., Kim, I.-

K., Cantoni, G. L. and Chiang, P. K. (1982) J. Med. Chem. 25, 626-629.

Ohno, H., Itoh, T., Nomura, A. and Mizuno, Y. (1984) Nucleosides & Nucleotides 3, 345-351.

Palmer, J. L. and Abeles, R. H. (1979) J. Biol. Chem. 254, 1217-1226.

Patel-Thrombre, U. and Borchardt, R. T. (1985) Biochemistry 24, 1130-1136.

Richards, H. H., Chiang, P. K. and Cantoni, G. L. (1978) J. Biol. Chem. 253, 4476-4480.

Schanche, J.-S., Schanche, T., Ueland, P. M., Holý, A. and Votruba, I. (1984) Mol. Pharmacol. 26, 553-558.

Shimizu, S., Shiozaki, S., Ohshiro, T., and Yamada H. (1984). Eur. J. Biochem. 141, 385-392.

White, E. L., Shaddix, S. C., Brockman, R. W. and Bennett, Jr., L. L. (1982) Cancer Res. 42, 2260-2264.

Zimmerman, T. P., Wolberg, G., Duncan, G. S. and Elion, G. B. (1980) Biochemistry 19, 2252-2259.

PROBES FOR EXAMINING THE STRUCTURE AND FUNCTION OF HUMAN

S-ADENOSYLHOMOCYSTEINE HYDROLASE, AND FOR ISOLATION OF cDNA

Michael S. Hershfield, V. Nambi Aiyar, Sara
Chaffee, Sylvia Curtis, Michael L. Greenberg

Duke University Medical Center
Durham, North Carolina USA 27710

The catalytic activity of AdoHcy hydrolase requires
formation of a stable complex with the cofactor NAD (Palmer
and Abeles, 1976). In addition to NAD, Hershfield and
Kredich (1978) identified AdoHcyase as the so-called
´cAMP-Ado´ or ´adenine analogue´ binding protein that had
been isolated by a number of investigators (Yuh and Tao,
1974; Sugden and Corbin, 1976; Ueland and Doskeland, 1977;
Olsson, 1978). The ability to form stable complexes with
NAD, Ado and its analogs, and cAMP raises questions
regarding the relationship of AdoHcyase to other proteins
that bind these ligands, and possible functions of ligand
binding, which might be related or unrelated to the role of
this enzyme in metabolism.

Gabriel (1978) has noted similarities in the mechanisms
of reactions catalyzed by a group of enzymes, including
AdoHcyase, that contain tightly bound NAD, which may
indicate an origin distinct from enzymes that catalyze
exogenous NAD dependent redox reactions. The cAMP binding
region of AdoHcyase might be related to the cAMP binding
sites of the regulatory subunits of cAMP dependent protein
kinase, which are the major cAMP binding proteins in
eucaryotic cells. We have shown that the loci for the
structural genes of AdoHcyase and ADA are linked, but
probably are not contiguous, on the long arm of chromosome
20 (Hershfield and Francke, 1982; Mohandas et al., 1984).
This finding, taken together with the evidence of the
functional dependence of AdoHcyase on ADA activity (Kredich

253

and Hershfield, 1983), has led us to postulate an
evolutionary relationship between the genes for these
enzymes, either that linkage of the evolving gene for
AdoHcyase to the ADA locus was an advantage during
evolution, or that the two genes arose from a common
sequence that encoded a primitive nucleoside binding domain
(Hershfield and Francke, 1982).

In order to address questions regarding the evolution
of AdoHcyase, its relatedness to other proteins that
interact with adenine nucleosides and nucleotides, and the
function of ligand binding, it will be necessary to develop
probes for the different binding sites on the enzyme, and to
obtain direct information regarding the sequence of the
enzyme and its structural gene(s). As a step toward
physical characterization of the Ado and cAMP binding sites
of AdoHcyase we have investigated the possibility of
covalently labeling the enzyme with photoactive derivatives
of these compounds, 8-azidoadenosine (8-N_3Ado) and
8-azidocAMP (8-N_3cAMP). We have isolated monoclonal
antibodies (MAb) directed toward sites on both native and
denatured AdoHcyase, which we have used to examine the
effect of ligand binding on enzyme conformation and
turnover, and which which we are using in the isolation of
cDNA for the mRNA of human AdoHcyase. The focus of this
meeting is on the biochemistry of AdoMet as a basis for drug
design. In that context we wish to describe an effect of
3-deazaaristeromycin, a potent inhibitor of AdoHcyase, on
the metabolism of AdoHcy.

                    PHOTOAFFINITY LABELING OF ADOHCYASE

We initially attempted to label AdoHcyase with
periodate oxidized Ado, but were unsuccessful in obtaining
acid or SDS stable binding, even with use of borohydride to
trap a Schiff base that this compound might form with a
lysine on the enzyme (Borchardt et al., 1982). We found,
however, that 8-N_3Ado caused slow inactivation of AdoHcyase,
which was enhanced by about 500 fold upon periodate
oxidation, suggesting that this compound interacted with the
enzyme active site. Consistent with this possibility was
the finding that 8-N_3Ado caused reduction of enzyme bound
NAD to NADH, though it did not serve as a substrate for
AdoHcy analog formation. Unirradiated placental AdoHcyase
bound [^{3}H]8-N_3Ado and [^{32}P]8-N_3cAMP noncovalently, as

Table 1

Additions	cpm bound
$[^3H]8-N_3-Ado$	38,990
$[^3H]8-N_3Ado$ + Ado, 40 uM	3,890
$[^3H]8-N_3Ado$ + cAMP, 50 uM	3,925
$[^{32}P]8-N_3-cAMP$	63,000
$[^{32}P]8-N_3cAMP$ + Ado, 170 uM	6,280
$[^{32}P]8-N_3cAMP$ + cAMP, 50 uM	2,270

Binding of $[^3H]8-N_3Ado$ and $[^{32}P]8-N_3cAMP$ by AdoHcyase. AdoHcyase, 0.2 mg/ml in 50 mM KPi, pH 6.8, 1 mM EDTA was incubated for 30 min at 37° with the indicated concentration of Ado or cAMP. Then $[^3H]8-N_3Ado$ or $[^{32}P]8-N_3-cAMP$ was added to a final concentration of 0.4 uM. Incubation was continued for 60 min in the dark, after which aliquots containing 10 ug of AdoHcyase were removed and chromatographed over PD-10 Sephadex G-25 (Pharmacia) gel filtration columns for measurement of radioactivity bound.

measured by gel filtration. The binding of each compound was inhibited >85% by preincubation with either excess unlabeled Ado or unlabeled cAMP (Table 1).

The above results results show that the 8-azido derivatives of both Ado and cAMP bind to specific Ado and cAMP sites on the enzyme, and thus they might be used as photoaffinity reagents for labeling these sites covalently. We found that from 5-14% of specifically bound, radiolabeled $8-N_3Ado$, periodate oxidized $8-N_3Ado$, or $8-N_3cAMP$ remained associated with AdoHcyase in an acid precipitable form following irradiation for 5-10 minutes at 0`, at a distance of 8 cm with a UVP mineralight at 254 nm. This yield, which is typical for photoincorporation of azido compounds, could not be improved by varying time of irradiation, or by use of high intensity irradiation at 320 nm. Of the label incorporated covalently, from 40-60% was blocked by unlabeled Ado or cAMP, but not by uridine, present at concentrations 100-200 fold in excess of the labeled azido analog. We observed no covalent photolabeling by

$[^3H]8-N_3Ado$ or its periodate oxidized derivative of
ovalbumin, ADA, or the Rl cAMP binding protein isolated from
human leukemic lymphoblasts. However, both ligands were
able to label proteins in crude placental extracts in a
nonspecific manner. Monoclonal antibodies to placental
AdoHcyase precipitated AdoHcyase photolableled with either
$8-N_3Ado$ or $8-N_3cAMP$, but did not precipitate proteins
labeled nonspecifically by these compounds, or Rl labeled
specifically with $[^{32}P]8-N_3cAMP$. We found no similarity in
the pattern of radioactive peptides generated by proteolytic
digestion of denatured AdoHcyase and Rl, each labeled with
^3H or ^{32}P $8-N_3cAMP$.

The finding that Ado and cAMP were both effective in
blocking the noncovalent binding and photoincorporation of
$8-N_3Ado$ and $8-N_3cAMP$ by AdoHcyase suggests that these
compounds interact at the same site or sites on the enzyme.
Consistent with this possibility, digestion with V8 protease
of AdoHcyase that had been photolabeled with $[^{32}P]8-N_3cAMP$
and $[^3H]8-N_3Ado$ yielded virtually identical patterns of
peptides (Figure 1). Competetive binding studies with
´adenine analogue´ or ´cAMP-Ado´ binding proteins that were
later identified as AdoHcyase (cited above) suggested that
Ado and cAMP occupied distinct sites, with Ado able to bind
to the cAMP site, but not the converse. However, another
interpretation of these data is possible. Abeles et al.
(1982) have suggested that Ado analogs with 3´OH groups,
which are able to reduce enzyme bound NAD to NADH, convert
AdoHcyase to a closed form that traps these ligands on the
enzyme. cAMP may bind to the same sites on AdoHcyase as
Ado, but lacking a 3´OH it cannot form a tight complex, and
it cannot prevent formation of a tight complex by Ado;
thus, cAMP will appear to only partially block Ado binding.

Our observations with 8-azido derivatives of Ado and
cAMP suggest that these compounds may indeed bind to the
same sites on the enzyme. However, our results must be
interpreted with caution since only about 50% of the
photolabelling we observed could be blocked with excess Ado
or cAMP in many experiments. It will be useful to develop
more efficient and specific affinity ligands, and to
physically define their binding sequences, to definitively
identify Ado and cAMP binding sites of AdoHcyase.

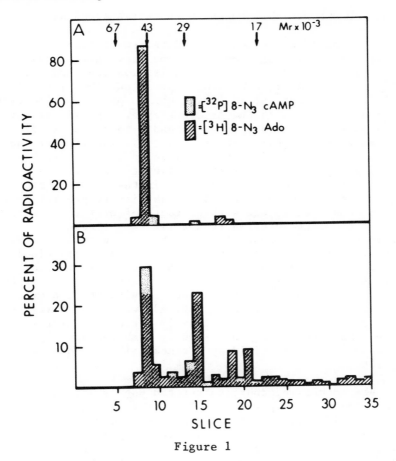

Figure 1

Comparison of 8-N$_3$Ado and 8-N$_3$cAMP binding sites of
AdoHcyase by proteolytic mapping. Enzyme was incubated in
the dark for 30 minutes at 37° with either 5 uM [^{3}H]8-N$_3$Ado
or 1.5 uM [^{32}P]8-N$_3$cAMP, followed by photolysis at 0° for 10
minutes. The samples were then denatured by boiling in SDS
PAGE sample buffer. Aliquots containing 16 ug of AdoHcyase
were incubated at 37° for 30 minutes in the absence (panel
A) or the presence (panel B) of 1 ug of V8 protease,
followed by SDS PAGE on a 15% slab gel. After
electrophoretic transfer to nitrocellulose, lanes containing
the labeled proteins were cut into 2 mm slices for
scintillation counting. Results are expressed as percent of
total cpm recovered in the lane.

MONOCLONAL ANTIBODIES TO PLACENTAL ADOHCYASE

Monoclonal antibodies (MAb) directed at distinct
epitopes can serve as probes for domains within proteins,
for examining cellular and tissue distribution, and for
isolation of cDNA for mRNA from expression libraries. In
our initial attempts at isolating MAb to placental AdoHcyase
we immunized mice with the native enzyme. Hybridomas were
generated as described by Scearce and Eisenbarth (1983)
using as donor the P3X63Ag8 myeloma cell line (Kohler and
Milstein, 1975). We identified 21 wells as positive by
screening supernatants for the ability to precipitate
preformed [^{3}H]Ado-AdoHcyase complex in the presence of
staphylococcus. Comparison of the ability to preciptate
similar complexes formed with extracts of erythrocytes from
a series of nonhuman primates identified at least 8
different specificities. None of these MAbs caused direct
inhibition of placental AdoHcyase catalytic or Ado binding
activity. We prepared high titer ascites fluid with one
clone, B2A3, which was found to react with human enzyme but
not with monkey or lemur AdoHcyase, or with the enzyme from
mouse or hamster cells. This antibody was used to screen a
series of human-rodent somatic cell hybrids for expression
of the human AdoHcyase gene product, enabling mapping of the
AdoHcyase gene (Hershfield and Francke, 1982; Mohandas et
al., 1984).

MAbs to native AdoHcyase reacted poorly with AdoHcyase
in immunoblotting experiments (Towbin et al., 1979), and did
not detect AdoHcyase in fixed tissue sections. We have used
these MAb's to probe for more subtle changes in enzyme
conformation that occur upon binding of nucleosides. The
B2A3 MAb coordinately precipitated the catalytic and Ado
binding activity of untreated purified AdoHcyase. After
treatment of AdoHcyase with deoxyadenosine, followed by
dialysis, we obtained a preparation that retained about 18%
of initial catalytic and 65% of initial Ado binding
activity. All of the residual catalytic, but only 50% of
the binding activity could be precipitated with B2A3.
Similarly, B2A3 and other MAbs to native AdoHcyase were
found to precipitate only about 50% of [^{3}H]Ado-AdoHcyase
complexes. These results suggest that the combining sites
for these antibodies on some, but not all enzyme molecules,
become buried upon ligand binding.

In order to obtain MAbs that would react with a wider
range of sites, we immunized a second group of mice with a
mixture of native and guanidine-denatured AdoHcyase, and
then prepared hybridomas. We screened in two ways, with the
precipitation assay described above, and with a solid phase
assay in which native or denatured AdoHcyase was adsorbed to
nitrocellulose. Using the latter procedure we have obtained
several MAbs that react with fully denatured AdoHcyase with
high avidity, and which display strong cytoplasmic
reactivity with tissue sections. A mixture of these MAbs
(isolated from ascites fluids) can detect as little as 0.5
nanogram of AdoHcyase in immunoblotting experiments when
used at a dilution of 1:40,000. This mixture identifies a
single band of Mr 47-50,000 in crude extracts of human cells
and species as distant as Xenopus.

We have used MAb to denatured AdoHcyase and a solid
phase assay to quantitate the total amount and specific
activity of AdoHcyase protein in crude extracts of nucleated
cells from the bone marrow of 2 children with inherited
deficiency of ADA. In each case we found the same amount of
AdoHcyase protein as was present in similar preparations
from 7 controls, 0.02-0.05% of total cytoplasmic protein.
However, the specific activity of the patients´ AdoHcyase
was in each case approximately 17% of control values; the
latter was virtually identical to the specific activity of
purified placental AdoHcyase (Hershfield et al., 1985).
These results strongly support our earlier conclusion that
low activity of AdoHcyase in ADA deficiency is caused by
inactivation of the enzyme by deoxyadenosine (Hershfield et
al., 1979).

Using MAb to denatured AdoHcyase we have begun to
screen human cDNA libraries constructed in the lambda GT11
expression vector (Young and Davis, 1983), which have been
made available to us by Drs. Paul Modrich and Jack Keene of
Duke University. We have isolated phage that encode a
fusion protein containing both E. coli -galactosidase and
human AdoHcyase immunoreactive sequences, which is expressed
under the control of the galactosidase promoter. The cDNA
inserts in these phage, which presumably contain AdoHcyase
sequences, are now being subcloned for further analysis and
sequencing. It is hoped that we will soon be able to
address definitively questions regarding the structure of
the AdoHcyase gene, the origin and function of of its ligand
binding sites, and the regulation of its expression.

ADAPTATION TO 3-DEAZAARISTEROMYCIN

In order to evaluate the role of AdoHcy hydrolase
inactivation in contributing to the growth inhibition caused
by adenine arabinoside and deoxyadenosine, we have used
mutant T and B lymphoblastoid cell lines that are deficient
in the enzymes that phosphorylate these nucleosides, Ado
kinase and deoxycytidine kinase (Hershfield et al.,
1982a,b). We found that inhibition of growth was associated
with a fall in the intracellular AdoMet:AdoHcy ratio from
values in untreated cells of >10, to values of <3 in the
presence of the nucleosides. Under these conditions we
noted a consistent increase in in the concentration of
AdoMet by 20-50%, which has also been observed in vivo in
the lymphoblasts of patients undergoing treatment for
leukemia with the ADA inhibitor deoxycoformycin (Hershfield
et al., 1983; Hershfield et al., 1984).

To characterize the long term effects of AdoHcy
accumulation we have grown a kinase deficient derivative of
the WI-L2 human B cell line in the presence of increasing
concentrations of 3-deazaaristeromycin (c_3Ari), a potent
inhibitor of AdoHcyase that is not a substrate for ADA
(Montgomery et al., 1982). The cell line was cloned by
limiting dilution in the presence of 75 uM c_3Ari, a
concentration that prolonged the doubling time of the
untreated cell line to >80 hours. Several independent
clones were then grown in increasing concentrations of the
drug, and were eventually maintained as stocks in 300 uM
c_3Ari. Under these conditions the clones displayed a c_3Ari
resistant (c_3Ari^r) phenotype. The doubling times of the
untreated parental line in the presence of 0, 10, 50 and 500
uM c_3Ari were 30, 48, 84 and 104 hours, respectively.
Doubling times of a c_3Ari^r clone in 0, 10 and 500 uM c_3Ari
were 38, 40 and 52 hours, respectively in a parallel
experiment.

The concentration of AdoMet in parental cells never
exposed to c_3Ari is 150-250 nmol/10^9 cells. During routine
growth in the presence of 300 uM c_3Ari, the resistant clones
were found to have strikingly elevated pools of AdoMet, 4-7
times that of the untreated cells, approaching the size of
the ATP pool. After growth for 2 weeks in the absence of
drug the clones still had 2-3 fold higher AdoMet content
than the parent. Exposure to c_3Ari caused essentially
identical increases in AdoHcy content in both the parental

and c_3Ari adapted cells. Thus, with exposure to any concentration of c_3Ari the drug-adapted clones maintained AdoMet:AdoHcy ratios that were 2-3 fold higher than in the parent, which may account for their c_3Ari^r phenotype. For example, in one clone during continuous culture in c_3Ari the AdoMet and AdoHcy concentrations were 1400 and 200 nmol/10^9 cells. In the parental cells exposed to 80 uM c_3Ari for 3 hours the concentrations of AdoMet and AdoHcy were 350 and 240 nmol/10^9 cells. The same exposure (3 hours, 80 uM drug) produced AdoMet and AdoHcy concentrations of 800 and 220 nmol/10^9 cells in a clone that had been grown in drug free medium for 2 weeks.

The basis for the effect on AdoMet pool size has not been determined. The specific activites of AdoMet synthetase and AdoHcy hydrolase, measured at saturating substrate concentrations, were virtually identical in extracts of the parental and c_3Ari adapted cells. We cannot exclude an effect (mutation, posttranslational modification) that might result in altered activity of AdoMet synthetase under conditions that exist in the intact cell, or some change that affects AdoMet turnover. The stability of the effect on AdoMet pools and cross resistance to other agents that inhibit AdoHcy degradation are now being examined. An understanding of this phenomenon may shed light on factors that may operate to regulate the size or turnover of the AdoMet pool, and may provide useful information in developing strategies for pharmacologic manipulation of AdoMet metabolism.

REFERENCES

Abeles, R. H., Fish, S. and Lapinskas, B. (1982) Biochemistry 21, 5557-5562.

Borchardt, R. T., Patel, V. G. and Bartel, R. L. (1982) in Biochemistry of S-Adenosylmethionine and Related Compounds (Borchardt, R. T., Usdin, E. and Creveling, C. R., Eds.) pp.645-652, MacMillan Company, London.

Gabriel, O. (1978) Trends in Biological Sciences 3, 193-195.

Hershfield, M. S., Aiyar, V. N., Premakumar, R. and Small, W. C. (1985) Biochemical J. in press.

Hershfield, M. S., Fetter, J. E., Small, W. C., Bagnara, A.S., Williams, S.R., Ullman, B., Martin, D.W. Jr., Wasson, D. B. and Carson, D.A. (1982a) J. Biol. Chem. 257, 6380-6386.

Hershfield, M. S. and Francke, U. (1982) _Science_ 216, 739-742.

Hershfield, M. S. and Kredich, N. M. (1978) _Science_ 202, 757-760.

Hershfield, M. S., Kredich, N.M., Koller, C. A., Mitchell, B.S., Kurtzberg, J., Kinney, T.R. and Falletta, J.M. (1983) _Cancer Res._ 43, 3451-3458.

Hershfield, M. S., Kredich, N.M., Ownby, D.R., Ownby, H. and Buckley, R. (1979) _J. Clin. Invest._ 63, 807-811.

Hershfield, M.S., Kurtzberg, J., Harden, E., Moore, J.O., Whang-Peng, J. and Haynes, B.F. (1984) _Proc. Natl. Acad. Sci. USA_ 81, 253-257.

Hershfield, M. S., Small, W. C., Premakumar, R., Bagnara, A. S. and Fetter, J. E. (1982b) in _Biochemistry of S-Adenosylmethionine and Related Compounds_ (Borchardt, R. T., Usdin, E. and Creveling C.R., Eds.) pp. 657-665, MacMillan Company, London.

Kohler, G. and Milstein, C. (1975) _Nature (London)_ 256, 495-497.

Kredich, N. M. and Hershfield, M. S. (1983) in _The Metabolic Basis of Inherited Disease_ (Stanbury, J. B., Wyngaarden, J.B., Fredrickson, D.S., Goldstein, J. and Brown, M., Eds.) pp. 1157-1201, McGraw-Hill, New York.

Mohandas, T., Sparkes, R. S., Suh, E. J. and Hershfield, M. S. (1984) _Hum. Genet._ 66, 292-295.

Montgomery, J. A., Clayton, C. J., Thomas, H. J., Shannon, W. M., Arnett, G., Bodner, A. J., Kion, I-K., Cantoni, G.L. and Chiang, P.K. (1982) _J. Med. Chem._ 25, 626-629.

Olsson, R. A. (1978) _Biochemistry_ 17, 367-375.

Palmer, J. L. and Abeles, R. H. (1976) _J. Biol. Chem._ 251, 5817-5819.

Scearce R. M. and Eisenbarth G. S. (1983) _Methods in Enzymology_ 103, 459-469.

Sugden, P. H. and Corbin, J. D. (1976) _Biochem. J._ 159, 423-437.

Towbin, H., Staehelin, T. and Gordon, J. (1979) _Proc. Natl. Acad. Sci. USA_ 76, 4350-4354.

Ueland, P. M. and Doskeland, S. O. (1977) _J. Biol. Chem._ 252, 677-686.

Young, R. A. and Davis, R. W. (1983) _Proc. Natl. Acad. Sci. USA_ 80, 1194-1198.

Yuh, K.-C. M. and Tao, M. (1974) _Biochemistry_ 13, 5220-5226.

DISPOSITION OF ENDOGENOUS
S-ADENOSYLHOMOCYSTEINE AND HOMOCYSTEINE
FOLLOWING EXPOSURE TO NUCLEOSIDE ANALOGUES
AND METHOTREXATE

P. M. Ueland, A. Svardal, H. Refsum. J.R. Lillehaug, J-S. Schanche and S. Helland.

From the Clinical Pharmacology Unit, Department of Pharmacology, University of Bergen, N-5016 Bergen, Norway

INTRODUCTION

S-Adenosylhomocysteine (AdoHcy) is a product from and an inhibitor of S-adenosylmethionine-dependent transmethylation reactions. This compound is degraded to adenosine and L-homocysteine (Hcy) in the cell through the action of the enzyme AdoHcy hydrolase (EC 3.3.1.1.) (de la Haba & Cantoni, 1959). The view is held that the AdoHcy hydrolase reaction is the only source of Hcy in vertebrates (Cantoni & Chiang, 1980). Hcy is converted to cystathionine or is salvaged to methionine. In all tissues, except liver and kidney, the latter pathway is catalyzed by a single enzyme, which requires 5-methyl - tetrahydrofolate as methyl donor (Mudd & Levy, 1983). These metabolic relations are depicted in figure 1.

Interest in AdoHcy metabolism was stimulated by the pioneering work of Chiang et al. (1977) and Hershfield (1979) demonstrating that AdoHcy hydrolase is inhibited by various adenosine analogues and some analogues serve as substrate for this enzyme. Consequently, these adenosine analogues may induce high level of intracellular

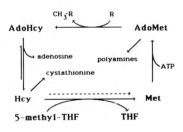

FIGURE 1: Metabolism of AdoHcy, Hcy and related compounds. THF, tetrahydrofolate.

263

nucleosidylhomocysteine, which in turn block AdoMet dependent methyltransfer reactions (for review, see Borchardt, 1980; Ueland, 1982). These observations form the basis for the concept of AdoHcy hydrolase as a target enzyme for adenosine analogues.

The first part of this article reviews data from our and other laboratories, on the effect of nucleoside analogues on AdoHcy catabolism *in vivo*. Because the biological consequences of AdoHcy accumulation have been thoroughly debated (Ueland, 1982), we have recently focused on the pharmacological perturbation of Hcy metabolism. This may be obtained by inhibitors of AdoHcy catabolism, but also by antifolate drugs leading to deprivation of reduced folates. Some recent data on this topic are presented.

INHIBITION OF ADOHCY CATABOLISM IN VIVO

Numerous nucleoside analogues function as inhibitors, inactivators (irreversible inhibitors) or substrates of isolated AdoHcy hydrolase (Ueland, 1982). However, effectiveness in cell free system does not ensure potent inhibition of AdoHcy catabolism in the intact cell. This is clearly demonstrated with 2-chloroadenosine and aristeromycin which are among the most effective inhibitors of AdoHcy hydrolase yet discovered (Chiang et al., 1981), but which have only a slight inhibitory effect on AdoHcy degradation in intact cells (Schanche et al., 1984b). Factors which may counteract the intracellular effect of an inhibitor of AdoHcy hydrolase, include slow transport, metabolic degradation, protection of the enzyme against inactivation by natural substrates and reactivation of inactivated enzyme (Schanche et al., 1984a,b). In addition, there may be species differences with respect to the response of AdoHcy hydrolase to a particular nucleoside analogue, as has been demonstrated for 3-deaza - adenosine (Kim et al., 1983) and neplanocin A (Borchardt et al., 1984; Glazer et al, 1984).

Some nucleosides, which are potent inhibitors of AdoHcy catabolism in intact cells, are listed in Table 1. Some properties assumed to be critical for their effectiveness *in vivo,* are also shown.

High affinity towards the target enzyme, AdoHcy hydrolase, and metabolic stability of the nucleoside analogue are factors which seem critical for inhibition of AdoHcy catabolism *in vivo*. This statement is supported by data listed in table 1. Active compounds include adenosine analogues modified in the purine and/or the sugar moiety. Substitution of the nitrogen in the 3 position of the purine skeleton with carbon seems to be well tolerated by the adenosine binding site of AdoHcy hydrolase, but the 3-deaza-analogues are not substrate of other adenosine metabolizing enzymes (Montgomery et al., 1982; Schanche et al., 1984b). Several active compounds modified in the ribose moiety are acyclic adenosine derivatives. These include D-eritadenine (Votruba & Holy, 1982;

Table 1

Some properties of nucleoside analogues acting as potent inhibitors of

AdoHcy catabolism in vivo [a]

Compound	Mode of action	Substrate of AK	ADA	Effect on cellular AdoHcy
c[3]Ado	Substrate and inhibitor ($K_i=4\mu M$)	NS	NS	marked increase
c[3]ara-A	Inhibitor	NS	NS	moderate increase
c[3]Ari	Inhibitor ($K_i=1nM, 4nM, 3\mu M$)	NS	NS	marked increase
ara-A	Inactivator and inhibitor ($K_i= 5\mu M$)	S	S	marked increase
D-Erit-A	Inactivator and inhibitor ($IC_{50}=7nM$)	NS	NS	marked increase
Neplanocin A	Inactivator and inhibitor ($K_i= 8\ nM$)	S	S	marked increase*
Ado-ox	Inactivator and inhibitor ($K_i= 3nM$)	S	S	marked increase

[a]Data taken from or quoted in the following articles: Patel-Thombre & Borchardt, 1985; Schanche et al.,1984a,b; Ueland, 1982; Votruba & Holy, 1982.
c[3]Ado, 3-deazaadenosine; c[3]ara-A, 3-deazaadenine arabinoside; c[3]-Ari, 3-deazaaristeromycin; ara-A, adenine arabinoside; D-Erit-A, D-eritadenine; Ado-ox, periodate oxidized adenosine; ADA, adenosine deaminase; AK, adenosine kinase; NS, not substrate; S, substrate;
*Inhibits AdoHcy catabolism in some cells (Borchardt et al., 1984).

Schanche et al., 1984a), adenosine dialdehyde (Hoffman, 1980; Bartel & Borchardt, 1984) and related compounds (Houston et al., 1985).

DISPOSITION OF ADOHCY IN CELLS EXPOSED TO NUCLEOSIDE ANALOGUES

Treatment of isolated cells or whole animals with adenosine analogues inhibiting AdoHcy hydrolase *in vivo*, leads to a massive accumulation of AdoHcy. This has been demonstrated for all compounds listed in table 1. Even in the presence of high concentrations of nucleoside analogues inactivating AdoHcy hydrolase, a small residual fraction of the intracellular enzyme seems to be protected from inactivation (Helland & Ueland, 1982a). The elevation of AdoHcy may be dependent on the degree of AdoHcy hydrolase inhibition. In addition, the elevation of AdoHcy is largely dependent on cell type or tissue under study. Inhibition of AdoHcy catabolism in whole liver or isolated hepatocytes leads to extremely high levels of AdoHcy, corresponding to a [AdoHcy]/[AdoMet] ratio higher than 1. The increase in AdoHcy in kidney is also pronounced, whereas in most other cell types, the AdoHcy content approaches but does not exceed the amount of AdoMet (Helland & Ueland, 1983). The marked AdoHcy response in liver and kidney is probably explained by the high turnover rate of AdoMet in these tissues (Hoffman, 1981), but may also partly be related to the presence of transmethylation reactions not sensitive to the inhibitory effect of AdoHcy (Helland & Ueland, 1983). The different AdoHcy response in different tissues explains the finding that some AdoMet dependent transmethylation reactions are nearly completely blocked in liver exposed to nucleoside analogues (Hoffman et al., 1980; Schanche et al., 1982), whereas only partial inhibition is observed in some cells (Bartel & Borchardt, 1984).

High intracellular level of AdoHcy induced by nucleoside analogues leads to AdoHcy egress into the extracellular medium. This has been demonstrated for isolated perfused liver (Hoffman et al., 1980), in whole animals (Helland & Ueland, 1983) and with isolated (Helland & Ueland,1982a) and cultured cells (Bartel & Borchardt, 1984; Carson et al.,1982; Helland & Ueland, 1982a). Cells exposed to a potent inhibitor of AdoHcy hydrolase for a few hours may release AdoHcy into the medium in amounts which equal that retained within the cells (Helland & Ueland, 1982a). Thus, a transport mechanism for AdoHcy may exist, which relieves the accumulation of AdoHcy under conditions where its catabolism is inhibited.

HOMOCYSTEINE IN TISSUES AND CELLS

Homocysteine is present in various tissues (Ueland et al., 1984). About 50 % could be extracted with acid and is referred to as free homocysteine whereas a portion is tightly associated with tissue proteins, probably via disulfide linkage. In the liver, free Hcy was localized to the soluble fraction, whereas bound Hcy was about equally distributed between the soluble and microsomal fractions (unpublished). Liver contained highest the level of Hcy; somewhat lower concentrations were observed in kidney and other tissues (Table 2).

Table 2
Distribution of homocysteine in rat tissues

Tissue	Free Hcy*	Bound Hcy*	Free/Bound*
	(nmol/g)	(nmol/g)	
Liver	4.57±1.09	3.04±0.28	1.47±0.25
Kidney	2.10±0.29	1.73±0.52	1.52±0.32
Spleen	1.62±0.31	0.53±0.02	3.15±0.90
Heart	1.70±0.24	1.10±0.12	1.60±0.20
Lung	1.87±0.18	1.40±0.12	1.36±0.13
Cerebellum	5.15±1.07	0.29±0.03	17.81±2.87
Cerebrum	0.78±0.17	0.33±0.05	2.72±0.70

*Mean of 6 determinations ± S.E.M.

The presence of homocysteine has been demonstrated in isolated hepatocytes (unpublished results), cultured fibroblasts (Ueland et al., 1985) and lymphocytes (German et al., 1983). In the hepatocytes, both free and bound Hcy could be demonstrated in proportions equal to those found in whole liver. Pulse-chase experiments with radioactive methionine labelled in the sulfur atom showed that there was isotope equilibrium between AdoHcy and free and bound Hcy in these cells. This finding is in accordance with the current view (Cantoni & Chiang, 1980) that AdoHcy is the source of Hcy and suggests that a rapid equilibrium exists between free and bound Hcy. When free and bound Hcy are regarded as a single pool, the half-life of Hcy in isolated rat hepatocytes was calculated to about 2 seconds.

Copious amounts of Hcy was released into the extracellular medium from both isolated liver cells and cultured cells, and the Hcy egress was greatly enhanced by addition of methionine to the cellular medium. Thus, the Hcy egress is probably dependent on the metabolic flux through the AdoHcy hydrolase pathway, which in turn is enhanced by the presence of excess methionine.

HOMOCYSTEINE IN TISSUES AND CELLS EXPOSED TO NUCLEOSIDE ANALOGUES

We have investigated the effect of injecting the drug combination ara-A plus 2'-deoxycoformycin into mice on free Hcy in various organs (Ueland et al., 1984). This treatment almost completely inactivated AdoHcy hydrolase in various tissues, and the amount of AdoHcy increased drastically. Notably, there was no decrease in the Hcy content in tissues, and in kidney a moderate increase in Hcy was in fact observed.

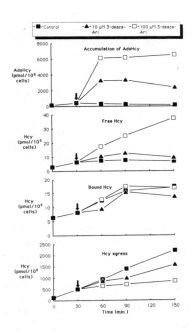

FIGURE 2: Disposition of endogenous Hcy by isolated hepatocytes following inhibition of AdoHcy catabolism by 3-deazaaristeromycin. Isolated rat hepatocytes (5×10^6 cells/ml) were preincubated with 200 μM methionine. After 30 minutes, the incubation medium was supplemented with either 10 μM or 100 μM 3-deaza-aristeromycin (arrow). Intracellular AdoHcy (upper panel), free Hcy, protein-bound Hcy and Hcy release into the extracellular medium were determined for the hepatocytes exposed to 3-deaza-aristeromycin and for control cells.

The observation that inhibition of AdoHcy degradation to Hcy is not associated with cellular depletion of Hcy (Ueland et al., 1984) raised several important questions on the source and metabolic fate of cellular Hcy. Answers to these questions were sought by investigating the effect of nucleoside analogues serving as inhibitors of AdoHcy hydrolase on the disposition of endogenous Hcy in isolated rat hepatocytes. The results obtained with 3-deazaaristeromycin are shown in figure 2. This compound is a potent inhibitor of intracellular AdoHcy hydrolase in these cells (Schanche et al., 1984b) and increases the AdoHcy content to extremely high levels in a dose dependent manner. Notably, 3-deaza-aristeromycin slightly increased both free and protein bound Hcy in isolated rat hepatocytes, and this effect was more pronounced in cells accumulating large amounts of AdoHcy. Furthermore, whereas control cells released Hcy into the medium, the Hcy egress was partly blocked in the presence of low levels of 3-deazaaristeromycin, and was almost totally inhibited by high levels of 3-deazaaristeromycin (Fig. 2). These data are in accordance with those obtained with whole animals injected with the drug combination ara-A plus 2'-deoxycoformycin (Ueland et al., 1984).

The amount of intracellular Hcy seems to be tightly regulated and to be under the influence of the cellular content of AdoHcy. When the production of Hcy is blocked this is compensated for by a reduction or total inhibition of export of Hcy into the extracellular medium. It is conceivable that intracellular Hcy is critical for some vital cellular function, and the Hcy export may be important for maintenance of cellular Hcy within certain limits. The Hcy egress may therefore be a measure of the intracellular balance between Hcy production and utilization.

Kim et al. (1982) have provided indirect evidence that the cytostatic activity of 3-deazaaristeromycin is mediated by inhibition of homocysteine synthesis required for the regeneration of tetrahydrofolate from 5-methyltetrahydro- folate. This conclusion was based on the observation that exogenous supplied homocysteine almost completely prevented the cytostatic activity of this nucleoside analogue.

HOMOCYSTEINE AND METHOTREXATE

Methotrexate is an antifolate drug which acts by inhibiting the enzyme dihydrofolate reductase; the enzyme responsible for regeneration of tetrahydrofolate from dihydrofolate (Jackson,1984). Methotrexate thereby induces cellular depletion of reduced folates, including 5-methyl - tetrahydrofolate, which serves as a methyl donor in the methionine synthase reaction (see figure 1). On the basis of these facts we investigated the effect of methotrexate on the disposition of endogenous homocysteine in cultured cells.

The mouse fibroblast cell line, C3H/10T1/2 Cl 8 (Cl 8) were less sensitive towards the cytotoxic effect of methotrexate than their malignant counterpart, MCA Cl 16 cells. Methotrexate increased the homocysteine secretion(up to 3 fold) from both cell types in a dose dependent manner, but about ten times higher concentrations were required for the enhancement of Hcy egress from the methotrexate resistant Cl 8 cells as compared with the sensitive Cl 16 cells. Thus, a correlation between Hcy egress and methotrexate cytotoxicity seems to exist. The effect of methotrexate on the release of Hcy into the extracellular medium was not associated with intracellular increase in AdoHcy. This suggests that intracellular Hcy is kept below the level required for reversal or inhibition of the AdoHcy hydrolase reaction. This is in accordance with the view that intracellular Hcy is tightly regulated.

The methotrexate dependent Hcy egress from Cl 16 cells is almost completely inhibited following "rescue" of these cells with 5-formyl - tetrahydrofolate, whereas a "rescue" therapy with thymidine plus

Ueland et al.

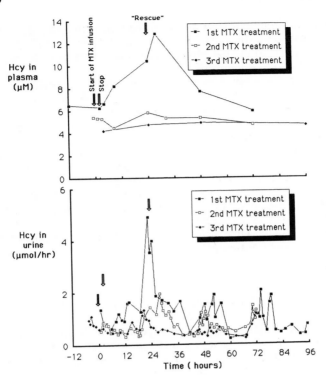

FIGURE 3: Total Hcy in plasma (upper panel) and urinary excretion of Hcy (lower panel) in a patient (K.A.L.) receiving high-dose treatment with MTX, followed by "rescue" with leucovorin (5-formyl-THF). The patient received infusion with high-dose MTX (220 mg/kg body weight) for 2 hours and "rescue" therapy with leucovorin (165 mg) at time 24 hours after initiation of MTX dosing. The treatment was repeated three times with 14 days of drug free intervals.

hypoxanthine (Jackson, 1984) had essentially no effect on the egress. Furthermore, cytotoxic agents other than methotrexate reduced rather than increased Hcy egress. These data show that stimulation of Hcy egress is not an effect of cytotoxic agents in general, but seems to be related to reduction of reduced folates relative to the metabolic demand.

Induction of homocysteine release from cells by methotrexate led us to investigate the homocysteine secretion in urine and Hcy content in plasma from patients receiving high-dose methotrexate treatment against malignant disease. The data obtained were compared with normal values (Refsum et al., 1985) for these parameters in humans.

In some patients a drastic increase of Hcy in plasma was observed a few hours after methotrexate infusion, and this plasma peak was often associated with the secretion of copious amounts of Hcy in the urine. The Hcy response declined progressively after each treatment. Typical data (from patient K.A.L.) are shown in figure 3. The Hcy response varied markedly from one patient to another; some patients showed an increase in plasma content whereas in others an increase in urinary secretion predominated. The amount of methionine in plasma from these patients did not show similar variations.

It is conceivable that the release of Hcy from cells into the extracellular media like culture medium, plasma or urine, is a measure of depletion of reduced folates in target cells and thereby the cytotoxic effects of methotrexate. In this case, monitoring the Hcy response may provide useful information on metabolic effects of methotrexate therapy. This possibility is further investigated.

PERSPECTIVES

There are increasing numbers of reports showing that biological effects of nucleoside analogues interacting with AdoHcy hydrolase can be dissociated from inhibition of AdoMet dependent transmethylation reactions, induced by nucleosidylhomocysteine. Such data have been provided for 3-deazaadenosine and 3-deazaaristeromycin (Aksamit et al., 1982,1983; Garcia-Castro et al., 1983; Zimmerman et al., 1984).

Competitive inhibitors, irreversible inactivators and substrates of AdoHcy hydrolase may have similar effects on the metabolism of AdoHcy; all these compounds induce massive accumulation of AdoHcy. However, it is conceivable that adenosine analogues which serve as substrates, may condense with endogenous Hcy, and thereby cause effects on Hcy metabolism quite different from those induced by compounds which merely block the conversion of AdoHcy to Hcy.

Inhibition of the AdoHcy hydrolase reaction may reduce the rate of formation of Hcy and thereby the metabolic reactions dependent on Hcy. These include the conversion of 5-methyltetrahydrofolate to tetrahydrofolate (Cantoni et al., 1981) and synthesis of methionine, cystathionine and cysteine (Fig. 1). Furthermore, Hcy or its protein-mixed disulfide may play a role in metabolic regulation, and inhibition of Hcy formation may therefore have biological effects not hitherto recognized.

Adenosine analogues interacting with AdoHcy hydrolase and antifolate drugs seem to have a common intracellular target, in that both classes of compounds interfere with Hcy metabolism, albeit in the opposite direction. This fact suggests interactions between adenosine analogues and antifolate drugs.

SUMMARY

1) Some adenosine analogues inhibit or inactivate the enzyme AdoHcy hydrolase. High affinity towards the intracellular enzyme and metabolic stability of the analogue are factors which seem critical for effectiveness *in vivo*.

2) Inhibition of AdoHcy hydrolase leads to accumulation of large amounts of intracellular AdoHcy, particularly in liver and kidney. Accumulation of AdoHcy is associated with release of copious amounts of AdoHcy into the extracellular medium.

3) Hcy is present in tissues as free Hcy and partly as Hcy associated with proteins (protein-bound Hcy). Hcy is exported into the medium from cultured cells or cells in suspension.

4) Inhibition of Hcy formation from AdoHcy by adenosine analogues is not associated with a reduction of the amount of Hcy in tissues or cells, but blocks the Hcy egress into the extracellular medium.

5) Hcy egress from cultured cells into the extracellular medium is greatly enhanced following exposure to the antifolate drug, methotrexate. The methotrexate dependent Hcy egress is probably related to cellular depletion of reduced folates, including 5-methyltetrahydrofolate required for the salvage of Hcy to methionine in most tissues.

6) The *in vitro* data (point 5) led us to investigate the amount of Hcy in extracellular media like plasma and urine from patients receiving high-dose methotrexate treatment against cancer. Both plasma content and urinary excretion of Hcy showed a transitory increase following methotrexate infusion. It is conceivable that the biological effects of methotrexate *in vivo* could be monitored from plasma and/or urinary Hcy.

REFERENCES

Aksamit, R.R., Backlund, P.S. and Cantoni, G.L. (1983) J. Biol. Chem. 258, 20-23.

Aksamit, R.R., Falk, W. and Cantoni, G.L. (1982) J. Biol. Chem. 257, 621-625.

Bartel, R.L. and Borchardt, R.T. (1984) Mol. Pharmacol. 25, 418-424.

Borchardt, R.T. (1980) J. Med Chem. 23, 347-356.

Borchardt, R.T., Keller, B.T., and Patel-Thombre, U. (1984) J. Biol. Chem. 259, 4353-4358.

Cantoni,G.L. and Chiang, P.K. (1980) in Natural Sulfur Compounds: Novel Biochemical and Structural Aspects (Cavallini, D., Gaull, G.E., and Zappia, V., Eds.) pp. 67-80, Plenum Press, New York and London.

Carson, D.A., Wasson, D.B., Lakow, E., and Kamatani, N. (1982) Proc. Natl. Acad. Sci. 79, 3848-3852.

Chiang, P.K., Guranowski, A. and Segall, J.E. (1981) Arch. Biochem. Biophys. 207, 175-184.

Chiang, P.K., Richard, H.H. and Cantoni, G.L. (1977) Mol. Pharmacol. 13, 939-947.

de la Haba, G. and Cantoni, G.L. (1959) J. Biol. Chem. 234, 603-608.

Garcia-Castro, I., Mato, J.M., Vasanthakumar, G., Wiesmann, W.P., Schiffmann, E. and Chiang, P.K. (1983) J. Biol. Chem. 258, 4345-4349.

German, D.C., Bloch, C.A. and Kredich, N.M. (1983) J. Biol.Chem. 258, 10997-11003.

Glazer, R.I. and Knode, M.C. (1984) J. Biol. Chem. 259, 12964-12969.

Helland, S. and Ueland, P.M. (1982a) Cancer Res. 42, 1130-1136.

Helland, S. and Ueland, P.M. (1982b) Cancer Res. 42, 2861-2866.

Helland, S. and Ueland, P.M. (1983) Cancer Res. 43, 1847-1850.

Hershfield, M.S. (1979) J. Biol. Chem. 254, 22-25.

Hoffman, J.L. (1980) Arch. Biochem. Biophys. 205, 132-135.

Hoffman, D.R., Marion, D.W., Cornatzer, W.E. and Duerre, J.A. (1980) J. Biol. Chem. 255, 10822-10827.

Houston, D.M., Dolence, E.K., Keller, B.T., Patel-Thombre, U. and Borchardt, R.T. (1985) J. Med. Chem. 28, 471-477.

Jackson, R.C. (1984) Pharmac. Ther. 25, 61-82.

Kim, I-K., Aksamit, R.R. and Cantoni, G.L. (1982) J. Biol. Chem. 257, 14726-14729.

Kim, I-K., Zhang, C-Y., Chiang, P.K. and Cantoni, G.L. (1983) Arch. Biochem. Biophys. 226, 65-72.

Montgomery, J.A., Clayton, S.J., Thomas, H.J., Shannon, W.M., Arnett, G., Bodner, A.J., Kim, I-K., Cantoni, G.L. and Chiang, P.K. (1982) J. Med. Chem. 25, 626-629.

Mudd, S.H. and Levy, H.L. (1983) in Metabolic Basis of Inherited Diseases (Standbury, J.B., Ed.) pp. 522-559, McGraw-Hill, New York.

Patel-Thombre, U. and Borchardt, R.T. (1985) Biochemistry 24, 1130-1136.

Refsum, H., Helland, S. and Ueland, P.M. (1985) Clin. Chem. 31, 624-628.

Schanche, J-S., Schanche, T. and Ueland, P.M. (1982) Biochim. Biophys. Acta 721, 399-407.

Schanche, J-S., Schanche, T., Ueland, P.M., Holy, A. and Votruba, I. (1984a) Mol. Pharmacol. 26, 553-558.

Schanche, J-S., Schanche, T., Ueland, P.M. and Montgomery, J.A. (1984b) Cancer Res. 44, 4297-4302.

Ueland, P.M. (1982) Pharmacol. Rev. 34, 223-253.

Ueland, P.M., Helland, S., Broch, O-J. and Schanche, J-S. (1984) J.Biol. Chem. 259, 2360-2364.

Ueland,. P.M., Refsum, H., Male, R. and Lillehaug, J.R. (1985) Cancer Res., submitted.

Votruba , I. and Holy, A. (1982) Collect. Czech. Chem. Commun. 47, 167-172.

Zimmerman, T.P., Iannone, M. and Wolberg, G. (1984) J. Biol. Chem. 259, 1122-1126.

REGULATION OF S-ADENOSYLMETHIONINE AND METHYLTHIOADENOSINE
METABOLISM IN METHYLTHIOADENOSINE PHOSPHORYLASE DEFICIENT
MALIGNANT CELLS

Dennis A. Carson
E. Olavi Kajander
Carlos J. Carrera
Hisashi Yamanaka
Taizo Iizasa
Masaru Kubota
Erik H. Willis
John A. Montgomery*

Scripps Clinic and Research Foundation
10666 North Torrey Pines Road
La Jolla, California 92037

*Southern Research Institute
Birmingham, Alabama 35255

The synthesis and metabolism of both polyamines and S-
adenosylmethionine (AdoMet) are important for cell growth
regulation. However, our understanding of the regulation
of polyamine and AdoMet metabolism in intact mammalian
cells is incomplete. 5'-deoxy-5'-methylthioadenosine
(abbreviated as MTA or MeSAdo) is the purine end product
of the polyamine biosynthetic pathway. Polyamines are
organic cations that all dividing cells produce in
abundance. Their exact metabolic functions are not known.
However, states of increased cellular proliferation, such
as cancer, are uniformly associated with accelerated rates
of polyamine synthesis (Pegg & McCann, 1982; Heby, et al.,
1976.

Exogenous MTA is cytostatic toward mammalian cells. The
nucleoside has been reported to have diverse effects on
cellular metabolism (Schlenk, 1983). Micromolar
concentrations of MTA inhibit spermine synthesis (Pajula

et al., 1979). Higher concentrations can interfere with transmethylation reactions, either directly or via inhibition of S-adenosylhomocysteine hydrolase (Ferro et al., 1981; Galletti et al., 1981). The relationship between the metabolic effects of MTA, and toxic effects of the nucleoside, are not clear.

Normally, mammalian cells degrade MTA via a specific enzyme, methylthioadenosine phosphorylase (MTAse) Pegg & Williams-Ashman, 1969). The two reaction products, adenine and 5-methylthioribose-1-phosphate, are reconverted to adenine nucleotides and methionine, respectively (Kamatani & Carson, 1981; Backlund & Smith, 1981).

Many human and murine leukemic cell lines, and some leukemia specimens taken directly from patients, entirely lack MTAse (Kamatani et al., 1981). In contrast, all normal cells and tissues are MTAse positive. Conceivably, the MTA that accumulates in the enzyme deficient neoplasms could alter polyamine and AdoMet metabolism.

With this background, our experiments have addressed the following issues: Is MTAse deficiency associated with a characteristic clinical syndrome or cytogenetic abnormality? What are the relationships between MTA, AdoMet, and polyamine metabolism in intact cells? How do MTAse deficient cells adapt to avoid the potential anti-proliferative effects of the nucleoside? Does resistance to MTA confer cross-resistance to other anti-metabolites?

Structural and Regulatory Aspects of the MTAse Enzyme.

In initial experiments, we (i) analyzed the expression of the enzyme deficient phenotype in intraspecies and interspecies somatic cell hybrids (Kamatani et al., 1984; Carrera et al., 1984), and (ii) mapped the structural gene for human MTAse (Carrera et al., 1984)

The murine L-1210 lymphoblastoid cell line, and the L cell fibroblast line, are both MTAse deficient (Toohey, 1977; Carson, D. unpublished). We selected azaguanine variants of L-1210 cells that lacked hypoxanthine phosphoribosyltransferase. These enzyme deficient cells were fused with normal nucleated murine spleen cells.

Somatic cell hybrids were selected in hypoxanthine-aminopterin-thymidine medium, according to standard techniques. Sixteen clones were selected and analyzed for chromosome number, and the activity of MTAse. Notably, all hybrid clones that contained a full complement of chromosomes from each parental cell line were enzyme positive. In contrast, most hybrid clones maintaining one or only a few extra chromosomes were enzyme negative. Thus, the MTAse deficient phenotype was expressed in a recessive fashion in intraspecies cell hybrids.

Subsequently, we measured levels of the enzyme in interspecies somatic cell hybrids prepared by fusing MTAse deficient mouse L cell lines with human fibroblasts (Carrera et al., 1984). In the hybrid clones, MTAse activity segregated concordantly with adenylate kinase-1, a marker for human chromosome 9, but not with enzyme markers for any other human chromosome. Importantly, among hybrid clones derived from human fibroblasts with a reciprocal translocation between chromosomes 9 and 17, MTAse activity was confined to cells containing the 9 pter ----> 9 q12 region. These results indicate that the structural gene for human MTAse, designated MTAP, can be assigned to the 9 pter ----> 9q12 region of human chromosome 9. They raise the possibility that deletions or translocations affecting this chromosomal region might be associated with the enzyme deficient state.

Selection and Characterization of MTAse Deficient Lymphoblasts.

The effects of the loss of MTAse on cell growth and metabolism cannot readily be ascertained by using naturally enzyme deficient cell lines that may differ in multiple ways from MTAse positive cells. Biochemical genetics provides a means to determine the exact metabolic consequences of MTAse deficiency. Therefore, we perfected a technique for the selection of MTAse deficient mutants, and characterized two MTAse deficient clones derived from the transplantable murine T lymphoma cell line R1.1 (Kubota et al., 1983).

Briefly, MTAse deficient clones were selected by "tritium suicide". Mutagenized cells were briefly suspended in a medium containing 5'-chloro-[2,8-^{3}H] adenosine, an MTA analog (Savarese et al., 1981). The treated cells were washed, frozen in liquid nitrogen for two weeks to allow radiation damage to accumulate, and finally were thawed and cloned. The death of cells incubated with 5'-Cl[2,8-^{3}H] adenosine requires: (i) the transport of the nucleoside into the cells, (ii) its cleavage by MTAse to yield [2,8-^{3}H] adenine, (iii) the conversion of adenine to AMP and (iv) the further phosphorylation and incorporation of [2,8-^{3}H] AMP into nucleic acid. Cells defective in any step of this pathway would be expected to survive the "tritium suicide" procedure. R1.1 variants deficient in each of the four steps listed above were obtained after the final cloning. Remarkably, MTAse deficiency was the most common abnormality, occurring in approximately one-third of the clones. By comparison adenine phosphoribosyltransferase deficient clones were ten-fold less frequent.

The MTAse deficient variants excreted substantial amounts of MTA into the culture medium (as much as 0.32 mol/hr/mg protein) (Kamatani & Carson, 1980; Kubota et al., 1983. The amount of MTA in the medium of MTAse deficiency lymphoma cells eventually rose to 3-5μM. This concentration of MTA was sufficient to impede eventually the growth of the lymphoma cells (Kubota et al., 1983). The synthesis and release of MTA was dose-dependently blocked by two inhibitors of polyamine synthesis, α-difluoromethylornithine (DFMO) and methylglyoxal-bis-guanylhydrazone (MGBG) (Kamatani & Carson, 1981).

A mutant lymphoblastoid cell line was selected that was deficient in adenine phosphoribosyltransferase (APRT). The APRT deficient cells generated adenine at a pace equivalent to the rate of MTA formation by cells lacking MTAse (Kamatani & Carson, 1981; Kamatani et al., 1984). Furthermore, cells deficient in MTAse and APRT did not produce adenine at all. These results established that mammalian cells generate adenine at a considerable rate, and only via the polyamine-MTAse pathway.

MTAse deficient cells maintained in tissue culture do not catabolize MTA generated endogenously, but rather excrete the thioether nucleoside into the extracellular space. MTAse deficient tumors in vivo would be expected to behave similarly. However, because only the tumor cells lack the specific phosphorylase, the plasma concentrations of MTA should be a function of (i) the rate of polyamine synthesis by the tumor, (ii) the rate of MTA cleavage by enzyme positive normal cells, and (iii) the rate of clearance of MTA from the intravascular space. In patients with a large tumor burden, or with a rapidly proliferating neoplastic clone, synthesis might exceed metabolism. In such circumstances, MTA should accumulate in the plasma and urine.

The results of pilot studies support this contention. A sensitive fluorometic assay was used for the detection of nanomolar concentrations of MTA in plasma and urine. It involves (i) the rapid fractionation of crude specimens on acetonitrile-activated disposable Sep-pak C_{18} columns, (ii) the derivatization of adenine containing compounds with 2-chloroacetaldehyde, as described by Leonard and Tolman (1975), and (iii) measurement of the resulting fluorescent etheno-MTA derivative following high performance liquid chromatography.

With this method, we compared plasma MTA levels during the in vivo growth of the R1.1 murine T lymphoma cell lines, and the MTAse deficient mutant selected in this laboratory. Plasma MTA levels increased progressively with time only in animals carrying the MTAse deficient lymphoma. In other experiments, the nucleoside was also detectable in the urine. Hence, as the tumor burden enlarges, the production of MTA exceeds the catabolic capacity of normal tissues.

Regulation of MTA and L-Homocysteine Production

The consumption of AdoMet during polyamine synthesis and transmethylation reactions yields stoichiometric amounts of MTA and S-adenosylhomocysteine, respectively. The S-adenosylhomocysteine subsequently is cleaved to adenosine plus L-homocysteine. Both pathways of AdoMet metabolism are essential for cell growth and function, and could play a role in malignant transformation.

Information concerning the regulation of AdoMet and polyamine metabolism in viable cells under changing growth conditions is meager. Intracellular polyamine levels, and the activities of ornithine decarboxylase and AdoMet decarboxylase, have been reported to change considerably during the cell growth cycle (Pegg & McCann, 1982). However, the intracellular polyamine content reflects a balance between synthesis, degradation, excretion, and uptake. Furthermore, measurements of enzyme activities in crude extracts provide only indirect information concerning metabolic rates in intact cells.

We demonstrated that both anchorage-dependent and anchorage-independent MTAse deficient malignant cells excreted MTA and L-homocysteine into the culture medium (Iizasa & Carson, 1985). In accord with earlier data (German et al, 1983; Kamatani & Carson, 1982), the cells did not catabolize either compound appreciably. MTA and L-homocysteine are products of polyamine synthesis and transmethylation reactions, respectively. Therefore, the measurement of the time-dependent accumulation of MTA and L-homocysteine in the culture medium enabled us to estimate for the first time the actual rates of both polyamine synthesis and transmethylation reactions under dynamic growth conditions.

The two AdoMet consuming pathways proceeded quickly, when compared to the cellular AdoMet content. The intracellular AdoMet sufficed for only 5-10 minutes of polyamine synthesis and transmethylation reactions.

The kinetics of polyamine synthesis and transmethylation reactions during the cell growth cycle were strikingly different. MTA production (polyamine synthesis) was maximal early after the release of malignant lymphoblasts from density dependent growth arrest. By contrast, L-homocysteine formation (transmethylation reactions) was porportional to the specific growth rate, and reached a peak during mid-exponential phase, at which time MTA excretion was falling.

Effects of MTA on polyamine and AdoMet metabolism in intact cells.

The factors that control the rate of polyamine synthesis in mammalian cells have been studied intensively, but are still not well understood (Pegg & McCann, 1982). Literally hundreds of papers have documented that growth promoting stimuli lead to a rapid increase in the activities of ornithine decarboxylase and AdoMet decarboxylase. However, when general protein synthesis increases, enzymes that have a high rate of synthesis and degradation always respond with a rapid and marked rise in activity (Schimke & Doyle, 1970). By contrast, proteins with a slow turnover rate increase less in activity, and at a much later time. Hence, the observed elevations in ornithine decarboxylase and AdoMet decarboxylase that are induced by growth stimuli are entirely expected, and reveal little specifically about the actual factors that influence the enzyme activities.

The end products of the polyamine biosynthetic pathway are spermidine and spermine, and MTA. The addition of spermidine to mammalian cells has been shown to decrease the activities of ornithine decarboxylase and AdoMet decarboxylase (Mamont et al., 1981). Initially, we noted that as little as 3 μM MTA increased putrescine levels in MTAse deficient lymphoma cells (Kamatani & Carson, 1980). However, we could not ascertain if the elevation reflected a block in putrescine consumption, or an increase in synthesis. Moreover, we needed to determine whether the accumulation was secondary to changes in spermidine and spermine pools.

To address these issues, we measured the time dependent effects of MTA on (i) ornithine decarboxylase and AdoMet decarboxylase activities, (ii) putrescine and polyamine levels, and (iii) decarboxylated AdoMet and S-adenosylhomocysteine levels in MTAse deficient cells (Kubota et al, 1985). In viable lymphoblasts, the addition of MTA elicited within one hour an increase in the activities of both decarboxylases, and a subsequent rise in putrescine and decarboxylated AdoMet levels. S-adenosylhomocysteine did not rise appreciably. The increased decarboxylase activities occurred prior to any detectable changes in intracellular polyamine pools, but simultaneously with a reduced velocity of spermine synthesis, as estimated by precursor-product incorporation studies with radioactive ornithine. DFMO, an inhibitor of ornithine decarboxylase, did not prevent the MTA triggered increase in AdoMet decarboxylase. MGBG, an inhibitor of S-adenosylmethionine decarboxylase, did not deter the MTA-induced rise in ornithine decarboxylase. The altered enzyme activities were not a non-specific consequence of

changes in cell growth kinetics, because (i) they were
completed several hours before cell proliferation
declined, and (ii) the same changes were observed in
secondary mutants impervious to the anti-proliferative
effects of MTA.

These experiments indicate that MTA-induced perturbations
in the velocity of spermine synthesis, and perhaps MTA
itself, can regulate ornithine decarboxylase and AdoMet
decarboxylase activities independently of growth state.
In the MTAse deficient leukemias, the accumulation of MTA
could inappropriately stimulate an increase in the
activities of both enzymes. Both ornithine decarboxylase
and AdoMet decarboxylase are thought to play a role in
the initiation of cell proliferation. Conceivably, the
induction of the two enzymes by MTA could provide a
natural pressure for the selection of MTAse deficient
leukemias.

AdoMet Metabolism in MTA-Adenosine Resistant Mutant Cells

Three to five µM MTA inhibited by 50% the growth of the
MTAse deficient mutant R1.1 lymphoblasts selected in our
laboratory (Kubota et al., 1983). In contrast, 30-100µM
MTA was required to inhibit similarly the proliferation of
naturally MTAse deficient murine and human leukemia cell
lines (White et al., 1983). These results emphasized a
distinct difference between the two types of MTAse
deficient malignant cell populations.

Information concerning the mechanism of MTA toxicity
toward mammalian cells is scanty. As discussed earlier,
MTA is a potent inhibitor of spermine synthase (Ki about
1-2 µM) (Pajula et al., 1979). These MTA concentrations
are routinely achieved during the growth of MTAse
deficient cells (Kamatani & Carson, 1980). One hundred to
1,000 fold higher concentrations of the thioether
nucleoside have been reported to block AdoMet-dependent
transmethylation reactions, either directly or indirectly
via inhibition of S-adenosylhomocysteine hydrolase (Ferro
et al., 1981; Galletti et al., 1981). The true importance
of these effects in viable cells has not been established.

Recently, we have selected and characterized an adenosine
resistant mutant of an adenosine kinase deficient murine

lymphoblastoid cell line (Kajander et al., manuscript in preparation). Surprisingly, the mutant is cross resistant to the anti-proliferative actions of MTA, 3-deaza-adenosine, adenine, and many adenine nucleosides. Moreover, the mutant cells are also resistant to cycloleucine, ethionine, (+)-2-aminobicyclo-[2.1.1]hexane-2-carboxylic acid (ABCHA), and other inhibitors of AdoMet synthesis (Sufrin & Lombardini, 1982). This phenotype has remained stable during more than one year of continuous passage in tissue culture.

Initial biochemical analyses of the resistant cells have shown that the membrane transport of nucleosides and methionine is entirely normal. However, when compared to MTA sensitive lymphoblasts, the mutant cells have 5-7 fold increased levels of AdoMet. This change reflects an augmented activity of methionine adenosyltransferase, the enzyme catalyzing the synthesis of AdoMet from methionine and ATP. These preliminary results suggest that the anti-proliferative effects of adenosine, MTA, and several other adenine nucleosides are related to AdoMet metabolism. Apparently, an increase in endogenous AdoMet pools can render mammalian cells cross-resistant to a variety of compounds that affect AdoMet-dependent pathways.

Summary.

Our results may be summarized as follows:

(i) MTAse activity is easily detectable in all normal human tissues. Some leukemic cell clones obtained directly from patients, as well as many human malignant cell lines, entirely lack the enzyme.

(ii) The structural gene for human MTAse is encoded in the 9pter----> 9q12 region of human chromosome 9, which is known to contain a heritable fragile site. The enzyme deficiency behaves as a recessive characteristic in intraspecies and interspecies somatic cell hybrids.

(iii) The loss of MTAse causes the rapid accumulation of MTA, at a pace equivalent to the quantitative rate of polyamine synthesis. MTAse positive cells, but not enzyme deficient tumors, recycle endogenously generated MTA to ATP and methionine. In dividing cells, the conversion of MTA to methionine is considerable, and may exceed in quantitative importance the homocysteine to methionine biosynthetic pathway.

(iv) In MTAse deficient leukemia cells, MTA can selectively augment the activities of ornithine decarboxylase and AdoMet decarboxylase, the rate limiting enzymes in the polyamine biosynthetic pathway.

(v) MTAse deficient mutant lymphoma cells selected in the laboratory are much more sensitive to the anti-proliferative effects of MTA than are naturally arising MTAse deficient leukemias. Secondary mutants, with an increased rate of AdoMet synthesis, are cross-resistant to the anti-proliferative effects of several different compounds, including adenosine, MTA, adenine, and cycloleucine.

Acknowledgment

This research was supported in part by grant GM 23200 from the National Institutes of Health and by grants CA 35048 and CA 41563 from the National Cancer Institute. This is publication number 3998BCR from the Scripps Clinic and Research Foundation.

References

Backlund, P.S. Jr. and Smith, R.A. (1981) J. Biol. Chem. 256, 1533.

Carrera, C.J., Eddy, R.L., Shows, T.B. and Carson, D.A. (1984) Proc. Natl. Acad. Sci. USA 81, 2665.

Ferro, A.J., Vandenbark, A.A. and MacDonald, M.R. (1981) Biochem. Biophys. Res. Commun., 100, 523.

Galletti, P., Oliva, A., Manna, C., Della Ragione, F. and Carteni-Farina, M. (1981) FEBS Lett 126, 236.

German, D.C., Block, C.A. and Kredich, N.M. (1983) J. Biol. Chem. 258, 7288.

Heby, O., Marton, L.J., Wilson, C.B., and Martinez, H.M. (1975) J. Cell. Physiol. 86, 511.

Iizasa, T. and Carson, D.A. (1985) Biochim. Biophys. Acta 844, 280.

Kamatani, N. and Carson, D.A. (1980) Cancer Res. 40, 4178.

Kamatani, N. and Carson, D.A. (1981) Biochim. Biophys. Acta 675, 344.

Kamatani, N. and Carson, D.A. (1982) Intl. Arch. Allergy Appl. Immunol. 68, 84.

Kamatani, N., Kubota, M., Willis, E.H., Frincke, L.A. and Carson, D.A. (1984) Adv. Exp. Med. Biol. 165B, 83.

Kamatani, N., Nelson-Rees, W.A. and Carson, D.A. (1981) Proc. Natl. Acad. Sci. USA 78, 1219.

Kubota, M., Kajander, E.O. and Carson, D.A. (1985) Cancer Res., in press.

Kubota, M., Kamatani, N. and Carson, D.A. (1983) J. Biol. Chem. 258, 7822.

Leonard, N.J. and Tolman, G.L. (1975) Ann. N.Y. Acad. Sci. 255, 43.

Mamont, P.S., Joder-Ohlenbusch, A-M, Nussli, M., Grove, J. (1981) Biochem. J. 196, 411.

Pajula, R.-L., Raina, A. and Eloranta, T. (1979) Eur. J. Biochem. 101, 619.

Pegg, A.E. and McCann, P.P. (1982) Am. J. Physiol. 243, C212.

Pegg, A.E. and Williams-Ashman, H.G. (1969) Biochem. J. 115, 241.

Savarese, T.M., Crabtree, G.W. and Parks, R.E., Jr. (1981) Biochem. Pharmacol., 30, 189.

Schimke, R.T. and Doyle, D. (1970) Ann. Rev. Biochem. 39, 929.

Schlenk, F. (1983) Adv. Enzym. 54, 195.

Sufrin, J.R. and Lombardini, J.B. (1982) Mol. Pharmacol.,
22; 752.

Toohey, J.I. (1977) Biochem. Biophys. Res. Com. 78, 1273.

White, M.W., Resiol, M.K. and Ferro, A.J. (1983) Biochim.
Biophys. Acta 762, 405.

PURIFICATION AND PROPERTIES OF MAMMALIAN 5'-METHYLTHIOADENOSINE PHOSPHORYLASE AND BACTERIAL 5'-METHYLTHIOADENOSINE NUCLEOSIDASE: PHARMACOLOGICAL IMPLICATIONS AND PERSPECTIVES.

Vincenzo Zappia, Fulvio Della Ragione and Maria Cartenì-Farina.
Department of Biochemistry of Macromolecules
I Medical School, University of Naples,
Via Costantinopoli 16, 80138, Napoli, Italy

A successful approach to antibacterial therapy is generally based on enzymatic and metabolic differences between eukaryotes and prokaryotes. Indeed comparative studies have yielded, so far, a rich harvest of clinically efficacious antibacterial drugs characterized by low toxicity.

In this respect, the well-defined differences between the catabolism of the sulfur nucleoside, 5'-methylthioadenosine (MTA), in eukaryotes and prokaryotes are of pharmacological interest, also considering the numerous biological effects of this thioether reported in Literature (Zappia et al., 1980; Wolford et al., 1981; Pegg et al., 1981; Williams-Ashman et al., 1982; Raina et al. 1982; Cartenì-Farina et al., 1983).

MTA, which is ubiquitously distributed in mammalian tissues and bacterial cells, is formed from S-adenosylmethionine (AdoMet) through several pathways. Among them polyamine biosynthesis represents the major pathway of MTA formation in eukaryotes (Kamatani and Carson, 1981), while in prokaryotes the synthesis of 7,8-pelargonic acid and 3-(3-amino-carboxypropyl)uridine are also relevant in this respect (Stoner and Eisenberg, 1975; Nishimura et al., 1974). Furthermore, in plant tissues the thioether is also produced during the synthesis of ethylene, a plant

287

Table 1.   MTA-cleaving enzymes in prokaryotes an eukaryotes

ENZYMATIC SOURCE	REACTION MECHANISM	PURIFICATION (fold)	REFERENCES
EUKARYOTES			
Human Placenta	Phosphorolytic (MTA)	372	G. Cacciapuoti et al., 1978
"	"	29,700	F. Della Ragione et al., 1985b
Human Prostate	"	341	V. Zappia et al., 1978
Human Lymphocytes	"	13	M. White et al., 1982
Rat Liver	"	112	A.J. Ferro et al., 1982
Rat Lung	"	30	D.L. Garbers, 1978
Bovine Liver	"	471	M.K. Riscoe and A.J. Ferro, 198∠
HL-60 Cells	"	35	T.M. Savarese et al., 1985
Drosophila melanogaster	Phosphorolytic (MTA)	24	L. Shugart et al., 1979
Ochromonas malhamensis	Hydrolytic (MTA)	-	Y. Sugimoto et al., 1976
Lupineus luteus seeds	Hydrolytic (MTA)	8,943	A.B. Guranowski et al., 1981
Vinca Rosea	"	15	C. Baxter et al., 1973
Tomatoes	"	-	Y.-B. Yu et al., 1979
PROKARYOTES			
Escherichia coli	Hydrolytic (MTA,AdoHcy)	160	J.A. Duerre, 1962
"	"	220	A.J. Ferro et al., 1976
"	"	9,810	F. Della Ragione et al., 1985a
ARCHAEBACTERIA			
Caldariella acidophila	Phosphorolytic (MTA)	320	M. Carteni-Farina et al., 1979

hormone (Adams and Yang, 1979).

The molecule does not accumulate in the cell (Della Ragione et al., 1981; Zappia et al., 1983a), since it is rapidly metabolized by very effective enzymatic systems (Table 1). A hydrolytic cleavage of the molecule occurs in prokaryotes, plants and protozoa (Shapiro and Mather, 1958; Sugimoto et al., 1976; Guranowski et al, 1981),while a phosphorolytic breakdown of the thioether, leading to 5-methylthioribose-1-phosphate (MTR-1-P) and adenine, is operative in mammals, insects and archaebacteria (Pegg and Williams-Ashman, 1969; Zappia et al., 1978; Shugart et al., 1979; Cartenì-Farina et al., 1979; Zappia et al., 1983b). It is noteworthy in this respect that prokaryotic MTA nucleosidase is also responsible for the cleavage of S-adenosyl-homocysteine (AdoHcy) (Duerre, 1962).

The potential role of these enzymes as specific targets for chemotherapeutic agents prompted us to investigate their molecular properties and catalytic mechanism. Thus, the purification to homogeneity of MTA phosphorylase from human placenta (Della Ragione et al., 1985a) and AdoHcy/MTA nucleosidase from Escherichia coli (Della Ragione et al., 1985b), recently performed in our laboratory, gave us the opportunity to identify and characterize selective inhibitors of potential pharmacological use.

BACTERIAL ADOHCY/MTA NUCLEOSIDASE

Historical Survey and Purification

AdoHcy/MTA nucleosidase has been reported to occur in E. coli as well as in other bacteria including S. typhymurium and A. aerogenes (Shapiro and Mather, 1958; Duerre, 1962; Ferro et al., 1976). However, at present no extensive studies on its distribution in bacteria have been carried out.

As reported in Table 1, the nucleosidase has been partially purified from E. coli by Duerre (1962) and Ferro et al. (1976). Recently, the enzyme has been purified to homogeneity in our laboratory by using, as key step,

Table 2.   Purification of E. coli AdoHcy/MTA nucleosidase

Step	Total Protein (mg)	Specific activity (units/mg)	Purification (fold)	Yield (%)
Supernatant at 15,000xg	12,000	0.038	1	100
Ammonium sulfate (40–60%)	8,300	0.045	1.2	81
DEAE Sephadex	500	0.7	15.5	76
Hydroxyapatite	70	4.2	110	64
Sephacryl S–200	15	15.3	400	50
SFH Sepharose	0.5	373	9,810	40

1 Unit is the amount of the enzyme which cleaves 1 μmole of MTA/min at 37°C
(Della Ragione et al. 1985a)

affinity   chromatography   on   S-formycinylhomocysteine(SFH)-
Sepharose (Della Ragione at al., 1985a) (Table 2).

Molecular and Kinetic Properties

Several physical and kinetic properties of the
homogeneous enzyme are reported in Table 3: the nucleosidase
has a molecular weight of 26,500 and is composed by a single
polypeptide chain. The Mr value is slightly lower than that
previously reported by Ferro et al. (1976) (31,000), with a
220-fold purified enzyme.

The specific activity of the pure enzyme (i.e. 373
μmoles of MTA and 156 μmoles of AdoHcy cleaved for min per
mg of protein) is more than 300-fold higher than that of
homogeneous mammalian AdoHcy hydrolase (Richards et al.,
1978; Palmer and Abeles, 1979; Ueland and Saebo, 1979;
Fujoka and Takata, 1981) and significantly higher than that
of highly purified eukaryotic MTA phosphorylase (Cacciapuoti
et al. 1978; Riscoe and Ferro, 1984; Della Ragione et al.
1985b).

The enzyme has a remarkably high affinity for MTA (Km

Table 3.   Molecular and catalytic properties of E. coli
            AdoHcy/MTA nucleosidase

Specific activity	373 units/mg of protein (MTA)
	156 units/mg of protein (AdoHcy)
Molecular weight	26,500
Turnover number	9.32×10^3 (MTA)
	3.9×10^3 (AdoHcy)
Stokes radius	2.1 nm
Protein structure	Monomeric
Isoelectric point	5.1
Kinetic constants	Km (MTA) 0.43 μM
	Km (AdoHcy) 4.3 μM
	Ki(Adenine) 210 μM

1 Unit is the amount of enzyme which cleaves 1 μmole of
substrate per min at 37° C

0.4 μM) as for AdoHcy (Km 4.3 μM) (Della Ragione et al.,
1985a). It is noteworthy that considerably higher Km values
for MTA (1.8 mM) and AdoHcy (3 mM) have been previously
reported by Duerre (1962). Such a discrepancy is probably
due to the different sensitivity of the employed assay
methods as well as to the extent of purification.
Conversely, the Michaelis constant for MTA extrapolated by
Ferro et al. (1976) (0.31 μM) agrees very well with the
kinetic constant of the homogeneous enzyme. Moreover the
Vmax/Km ratio, which is a useful probe to evaluate the
relative efficiency towards the two substrates, is 867 for
MTA and 36 for AdoHcy, thus suggesting that the
nucleosidase is more effective towards MTA. However, the
lack of information on the cellular content of AdoHcy and
MTA in bacteria prevents conclusive inferences regarding the
in vivo efficiency of the system.
    The reaction is virtually irreversible both when
tested with a partially purified enzyme (Duerre, 1962) and
with the homogeneous enzyme (Della Ragione et al., 1985c).
    The enzyme is highly specific as far as substrate
requirements are concerned. Among the analogs tested, only

Table 4. <u>Inhibitors of E. coli AdoHcy/MTA nucleosidase</u>

Analog	I_{50} (μM)	Ki (nM)
5'-Methylthioformycin	0.06	28
5'-Chloroformycin	0.4	32
S-Formycinylhomocysteine	0.02	9.8
5'-Methylthiotubercidin	7.6	4,100
S-Tubercidinylhomocysteine	3.3	1,900
5'-Methylthio-3-deazaadenosine	80	33,000
5'-Isobutylthio-3-deazaadenosine	15	8,100

The I_{50} values were calculated employing MTA as substrate at a concentration of 0.8 μM. The Ki were extrapolated using MTA as variable substrate (Della Ragione <u>et al.</u>, 1985a).

5'-isobutylthioadenosine and 5'-n-butylthioadenosine are actively cleaved. These data are in good agreement with those reported by Ferro <u>et al.</u> (1976) on a number of 5'-modified analogs. Conversely, the replacement of N(7) or N(3) by a methinic radical as well as the substitution of the imidazole moiety by a pyrazole ring results in a complete loss of activity. These data indicate that the structural integrity of adenine is required for the catalytic activity, while the chemical nature of 5'-substituent is less relevant.

The analogs resistant to the enzymatic cleavage have been tested as inhibitors and the results are reported in Table 4. The tubercidinyl analogs exert a significant competitive inhibition, thus suggesting that N(7) is not relevant in the recognition process, while it is critical in the catalytic mechanism. This result indicates that the catalytic mechanism requires as essential step the protonation of the N(7) atom of the substrate in analogy with the mechanism postulated for acid hydrolysis of adenosine (Garrett and Mehta, 1972). The powerful inhibition exerted by the formycinyl derivatives is probably related to the occurrence in their purine moiety of a N(7) protonated at a physiological pH (Ward <u>et al.</u>, 1969), thus resembling the hypothesized transition-state.

EUKARYOTIC MTA PHOSPHORYLASE

Distribution in tissues and cells

MTA phosphorylase is distributed in a large number of eukaryotic tissues (Table 1). The enzyme has been identified for the first time by Pegg and Williams-Ashman in rat ventral prostate (1969): the cleavage of MTA was found to be dependent upon orthophosphate and the arsenate was able to replace phosphate, thus suggesting a phosphorolytic mechanism.

Following this report, MTA phosphorylase has been described and partially characterized in several human (Cacciapuoti et al., 1978; Zappia et al., 1978) and rat tissues (Garbers, 1978; Ferro et al., 1979), in human and murine cultured cell lines (Toohey, 1978; White et al., 1982) and in Drosophila melanogaster (Shugart, 1979). More recently, the product of the reaction was identified as 5-methylthioribose-1-phosphate, thus confirming the phosphorolytic nature of the reaction (Ferro et al., 1979).

It is noteworthy that several malignant cell lines lacking this activity have been identified (Toohey, 1978; Kamatani and Carson, 1981).

Purification and properties of MTA phosphorylase

In spite of the large number of the studies on MTA phosphorylase, the enzyme has been purified to homogeneity only recently (Della Ragione et al., 1985b). The procedure, developed in our laboratory, employs, as essential steps, covalent chromatography on organomercurial-agarose and anion exchange on Mono Q (Table 5).

As indicated in Fig. 1a, the molecular weight of the enzyme is 98,000. This value is in excellent agreement with previously reported data (Cacciapuoti et al., 1978; Ferro et

Table 5. Purification of human placenta 5'-methylthioadenosine phosphorylase

STEP	PROTEIN (mg)	SPECIFIC ACTIVITY (units/mg)	PURIFICATION (fold)	YIELD (%)
Supernatant at 15,000 g	29,000	0.00035	1	100
Ammonium sulfate (55-75%)	16,000	0,00061	1,8	97
Acetone (40-60%)	3,045	0,0031	8,8	93
DEAE Sephacel	725	0.077	220	55
Hydroxyapatite	10.38	0.43	1,245	44
Agarose organomer-curial	0.487	5.7	14,800	25
Mono Q	0.22	10.2	29,700	23

1 unit of enzyme is the amount of protein which cleaves 1 μmol of MTA/min

al. 1979) with the only exception of rat lung (45,000)
(Garbers, 1978).

Polyacrylamide gel electrophoresis under denaturating
conditions indicates that the enzyme is composed by three
apparently identical subunits (Mr 32,500) (Fig 1b).

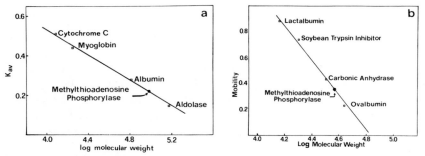

Fig. 1. Determination of the molecular weight of MTA
phosphorylase by gel filtration (a) and by sodium
dodecylsulfate/polyacrylamide gel electrophoresis (b).

It is worth noting in this respect that the homologous enzyme, purine nucleoside phosphorylase, has a similar molecular structure (Kim et al., 1968) which leads to the hypothesis of a common gene for the two phosphorylases.

The enzyme does not require for its activity any specific ion or cofactor and reducing agents, i.e. dithiothreitol, mercaptoethanol or glutathione are necessary for maximal activity. Moreover, it is effectively inhibited by sulphydryl-blocking agents, thus suggesting the involvement of -SH groups in the substrate binding or in the catalytic mechanism (Cacciapuoti et al., 1978; Zappia et al., 1978).

The rate of phosphorolysis is markedly increased by temperature. Up to 67°C the reaction was linear throughout 30 min incubation, whereas at 77°C the velocity is linear only for 15 min. These results, in excellent agreement with those reported by White et al. (1982) on the enzyme from human lymphocytes, probably depend on a significant protection exerted by MTA against thermal inactivation. Indeed, as reported in Fig. 2, preincubation at temperature higher than 55°C results in a loss of enzymatic activity, while 1 mM MTA significantly protects the enzyme.

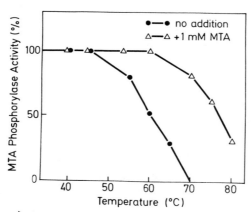

Fig. 2. Effect of MTA on the thermal inactivation of MTA phosphorylase. The enzyme was preincubated at the indicated temperatures for 15 min in absence (●—●) and presence of 1 mM MTA (△—△) and then assayed at 37°C.

Equilibrium studies and kinetic parameters

The equilibrium constant of the reaction has been calculated by incubating the enzyme with different amounts of MTA and phosphate. The reaction was monitored in the direction of phosphorolysis until no further production of MTR-1-P or adenine was detectable.From the concentration of substrates and products at equilibrium a Keq of 1.39×10^{-2} at 37°C was extrapolated.

The reversibility of the reaction has been directly demonstrated by incubating adenine and MTR-1-P in the presence of the purified MTA phosphorylase (Fig. 3).

The kinetic constants for the phosphorolytic and synthetic reaction are reported in Table 6. The Km for MTA, calculated at saturating level of phosphate, is 5 μM, in good agreement with the value reported for the enzyme from other sources (Ferro et al., 1979; White et al., 1982; Savarese et al. 1985). The affinity for phosphate is somewhat lower (Ki=320 μM) and in accord with that reported for the enzyme from rat liver (Ferro et al., 1979).

In spite of the equilibrium constant favouring the synthesis of MTA and the high affinity of the enzyme for MTR-1-P and adenine, it is unlikely that the synthetic reaction is operative in vivo mainly for the rapid enzymatic

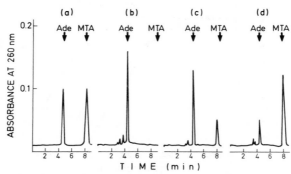

Fig. 3 a) Separation of adenine (Ade) and MTA by HPLC (Della Ragione et al.,1981); b,c,d) Chromatograms of assay mixtures containing 100 μM MTR-1-P, 50 μM adenine and 0 units (b), 0.001 units (c) and 0.002 units (d) of MTA phosphorylase.

Table 6. Kinetic constants of human placenta MTA phosphorylase

SUBSTRATE	Km
5'-Methylthioadenosine	5 μM
Orthophosphate	320 μM
Adenine	23 μM
5-Methylthioribose-1-phosphate	8 μM

removal of adenine and MTR-1-P. However, it is possible that the exposure of cells to adenine analogs or antimetabolites blocking adenine recycling may result in the reversal of the phosphorolytic reaction.

CONCLUDING REMARKS

The reported data on the catalytic mechanism and inhibition of E. coli AdoHcy/MTA nucleosidase indicate the 5'-modified formycinyl analogs as potential antibacterial agents. Indeed, this class of compounds may increase the cellular content of AdoHcy and MTA in bacteria, thus indirectly inhibiting both methylation reactions and polyamine biosynthesis.

Among the formycinyl derivatives assayed, 5'-methylthioformycin (MTF) is the most promising, since it permeates the eukaryotic cell membrane and is metabolically stable as results from studies on human red cells and erythroleukemic cells (Cartenì-Farina et al., 1984).

The compound shares the same transport system as MTA (Cartenì-Farina et al., 1983) and a facilitated diffusion mechanism with high capacity and low affinity has been demonstrated. Moreover, the in vivo studies on the metabolic stability of the molecule confirm the resistance of MTF to the phosphorolytic attack by purified MTA phosphorylase (Cartenì-Farina et al., 1984). Although the molecule is not recognized as substrate by the phosphorylase, it inhibits competitively this enzyme with a Ki (2 μM) two orders of magnitude higher than the Ki towards the bacterial nucleosidase (Ki 28 nM). This difference also argues in favour of the pharmacological use of MTF.

Two different procedures for the synthesis of MTF have recently been developed in our laboratory : one method employs as key step the enzymatic condensation of formycin and homocysteine (Cacciapuoti et al., 1984), while the alternative procedure requires the synthesis of 5'-chloroformycin as intermediate (Pontoni et al., 1985).

The support by the C.N.R. project "Oncologia" is gratefully acknowledged.

REFERENCES

Adams, D.O. and Yang, S.F. (1979) Proc. Natl. Acad. Sci. USA 76, 170-174.

Baxter, C. and Coscia, C.J. (1973) Biochem. Biophys. Res. Commun. 54, 147-154.

Cacciapuoti, G., Oliva, A. and Zappia V. (1978) Int. J. Biochem. 9, 35-41.

Cacciapuoti, G., Porcelli, M., Della Ragione, F. and Cartenì-Farina, M. (1984) Bull. Mol. Biol. Med. 8, 199-209.

Cartenì-Farina, M., Oliva, A., Romeo, G., Napolitano, G., De Rosa, M., Gambacorta, A. and Zappia, V. (1979) Eur. J. Biochem. 101, 317-324.

Cartenì-Farina, M. Della Ragione, F., Cacciapuoti, G., Porcelli, M. and Zappia, V. (1983a) Biochim. Biophys. Acta 727, 221-229.

Cartenì-Farina, M., Porcelli, M., Cacciapuoti, G., Zappia, V., Grieco, M. and Di Fiore, P.P. (1983b) in Advances in Polyamine Research (Bachrach, U., Kaye, A. and Chayen, R. eds.) vol. 4, pp. 779-792, Raven Press, New York.

Cartenì-Farina, M., Cacciapuoti, G., Porcelli, M., Della Ragione, F., Lancieri, M., Geraci, G. and Zappia, V. (1984) Biochim. Biophys. Acta 805, 158-164.

Della Ragione, F., Cartenì-Farina, M., Porcelli, M.,

Cacciapuoti, G. and Zappia, V. (1981) J. Chromatogr. 226, 243-247.

Della Ragione, F., Porcelli, M., Cartenì-Farina, M., Zappia, V., Pegg, A.E. (1985a) Biochem. J. in press.

Della Ragione, F., Cartenì-Farina, M., Gragnaniello, V., Schettino, M.I. and Zappia, V. (1985b) It. J. Biochem. in press.

Della Ragione, F., Porcelli, M., Cartenì-Farina, M., Zappia, V., Pegg, A.E. (1985c) in Recent Progress in Polyamine Research (Selmeci, L., Brosnan, M.E. and Seiler, N.) Akadèmiai Kiadò, Budapest and VNU, The Netherlands in press

Duerre, J. (1962) J. Biol. Chem., 237, 3737-3741.

Ferro, A.J., Barrett, A. and Shapiro, S.K. (1976) Biochim. Biophys. Acta 487-494.

Ferro, A.J., Wrobel, N.C. and Nicolette, J. (1979) Biochim. Biophys. Acta 570, 65-73.

Fujioka, M. and Takata, Y. (1981) J. Biol. Chem. 256, 1631-1635.

Garbers, D.L. (1978) Biochim. Biophys. Acta 523, 82-93.

Garrett, E.R. and Mehta, P.J. (1972) J. Am. Chem. Soc. 94/24, 1228-1237.

Guranowski, A.B., Chiang, P.K. and Cantoni, G.L. (1981) Eur. J. Biochem. 114, 293-299.

Kamatani, N. and Carson, D.A. (1981) Biochim. Biophys. Acta 675, 344-350.

Kim., B.K., Cha, S. and Parks, R.E., Jr. (1968) J. Biol. Chem. 243, 1763-1770.

Nishimura, S., Taya, Y., Kuchino, Y. and Ohashi, Z. (1974) Biochem. Biophys. Res. Commun. 57, 702-708.

Palmer, J.L. and Abeles, R.H. (1979) J. Biol. Chem. 254, 1217-1226.

Pegg, A.E. and Williams-Ashman, H.G. (1969) Biochem. J. 115, 241-247.

Pegg, A.E., Borchardt, R.T. and Coward, J.K. (1981) Biochem. J. 194, 79-89.

Pontoni, G., Gennari, F., Parrella, G., Cacciapuoti, G. and Della Ragione, F. (1985) It. J. Biochem. 34, 175-176.

Raina, A., Tuomi, K. and Pajula, R.L. (1982) Biochem. J. 204, 697-703.

Riscoe, M.K. and Ferro, A.J. (1984) J. Biol. Chem. 259,
    5465-5471.
Savarese, T.M., Chu, S.-H., Chu, M.-Y. and Parks, R.E., Jr.
    (1985) Biochem. Pharmacol. 34, 361-367.
Shapiro, S.K. and Mather, A.N. (1958) J. Biol. Chem. 233,
    631-633.
Shugart, L., Taucer, M. and Moore, J. (1979) Int. J.
    Biochem. 10, 901-904.
Stoner, G.L. and Eisenberg, M.A. (1975) J. Biol. Chem. 250,
    4029-4036.
Sugimoto, Y., Toraya, T. and Fukui, S. (1976) Arch. Microb.
    108, 175-182.
Toohey, J.I. (1978) Biochem. Biophys. Res. Commun. 83, 27-
    35.
Ueland, P.M. and Saebo, J. (1979) Biochemistry, 18, 4130-
    4135.
Ward, D.C., Reich, E. and Stryer, L. (1969) J. Biol. Chem.
    244, 1228-1237.
White, M.W., Vandenbark, A.A., Barney, C.L. and Ferro, A.J.
    (1982) Biochem. Pharmacol. 31, 503-507.
Williams-Ashman, H.G., Seidenfeld, J. and Galletti, P.
    (1982) Biochem. Pharmacol. 31, 277-288.
Wolford, R.W., MacDonald, M.R., Zehfus, B., Rogers, T.J. and
    Ferro, A.J. (1981) Cancer Res. 41, 3035-3039.
Yu, Y.-B., Adams, D.O. and Yang, S.F. (1979) Arch. Biochem.
    Biophys. 198, 280-286.
Zappia, V., Oliva, A., Cacciapuoti, G., Galletti, P.,
    Mignucci, G. and Cartenì-Farina, M. (1978) Biochem. J.
    175, 1043-1050.
Zappia, V., Cartenì-Farina, M., Cacciapuoti, G., Oliva, A.
    and Gambacorta, A. (1980) in Natural Sulfur Compounds:
    Novel Biochemical and Structural Aspects (Cavallini,
    D., Gaull, G.E. and Zappia, V., eds.) pp. 133-148,
    Plenum Press, New York.
Zappia, V., Cartenì-Farina, M., Galletti, P., Della Ragione,
    F. and Cacciapuoti, G. (1983a) Methods in Enzymology
    94, 57-66.
Zappia, V., Cartenì-Farina, M., Romeo, G., DeRosa, M. and
    Gambacorta, A. (1983b) Methods in Enzymology 94, 355-
    361.

UNCOUPLING OF GRANULOPOIETIC CELL PROLIFERATION AND DIFFERENTIATION BY METHYLTHIOADENOSINE

J.H. Fitchen, M.K. Riscoe and A.J. Ferro

Medical Research Service, Portland VAMC,

Portland, Oregon and Dept. of Microbiology,

Oregon State University, Corvallis, Oregon

The human bone marrow exhibits remarkable precision and flexibility, both in meeting steady-state blood cell requirements and in responding to hematopoietic stress. Despite production by the bone marrow of massive numbers of terminally differeniated cells (more than 10^{11} granulocytes per day), levels of circulating blood cells are maintained within remarkably narrow limits. In addition, the bone marrow has the ability to expand production dramatically in response to stress. This increased production is largely restricted to the specific cell type appropriate to a particular stress (e.g., increased granulopoiesis in response to bacterial infection). Taken together, these observations imply that proliferation and differentiation within the bone marrow are modulated by sensitive biological regulatory systems.

Because of the pyramidal nature of hematopoiesis, with large numbers of differentiated cells derived from relatively few stem cells, stimulatory or inhibitory influences applied to primitive cells can have profound effects on overall production. Study of the regulation of these primitive cells has been facilitated by the development of in vitro clonogenic assays for hematopoietic progenitor cells. Under appropriate experimental conditions, these progenitor cells can be stimulated to proliferate and form colonies of

301

differentiated progeny when grown in semi-solid medium.
For example, the granulocyte-macrophage progenitor cell
(colony forming unit-granulocyte, macrophage; CFU-GM)
gives rise to colonies of granulocytes and macrophages
when stimulated by colony-stimulating activity (CSA;
Quesenberry and Levitt, 1979). Since several thousand
mature granulocytes can be derived from a single CFU-GM,
it is evident that the relationship between proliferation
and differentiation of these progenitor cells is crucial
to overall production of granulocytes.

The progression of many types of cells from a
quiescent to a proliferating state is accompanied by
marked increases in the cellular levels of polyamines and
the activities of enzymes involved in their biosynthesis
(Rupniak and Paul, 1978; Morris, 1978). 5'-Deoxy-5'-
methylthioadenosine (MTA) is a co-product of the synthesis
of polyamines (Pegg and Williams-Ashman, 1969a) but does
not normally accumulate in cells. Its rapid degradation
is accomplished by the enzyme MTA phosphorylase (Pegg and
Williams-Ashman, 1969b). Although the biological
occurrence of MTA has been recognized for nearly 75 years
(Mandel and Dunham, 1912), it has only recently become
apparent that MTA may play a role in the control of cell
division. For example, MTA has been shown to inhibit the
transformation of chick embryo fibroblasts by Rous sarcoma
virus (Robert-Gero et al., 1975), antigen- and
lectin-induced blastogenesis of human lymphocytes
(Vandenbark et al, 1980), and the growth of several
malignant murine cell lines (Wolford et al., 1981).

Because of these demonstrated effects of MTA on
various types of proliferating cells, we wondered what
effect MTA might have on normal human CFU-GM. We found
that MTA potently inhibited colony formation by these
cells. Since colony formation is dependent upon both
proliferation and differentiation, we were interested in
determining whether inhibition was attributable to effects
on proliferation or differentiation or both. To address
this question, we studied the effect of MTA in two cell
systems which can be induced to undergo granulocytic
differentiation in vitro: the human promyelocytic-leukemia
cell line HL-60 and suspension cultures of normal human
bone marrow enriched for granulocytic precursors. We
found that MTA completely inhibited cell proliferation but
did not interfere with differentiation in either system.

MATERIALS AND METHODS

Cells

Normal human bone marrow was obtained from informed and consenting healthy adult volunteers by aspiration from the posterior iliac crest into preservative-free heparin. Low-density cells to be used for CFU-GM assays (see below) were prepared with Ficoll-Paque centrifugation (Boyum, 1976). Low-density marrow cell suspensions to be used in liquid culture experiments were further enriched for granulocytic precursors by sequential depletion of other cell types as follows. T-lymphocytes were removed by formation of E-rosettes with sheep red blood cells and a second centrifugation on Ficoll-Paque (Mendes et al., 1973). The residual buoyant cells were then depleted of monocytes and macrophages by selective adherence to serum-coated plastic dishes (Kunagai et al., 1979). B-lymphocytes were then removed from the non-adherent cell population by adherence to nylon fibers (Julius et al., 1973). The resulting "maximally depleted" cell suspension contained primarily immature lymphoid appearing cells, granulocytic precursor cells and a residual contamination of less than 10% mature graunulocytes.

HL-60 cells were the generous gift of Dr. H.P. Koeffler (UCLA School of Medicine). This cell line was derived from a patient with acute promyelocytic leukemia (Collins et al., 1978) and can be induced to undergo granulocytic differentiation by retinoic acid (RA; Breitman et al., 1980). We analyzed MTA phosphorylase activity in these cells by two different methods as previously described (Ferro et al., 1976; White et al., 1982) and found that HL-60 cells contain significant (7.4 nmol/10^7 cells/min).

CFU-GM Assay

CFU-GM were assayed as previously described (Fitchen et al., 1980). Briefly, low-density bone marrow cells were plated in 1 ml of 0.3% agar containing McCoy's 5A medium, 15% heat-inactivated fetal calf serum (FCS), antibiotics and 10% (vol/vol) human placenta-conditioned medium (HPCM) as a source of CSA (Schlunk and Schleger, 1980). Plates were incubated at 37°C in a humidified atmosphere of 7.5% CO_2 in air for 7 days and colonies containing 40 or more cells were enumerated under a dissecting microscope

Suspension Cultures

HL-60 cells in logarithimic growth phase were cultured in RPMI-1640 containing 10% FCS. Total and viable cells (those which excluded trypan blue) were counted on a hemacytometer at 1-2 day intervals. Growth in control cultures (no additions) was compared to growth in cultures added with 1uM cis-retinoic acid (Roche), 0.5mM MTA (Sigma), or both.

Suspension cultures of "maximally depleted" normal human bone marrow cells (see above) were seeded at 3 X 10^5 cells/ml in RPMI-1640 medium containing 10% FCS with or without 10% HPCM. MTA (50uM final concentration) was added to these cultures 24 hours after the addition of HPCM; a time when early granulopoiesis was at its peak (i.e., more than 50% of the total cell population contained azurophilic granules characteristic of promyelocytes). Growth in control cultures (HPCM only) was compared to growth in cultures to which both HPCM and MTA had been added. Cell viability was determined by hemacytometer and was greater than 90% in each culture over the 7-day period.

Analysis of Differentiation

The percent of cells with mature granulocytic morphology was assessed by enumerating the number of cells with band or segmented nuclei in differential counts of at least 300 cells on Wright-Giemsa stained cytopreps. Two functions characteristic of mature granulocytes (phagocytosis and superoxide generation) were examined by the NBT assay as described by Luk et al. (1982). In these assays, 3×10^5 cells suspended in 1ml of saline were incubated with 1ml of 0.2% NBT for 25 min at 37° C. The cells were then centrifuged onto microscope slides, stained with Wright-Giemsa, and examined for the presence of intracellular formazin deposits. Cells containing these black deposits (NBT-positive cells) are capable of both ingesting NBT particles and reducing them through the generation of superoxide. Chloroacetate esterase assays (histochemical stain specific for mature granulocytes) were performed as described by Yam et al. (1974).

RESULTS

MTA vs. CFU–GM

The effect of MTA on colony formation by normal human CFU–GM is shown in Fig. 1. Greater than 90% inhibition occurred at an MTA concentration of 10^{-4}M with an ID_{50} of 10^{-5}M and demonstrable inhibition at concentrations as low as 10^{-7}M. Since colony formation by CFU–GM requires both proliferation and differentiation, the inhibitory effect of MTA in this system could not be clearly ascribed to a specific effect on either process. Experiments with HL-60 cells and bone marrow cells in suspension culture were therefore carried out to make this distinction.

MTA vs. HL-60 Cells

The effect of MTA on the proliferation and RA-induced differentiation of HL-60 cells is shown in Figs. 2 and 3. After 7 days of culture, control cells (no additions) had undergone 2.5 doublings. In contrast, no increase in cell numbers was observed in cultures treated with 0.5mM MTA

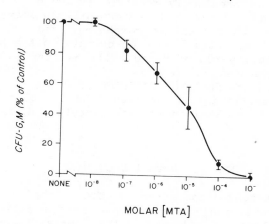

Figure 1: Effect of MTA on colony formation by human CFU–GM.

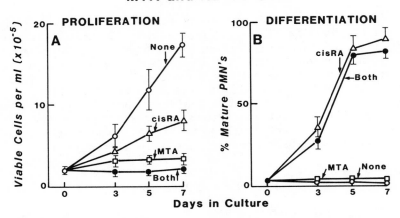

Figure 2: The effect of MTA on proliferation and
          differentiation of HL-60 cells.

(Fig. 2A). As previously reported by others (Breitman et
al., 1980), RA-treated cells underwent granulocytic differentiation as determined by morphology and NBT reduction
(Fig. 2B). Thus, after 7 days of culture in the presence of
RA, approximately 90% of HL-60 cells had the morphology of
band and segmented neutrophils (Fig. 3B) and were able to
ingest and reduce NBT. The addition of 0.5mM MTA to cultures also containing RA abolished cell proliferation but
did not affect RA-induced granulocytic differentiation
(Fig. 3D).

MTA vs. Normal Bone Marrow

We next tested the effect of MTA on the proliferation
and differentiation of human bone marrow cells grown in
liquid   culture.   These   cells   were   depleted   of
erythrocytes, T and B lymphocytes and monocyte/macrophages
and cultured in the presence of HPCM for 24 hours to
enrich for granulocytic precursor cells. As shown in Fig.
4A, cell numbers increased 5-fold over 7 days in control

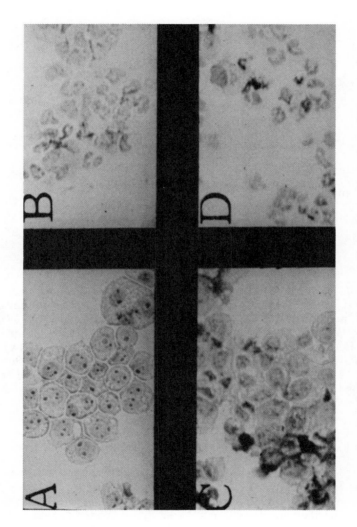

Figure 3: Morphologic appearance of HL-60 cells after 7 days of culture with no additions (A), 1uM RA (B), 0.5mM MTA (C), both RA and MTA (D).

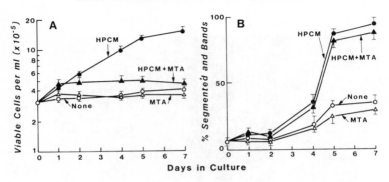

Figure 4: Effect of MTA on the proliferation and
          differentiation of normal human bone
          marrow grown in suspension culture.

cultures (HPCM alone). As expected, the cells generated
in the presence of HPCM were largely granulocytic (Figs.
4B and 5A). With the addition of MTA, cell growth ceased
(Fig. 4A). However, as noted with HL-60 cells, MTA did
not interfere with differentiation. By day 7, over 90% of
the cells developed the distinctive chloroacetate esterase
staining pattern and appeared as mature band and segmented
neutrophils in Wright-stained preparations (Fig. 5B).

                            DISCUSSION

     Our results indicate that MTA inhibits growth but not
induced differentiation of normal and leukemic granulopoietic cells in vitro. A linkage between cell division
and cell differentiation has been described in fetal mouse
liver (Gross and Goldwasser, 1970) and in chick embryo
erythroblasts (Sun and Green, 1976). In contrast, others
have found no effect on differentiation when cell division
is blocked by synthetic compounds that inhibit DNA
synthesis (Rovera et al., 1980; Territo and Koeffler,

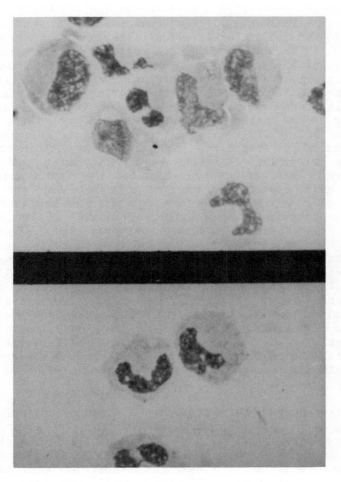

Figure 5: Morphologic appearance of normal human bone marrow after 7 days of culture with HPCM alone (A) or HPCM plus 0.1mM MTA (B).

1981). Our results obtained with MTA show that
differentiation of HL-60 cells and of normal human granulocytic precursor cells occur in the absence of cell growth.
    The finding that MTA does not interfere with granulo-
cytic differentiation contrasts with work by others on the
effects of MTA on erythroid differentiation. DiFiori et al
(1984) and Shafman et al. (1984) have reported that MTA prevents DMSO-induced differentiation of murine erythroleukemia cells. The reason for the contradictory results is
not clear but may reflect differences in the metabolism or
site of action of MTA in erythroid and granulocytic cells.
    That MTA is capable of dissociating the events of
cell proliferation and differentiation suggests a possible
role for this naturally-occurring nucleoside in the
regulation of normal granulopoietic growth and differentiation. One might speculate, for example, that changes in
biosynthesis and/or degradation of MTA could regulate
granulocytic production by altering the proliferative
state of granulopoietic progenitor cells. Indeed, MTA has
recently been implicated as an intracellular mediator of
the anti-proliferative activity of α and β interferon
(deFerra and Baglioni, 1984). Whatever the potential
biological roles of MTA, it may prove to be a useful laboratory reagent for studying the processes of proliferation
and differentiation independently in granulopoietic cells.
    Finally, since MTA selectively perturbs cell
proliferation without interfering with differentiation,
MTA (or structural analogs of MTA) might have therapeutic
efficacy. Treatment programs aimed at both inhibiting
proliferation (with MTA) and inducing differentiation
(e.g., with retinoic acid) may be useful in the management
of promyelocytic and other leukemias.

Acknowledgements: We are indebted to Linda Johnson for
excellent technical assistance and to Ruth Weidenaar for
typing the manuscript. This work was supported by V.A.
Research Funds and grants from the Medical Resarch Foundation of Oregon and the American Cancer Society. A.J.
Ferro is a recipient of a NIH Career Development Award.

REFERENCES

Boyum, A. (1976) Scand. J. Immunol 5 (suppl 5), 9.

Breitman, T. R., Selonick, S. E. and Collins, S. J. (1980) Proc. Natl. Acad. Sci. U.S.A. 77, 2936.

Collins, S. J., Gallo, R. C. and Gallagher, R. E. (1977) Nature 270, 347.

deFerra, F. and Baglioni, C. (1984) Cancer Res. 44, 2297.

DiFiore, P. P., Grieco, M., Pinto, A., et al. (1984) Cancer Res. 44, 4096.

Ferro, A. J., Barrett, A. and Shapiro, S. K. (1976) Biochem. Biophys. Acta 438, 487.

Fitchen, J. H., Ferrone, S., Quaranta, V., Molinara, G. A. and Cline, M. J. (1980) J. Immunol. 125, 2004.

Gross, M. and Goldwasser, E. (1970) J. Biol. Chem. 245, 1632.

Julius, M. H., Simpson, E. and Herzenberg, L. A. (1973) Eur. J. Immunol. 3, 645.

Kunagi, K., Itoh, K., Hinuma, S., and Tada, M. (1979) J. Immunol. Meth. 29, 17.

Luk, G. D., Civin, C. I., Weissman, R. M., and Baylin, S. D. (1982) Science 216, 75.

Mandel, J. A. and Durham, K. (1912) J. Biol Chem. 11, 85.

Mendes, N. F., Tonai, M. E. A., Silveira, N. P. A., et al. (1973) J. Immunol. 111, 860

Morris, D. R. (1978) in Advances in Polyamine Resarch (Campbell, R.A., Ed.) p. 105, Raven Press, New York.

Pegg, A. E. and Williams-Ashman, H. G. (1969a) J. Biol. Chem. 244, 682.

Pegg, A. E. and Williams-Ashman, H. G. (1969b) Biochem. J. 115, 241.

Quesenberry, P. and Levitt, L. (1979) N. Engl. J. Med. 301, 755.

Rovera, G., Olashaw, N. and Meo, P. (1980) Nature 284, 69.

Robert-Gero, M., Lawrence, F., Farrugia, G., et al. (1975) Biochem. Biophys. Res. Commun. 65, 1242.

Rupniak, H. T. and Paul, D. (1978) in Advances in Polyamine Research (Campbell, R.A., Ed.) p. 117, Raven Press, New York.

Shlunk, T. and Schleyer, M. (1980) Exp. Hematol. 8, 179.

Shafman, T. D., Sherman, M. L. and Kufe, D. W. (1984) Biochem. Biophys. Res. Commun. 124, 172.

Sun, T. T. and Green, H. (1976) Cell 9, 511.

Territo, M. C. and Koeffler, H. P. (1981) Br. J. Haematol. 47, 479.

Vandenbark, A. A., Ferro, A. J. and Barney, C. L. (1980) Cell Immunol. 49, 26.

White, M. W., Vandenbark, A. A., Barney, C. L., Ferro, A. J. (1982) Biochem. Pharmacol. 31, 503.

Wolford, R. W., MacDonald, M. R., Zehfus, B., Rogers, T. J. and Ferro, A. J. (1981) Cancer Res. 41, 3035.

Yam, L. T., Cy, L., Wolfe, H. J., and Moy, P. W. (1974). Arch. Pathol. 97, 129.

D. Clinical Aspects of S-Adenosylmethionine

ADOMET AS A DRUG

PHARMACOKINETIC AND PHARMACOLOGICAL ASPECTS

GIORGIO STRAMENTINOLI

BIORESEARCH S.p.A. Research Laboratories

LISCATE, MILANO, ITALY

INTRODUCTION

S-Adenosyl-L-methionine (AdoMet), an important molecule in cell biochemistry, has been the subject of many experimental (Curcio et al.,1978; Stramentinoli et al.,1980; Boelsterli et al.,1983; Gualano et al.,1983; Schreiber et al.,1983; Cimino et al.,1984; Gualano et al.,1985) and clinical (Agnoli et al.,1976; Carney et al.,1983; Di Padova et al.,1984; Frezza et al.,1984; Lipinsky et al.,1984; Capretto et al.,1985; Marcolongo et al.,1985; Oriente et al.,1985) investigations. Experiments reported here refer to the evaluation of pharmacokinetic parameters of the drug in experimental animals and in man and to some pharmacological effects observed after its administration. In particular, central effects of AdoMet are described, such as the increase of 5-hydroxyindolacetic acid (5-HIAA) and 5-hydroxytriptamine (5-HT) in some regions of rat brain after treatment with various doses of the drug (Curcio et al.,1978), and its ability to prevent decrease of brain membrane fluidity in aging rats when administered chronically (Cimino et al.,1984). Results are also reported showing that AdoMet after both parenteral (Gualano et al.,1983) and oral (Gualano et al.,1985) treatment, has an anti-inflammatory activity, possibly due to its interference with the eicosanoid system.

315

PHARMACOKINETICS

Pharmacokinetics of AdoMet was previously studied in rats and at low doses (0.5 mg/Kg) in man (Stramentinoli & Catto,1976). In order to investigate the possible saturation of metabolism and excretion of the drug, plasma decay of AdoMet was studied (Giulidori et al.,1984a) after i.v. administration of 1.5 and 7.5 mg/Kg to six healthy volunteers (fig.1) . A biexponential decay was noted with a terminal disposition phase starting about 1 h after the administration. The apparent volumes of distribution after the low and high doses were 407 ± 27 and 443 ± 36 ml/Kg (mean ± SEM), respectively. Terminal half lives were 81 ± 8 and 101 ± 7 min and body clearances 3.7 ± 0.5 and 3.1 ± 0.2 ml/min per Kg.

The total urinary excretion of the drug was 30 ± 3 and 34 ± 3 mg at 8 and 24 h after the administration of the 1.5 mg/Kg dose; at the same times after the 7.5 mg/Kg dose 189 ± 11 and 201 ± 10 mg of the drug were excreted in urine. Urinary excretion of endogenous AdoMet was 6.1 ± 0.7 mg/24 h. Both drug disposition and renal excretion were almost

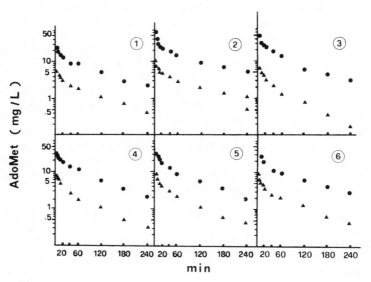

Fig. 1 <u>Plasma decay of AdoMet after its administration to healthy volunteers</u>. Plasma levels were determined by a radio-enzymatic method.
● = 7.5 mg/Kg; ▲ = 1.5 mg/Kg.

complete within 24h. These data show that no dose-dependent
change occurs, differently from the previous finding that
in rats the drug clearance is proportional to the
administered dose (Giulidori et al.,1984b).The ratio
between renal and total clearances indicated that at both
doses more than half of the given AdoMet was metabolized.
The results obtained in healthy volunteers are of relevance
for clinical use of the drug because they suggest that
body accumulation of AdoMet is unlikely, at least up to the
highest tested dose.

From the plasma levels of unmodified AdoMet after its
oral administration (200 mg) to healthy volunteers, the
systemic availability appeared to be very low (<1%).
However, previous works in the rat showed that AdoMet can
cross the intestinal barrier (Stramentinoli et al.,1979)
and metabolism of the compound is very rapid (Giulidori et
al.,1984b). Experiments in three healthy volunteers were
therefore carried out administering labelled AdoMet (10
μCi, 200 mg). The time-course of total radioactivity in
plasma is shown in fig. 2. The percent of the dose excreted
in urine was 15 ± 3.5 in 72 h. In these experiments AdoMet
was administered in gastroresistant capsules because in
rats much higher portal plasma levels were obtained after
intraduodenal than after oral treatment (fig.3).

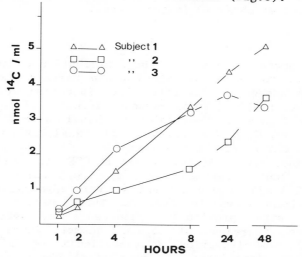

Fig. 2 Time-course of total plasma radioactivity in
subjects treated with methyl-labelled AdoMet (0.05 μCi/mg).
The drug was administered in gastroresistant capsules.

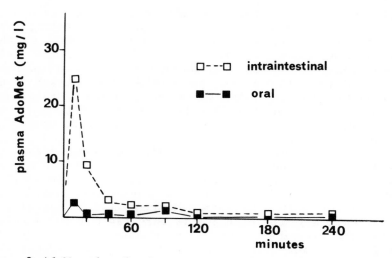

Fig. 3 <u>AdoMet levels in portal plasma of rats after oral</u>
<u>and intraduodenal treatment.</u> Intraduodenal treatment:
AdoMet (32 mg/Kg) in a gelatine capsule was inserted into
the intestine. Oral treatment: AdoMet (32 mg/Kg) was given
orally as an aqueous solution; animals were operated and an
empty capsule was inserted into the intestine. Results are
the mean values obtained in three rats.

An important feature of the distribution of AdoMet is
its ability to cross the blood brain barrier. Levels of
unmodified AdoMet in CSF after i.v. injection of 8 mg/Kg
of the drug, followed by intravenous infusion of 12 mg/Kg.h
for 6 h in dogs were 20–40 folds the basal values. Figure 4
shows the results obtained from the analysis of AdoMet
plasma and CSF levels in two dogs.
     The increase of AdoMet levels in CSF was confirmed in
man after acute treatment (200 mg i.v.) collecting CSF
samples (0.5 ml) from a patient with an epidural catheter
at the times shown in fig. 4. These results are in
agreement with previously reported data ·showing a
significant increase of brain AdoMet levels after
parenteral administration (Stramentinoli et al.,1978).
Moreover, a significant increase of AdoMet in CSF was
recently demonstrated in patients receiving a daily i.v.
injection of AdoMet (200 mg) for 14 days (Bottiglieri et
al.,1984).

EFFECTS ON THE CNS

Serotoninergic System

Previous works demonstrated that AdoMet administration causes a prolongation of the reaction time in the hot plate test for analgesia (Gualano et al.,1983) and of the sleeping time induced by hexobarbital (unpublished data) in laboratory animals. Moreover the effectiveness of AdoMet in releiving depression symptoms had been suggested from the results of clinical trials (Agnoli et al.,1976; Carney et al.,1983; Lipinsky et al., 1984).

Because serotoninergic neurons are involved both in sleep and analgesia (Samanin & Bernasconi,1972; Harvey et al.,1975) and modification of the CNS catecholamine and indolamine metabolism has been suggested as the biochemical basis of depression (Asberg et al.,1976), we became interested in studying whether AdoMet administration may cause changes of 5-HT and 5-HIAA brain levels (Curcio et al.,1978). To this purpose AdoMet was administered to male Sprague-Dawley rats. Levels of 5-HT and 5-HIAA were determined in the brainstem and forebrain.

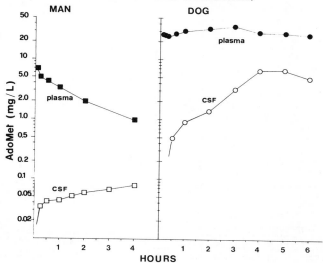

Fig. 4 <u>Levels of AdoMet in plasma and CSF after administration to dogs and man</u>. Results in dogs represent mean values in two animals whereas those in man were obtained in the CSF of a patient with an epidural catheter.

The results show that a repeated AdoMet administration induces a significant increase in the levels of both compounds in the forebrain (fig. 5A). A slight increase was also observed in the brainstem even if statistical significance was not reached in this area (fig. 5B). These results were confirmed by experiments carried out in depressed patients (Agnoli et al.,1977). AdoMet administration (100 mg, i.v.) after probenecid treatment induced an increase of 5-HIAA levels in CSF which was significantly higher than that obtained in control patients treated only with probenecid (fig. 6). The specificity of the effect was demonstrated by the lack of increase of homovanillic acid (HVA) levels by AdoMet (fig.6).

Dopaminergic and β-Adrenergic Systems

The effects of AdoMet on dopaminergic and β-adrenergic receptor systems were studied in aging rats. Earlier studies demonstrated that membrane fluidity and β-adrenergic

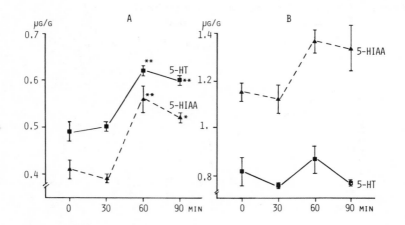

Fig. 5 **5-HT and 5-HIAA concentration in forebrain (A) and brainstem (B) of AdoMet treated rats.** Animals were injected twice with 50 mg/Kg i.m. and once with 100 mg/Kg i.v. at 12 h intervals and were killed at the shown times after the last injection. The results are expressed as $\mu g/g$ tissue and are the mean $\pm$ SEM for seven animals. Significance vs zero time was evaluated by the Duncan's New Multiple Range test. * = $p < 0.01$; ** = $p < 0.001$.

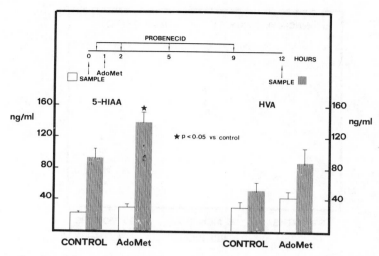

Fig. 6 <u>Levels of 5-HIAA and HVA in the CSF after AdoMet</u>
<u>treatment of depressed patients</u>. Results are the mean ± SEM
for nine patients.

and dopaminergic receptor properties are modified during
aging. Furthermore, membrane fluidity seems to be related
to phospholipid methylation (Hirata et al.,1978;
Strittmatter et al.,1979) which, in turn, may be stimulated
by AdoMet (Hirata et al.,1978). In this study, 27-month-old
rats were treated for three months with either AdoMet (50
mg/Kg.day, s.c.) or the vehicle. Three-month-old animals
were used as controls (Cimino et al.,1984). The viscosity
of the striatal membranes in 30-month-old rats was
significantly higher than in adult animals, as determined
by fluorescence polarization which gives a general index
of membrane fluidity (fig. 7). The modifications of
membrane fluidity were confined to the hydrofobic core, as
indicated by the higher viscosity of the core of the lipid
bilayer (fig.7). In the cortex, no change of membrane
viscosity was observed. The effects of aging on membrane
viscosity were reversed by AdoMet administration (fig.7).
    The effects on the β-adrenergic and dopaminergic
systems were evaluated labelling the specific sites with
labelled dihydroalprenolol (DHA) (Bylund & Snyder,1975) and
spiperone (Burt et al., 1976), respectively. The decrease

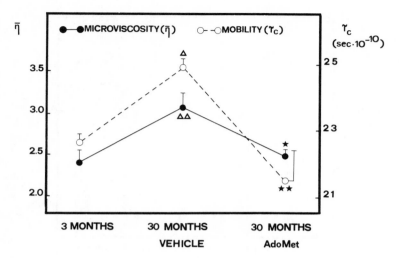

Fig.7 <u>Effect of AdoMet on the microviscosity of striatal</u>
<u>membranes.</u>   Viscosity $(\bar{\eta})$ was   calculated   from   the
fluorescence polarization (P) (Shinitzky & Barenholz,1978)
according to the empirical relation $\bar{\eta} = 2P/0.46-P$. Mobility
(τ) was determined using N-oxyl-4,4'-dimethyl oxazolidine
derivative of 16-ketostearic acid as spin label (Cimino et
al.,1984). Results are the mean ± SEM for five rats.
Δ = p<0.05,   ΔΔ = p<0.01 vs 3-month-old rats
* = p<0.05,   ** = p<0.01 vs 30-month-old rats.

in β-adrenergic binding sites induced by aging was
antagonized by administration of AdoMet (fig.8), suggesting
that a deficit in this brain area of senescent animals can
be antagonized by chronic treatment with the drug. Pineal
gland showed the same pattern of β-adrenergic receptor
changes as striatum: a decrease with age and restoration to
control values after chronic AdoMet administration. In
contrast, the treatment had no effect on tritiated DHA
binding in the cortex (Curcio et al.,1978) where also on
membrane fluidity AdoMet had no effect . Furthermore, in
striatum the dopaminergic system did not seem to be
modified by chronic AdoMet administration since neither
spiperone binding nor basal and dopamine-stimulated
activity of adenylate cyclase were affected by treatment.
    The above reported results demonstrate that AdoMet is

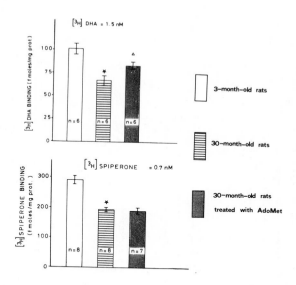

Fig.8 Effects of AdoMet on DHA and spiperone binding in
striatal membranes. Results represent the mean $\pm$ SEM of 6-8
replications. Significance of the difference was evaluated
by the Duncan's New Multiple Range test. * = $p<0.01$ vs
3-month-old rats; Δ = $p<0.05$ vs 30-month-old rats.

able to antagonize the age-related changes in membrane
fluidity and β-adrenergic receptor activity. They also
show, however, the heterogeneity of these biochemical
modifications in relation to the considered brain area, and
provide an insight into the different mechanisms regulating
the activity of various receptor systems and the
relationship between receptor systems and synaptic membrane
conditions.

ANTI-INFLAMMATORY EFFECTS OF ADOMET

The anti-inflammatory and antalgic properties of
AdoMet in the experimental animals (Gualano et al.,1983;
Gualano et al.,1985) and the therapeutic action on symptoms
of degenerative arthropaties (Capretto et al.,1985;
Marcolongo et al.,1985; Oriente et al.,1985) were reported.
The results here described give evidence that the activity

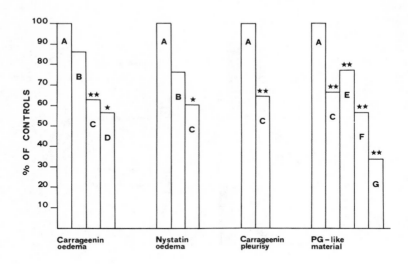

Fig.9 <u>Anti-inflammatory effects of AdoMet by parenteral and</u>
<u>oral route</u>. Results are expressed as % of controls. A =
controls; B = 50 mg/Kg AdoMet (i.m. in nystatin oedema and
s.c. elsewhere); C = 100 mg/Kg AdoMet (same route as in B);
D, E, F, G = 50, 60, 120, 240 mg/Kg AdoMet administered
intraduodenally in gelatine capsules. Details on the
experimental design have been described (Gualano et
al.,1983,1985).Statistical differences were evaluated by
the analysis of variance for randomized blocks of animals,
followed by the Dunnett's test.
* = p<0.05;   ** = p<0.01 vs controls.

of AdoMet in controlling acute inflammation reaction may be
connected with its ability to interact with the eicosanoid
system by both parenteral and oral administration.
     The results obtained in the tests used to determine
the effects of AdoMet (fig. 9) show the anti-inflammatory
activity of AdoMet after parenteral or intestinal
administration. It is interesting to note that in
experimental pleurisy AdoMet significantly reduces the
number of leukocytes present in the inflammed area (Gualano
et al.,1985). This is of particular importance considering
the role played by those cells in the phlogistic process.

The measurement of PG-like material in inflammatory exudates (Gualano et al.,1985) shows the capability of AdoMet to inhibit the cyclooxygenase metabolic pathway of arachidonate. Despite this evidence, AdoMet can hardly be classified among steroidal and non-steroidal anti-inflammatory drugs, because it is free from the well known gastrointestinal side-effects proper of those drugs. Its mechanism of action should be therefore investigated further, particularly for the metabolism of arachidonate to leukotrienes. Also noteworthy is AdoMet role in cell physiology by transsulfuration process. A possible involvement of AdoMet in the biochemistry of cartilage, where an altered sulfatation occurs in the presence of inflammatory degenerative osteoarthropathy, might also account for the anti-inflammatory activity of the compound.

REFERENCES

- Agnoli, A., Andreoli, V., Casacchia, M. & Cerbo, R. (1976) J. Psychiatr. Res. 13, 43-54.
- Agnoli, A., Ruggieri, S., Cerone, G., Aloisi, P., Baldassarre, M. & Stramentinoli, G. (1977) in Depressive Disorders (Garattini, S., Ed.) pp 447-458, F.K. Schattauer Verlag, Stuttgart-New York.
- Åsberg, M., Thoren, P., Träskman, L., Bertilsson, L. & Ringberger, V. (1976) Science, 191,478-480.
- Boelsterli, U.A., Rakhit, G. & Balazs, T. (1983) Hepatol. 3, 12-17.
- Bottiglieri, T., Laundy, M., Martin, R., Carney, M.W.P., Nissenbaum, H., Toone, B.K., Johnson, A.L. & Reynolds, E.H. (1984) Lancet II, 224.
- Burt, D.R., Creese, I. & Snyder, S.H. (1976) Science 196, 326-328.
- Bylund, D.B. & Snyder, S.H. (1975) Mol. Pharmacol. 12, 568-580.
- Carney, M.W.P., Martin, R., Bottiglieri, T., Reynolds, E.H., Nissenbaum, H., Toone, B.K. & Sheffield, B.F. (1983) Lancet I, 820-821.
- Capretto, C., Cremona, C. & Canaparo, L. (1985) Clin. Trials J. 22, 15-24.
- Cimino, M., Vantini, G., Algeri, S., Curatola, G., Pezzoli, C. & Stramentinoli, G. (1984) Life Sciences 34, 2029-2039.
- Curcio, M., Catto, E., Stramentinoli, G. & Algeri, S. (1978) Prog. Neuro-Psychopharmac. 2, 65-71.

- Di Padova, C., Tritapepe, R., Di Padova, F., Frezza, M. & Stramentinoli, G. (1984) Am. J. Gastroenterol. 79, 941–944.
- Frezza, M., Pozzato, G., Chiesa, L., Stramentinoli, G. & Di Padova, C. (1984) Hepatology 4, 274–278.
- Giulidori, P., Cortellaro, M., Moreo, G. & Stramentinoli, G. (1984a) Eur. J. Clin. Pharmacol. 27, 119–121.
- Giulidori, P., Galli Kienle, M., Catto, E. & Stramentinoli, G. (1984b) J. Biol. Chem., 259, 4205–4211.
- Gualano, M., Stramentinoli, G. & Berti, F. (1983) Pharm. Res. Commun. 15, 683–696.
- Gualano, M., Berti, F. & Stramentinoli, G. (1985) Int. J. Tiss. Reac. VII, 41–46.
- Harvey, J.A., Schlosberg, A.J. & Yunger, L.M. (1975) Fed. Proc. 34, 1796–1801.
- Hirata, F., Viveros, H.O., Diliberto, E. Jr. & Axelrod, J. (1978) Proc. Natl. Acad. Sci. USA 75, 1718–1721.
- Lipinski, J.F., Choen, B.M., Frankenburg, F., Tohen, M., Waternaux, C., Altesman, R., Jones, B. & Harris, P. (1984) Am. J. Psychiatry 141, 448–450.
- Marcolongo, R., Giordano, N., Colombo, B., Chériè-Lignière, G., Todesco, S., Mazzi, A., Mattara, L., Leardini, G., Passeri, M. & Cucinotta, D. (1985) Curr. Ther. Res. 37, 82–94.
- Oriente, P., Scarpa, R., Biondi, C., Riccio, A., Farinaro, C. & Del Puente, A. (1985) Clin. Rheumatol. 4, in press.
- Samanin, R. & Bernasconi, S. (1972) Psychopharmacologia 25, 175–182.
- Schreiber, A.J., Warren, G., Sutherland, E. & Simon, F.R. (1983) Clin. Res. 31, 86A.
- Shinitzky, M. & Barenholz, Y. (1978) Biochim. Biophys. Acta 515, 367–394.
- Stramentinoli, G. & Catto, E. (1976) Pharm. Res. Commun. 8, 211–218.
- Stramentinoli, G., Catto, E. & Algeri, S. (1978) in Transmethylations and the Central Nervous System (Andreoli, V.M., Agnoli, A. & Fazio, C., Eds.) pp 111–113, Springer Verlag, Berlin Heidelberg New york.
- Stramentinoli, G., Gualano, M. & Galli Kienle, M. (1979) J. Pharmac. exp. Ther. 209, 323–326.
- Stramentinoli, G., Di Padova, C., Gualano, M., Rovagnati, P. & Galli Kienle, M. (1981) Gastroenterology 80, 154–158.
- Strittmatter, W.J., Hirata, F. & Axelrod, J. (1979) Biochem. Biophys. Res. Commun. 88, 147–153.

A BIOCHEMICAL STUDY OF DEPRESSED PATIENTS RECEIVING S-ADENOSYL-L-METHIONINE (SAM)

T. BOTTIGLIERI, M. W. P. CARNEY, J. EDEH, M.
LAUNDY, R. MARTIN, E. H. REYNOLDS, C. THOMAS,
B. K. TOONE.
Departments of Psychiatry, Northwick Park and
Kings College Hospital London, and Departments
of Neurology, Institute of Psychiatry and
King's College Hospital, London (U.K.).

INTRODUCTION

It was Fazio et al (1974) who, whilst investigating the transmethylation hypothesis, inadvertently noted that SAM had antidepressant properties. Since then numerous clinical trials have supported this initial observation. The mechanism of the anti-depressant effect of SAM is unknown and previous trials did not include biochemical measures during treatment to relate to any clinical effects.

Our interest in SAM and depression was heightened by the association of folate deficiency commonly found in affective states (Carney 1970, Ghadrian et al 1980, Reynolds et al 1984) and the close relationship of the two compounds in the one-carbon cycle. During the course of a double-blind placebo controlled trial of SAM in depression we had the opportunity to investigate levels of SAM, folate, methionine, neurotransmitter metabolites and neuroendocrine measures in blood and spinal fluid. In this paper we present biochemical results from trial patients and the first study of SAM levels in CSF from depressed and neurological patients.

327

PATIENTS AND METHODS

Patients selected were all suffering from a major
depressive disorder according to Feighner criteria
sufficient to warrant in-patient treatment. All scored 20
or more points on the Hamilton rating scale for depression
Patients with physical illness, organic brain disease,
alcoholism, drug withdrawal states or other forms of
mental illness were excluded. Any previous medication was
withdrawn for at least one week prior to entry to the
study. The only medication permitted was a mild benzo-
diazepine hypnotic if required. The study was approved by
the Ethical Committees of Northwick Park and King's
College Hospitals.

Patients were randomly and blindly allocated to treatment with daily injections of I.V. SAM 200 mg or I.V. placebo
(saline) for 14 days. On day 0 of the trial venous blood
was withdrawn for wholeblood and plasma SAM estimations,
serum folate and plasma prolactin. In consenting patients
CSF examinations were carried out between 9 and 10 am, the
patient having fasted in the recumbant position since 10 pm
the previous evening. 13 mls was withdrawn and collected
in tubes on ice. 2 mls were immediately deproteinized with
perchloric acid for SAM estimation. CSF for folate
estimation was diluted 1:10 with 0.1 mM phosphate buffer
(pH 6.70) containing 0.15% ascorbic acid. The remaining
sample was aliquoted out and stored at −70°C for the assay
of methionine and monoamine metabolites. On day 14, 24 hrs
after the final injection of SAM or placebo, blood plasma,
serum and CSF examinations were repeated for comparison
with baseline metabolic variables. In addition blood
samples from normal subjects were collected in the same
manner as the trial patients. CSF was also obtained from
neurological patients undergoing routine CSF examinations.

Assay Methods

SAM was assayed by the enzymatic double isotope
method of Baldessarini and Kopin as modified by Giulidori

and Stramentinoli (1984). Folate was determined microbio-
logically utilizing Lactobacillus Casei as the assay
organism. CSF 5-hydroxyindole acetic acid (5HIAA), homo
vanillic acid (HVA) and 3-methyoxy-4-hydroxyphenylglycol
(MHPG) were determined by high performance liquid
chromatography (HPLC) using an isocratic separation method
(Bottiglieri et al 1984) employing electrochemical detection. CSF methionine was determined by pre-column derivatization with O-phthalaldehyde using fluorescence detection
after HPLC separation (Joseph et al 1983). Plasma prolactin
were determined by radioimmunoassay kits (Amersham
International plc, U.K.). All assays were carried out
blind to treatment groups. Adequate sensitivity and good
reproducibility in all methods employed were observed.

Statistical Methods. The students t-test was applied
for comparison of changes between groups and also individual variables. Where the data was found not to follow
Normal distribution they were log. transformed prior to
statistical analysis. Correlations were performed using
the Pearson product moment correlation coefficient.

RESULTS

Levels of SAM in whole blood were found to be significantly lower in females in both normal and depressed
patients (p<0.001) (Fig. 1). This was significant even
after correcting for the haematocrit value which is lower
in females. We found no correlation with age in both groups
and a normal distribution was observed. No difference
between normal and depressed groups were observed for
females, however depressed males were significantly lower
than the male normal group. Compared to erythrocyte levels
plasma SAM is considerably lower, males 35.0 $\pm$ 5.3 ng/ml
(n=19), females 28.4 $\pm$ 6.8 ng/ml (n=31). During the course
of SAM treatment (blood and plasma SAM estimated at day 7
and 14) SAM levels did not alter from the initial baseline
mean values.

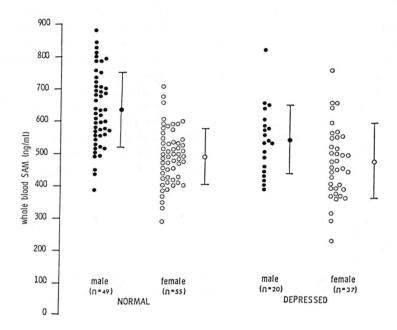

Fig. 1.   Whole blood SAM levels in normal and depressed
          patients (vertical bars indicate mean ± SD).

CSF SAM may be a better indicator of a deficit from a cent-
tral origin. Comparing baseline values from trial patients
with a group of neurological controls there was a trend
which was not significant, 10 depressed patients had values
below the control range (Fig. 2). The group of neurological
controls consisted of three patients with peripheral
neuropathies, three with motor neurone disease and one with
intracranial hypertension. No sex differences were observed
in the larger group of 25 depressed patients. In depressed
patients we noted a significant increase in CSF SAM after
drug treatment. Patients treated with placebo showed no
significant changes (Table 1). Levels of the substrate
methionine were not increased after 14 days in both
treatment groups.

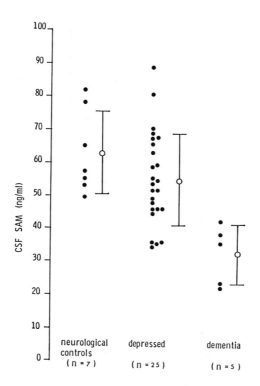

Fig. 2.   CSF SAM in depressed and neurological patients
(vertical bars indicate mean $\pm$ SD).

In a group of patients with dementia CSF SAM levels
were significantly lower than the neurological control
group and depressed patients ($p < 0.001$). One patient with a
severe memory impairment was also B_{12} deficient. Bone
marrow examination showed megaloblastic changes. Another
patient in that group had a multi-infarct dementia and the
remaining three patients who had the lowest CSF SAM levels
had senile dementia of the Alzheimers type. Red cell folate
was below the normal range or border-line in each case.

The folate status in trial patients revealed that 31%

Variable	Group (n)	Baseline	14 days	P+
CSF SAM ng/ml	SAM (13)	52.4 (48.2,55.7)	62.8 (58.8,67.1)	0.02
	PLACEBO (11)	54.8 (51.1,58.9)	55.9 (52.1,60.0)	
CSF Methionine µmoles/L	SAM (12)	2.43 (2.07,2.86)	2.67 (2.28,3.14)	N.S.
	PLACEBO (10)	3.18 (2.62,3.86)	2.82 (2.32,3.42)	
CSF Folate ng/ml	SAM (12)	17.9 (15.0,21.4)	17.3 (14.5,20.7)	N.S.
	PLACEBO (11)	14.2 (11.0,17.0)	15.8 (13.2,19.0)	
CSF 5HIAA nmoles/L	SAM (12)	77.6 (70.4,85.6)	101.2 (91.7,111.6)	0.10
	PLACEBO (11)	88.9 (80.2,98.5)	98.2 (88.6,108.8)	
CSF HVA nmoles/L	SAM (12)	160 (146,174)	200 (183,218)	N.S.
	PLACEBO (11)	166 (151,182)	194 (177,213)	
CSF MHPG nmoles/L	SAM (9)	51.1 (45.6,57.4)	55.5 (49.4,62.2)	N.S.
	PLACEBO (11)	48.3 (43.5,53.6)	51.2 (46.2,56.9)	
PLASMA PROLACTIN µIU/ml	SAM (9)	63.4 (48.7,82.6)	5.7 (4.2, 7.7)	0.0014
	PLACEBO (11)	26.6 (20.8,33.9)	38.1 (29.9,48.5)	

Table 1. Figures presented are backtransformed (antilog) means and 95% confidence intervals based on within patient variation in analysis of variance. P+ Comparison of changes between baseline and 14 days in SAM and placebo treated groups.

had a red cell folate value of less than 150 ng/ml. CSF folate was also low, 35% with a value of less than 15.0 ng/ml. We did not find any correlations in red cell, serum and CSF folate with SAM or methionine either pre-treatment or post-SAM treatment and CSF folate levels were unaffected (Table 1). However an interesting finding in the trial patients is a significant correlation of baseline red cell folate and CSF 5HIAA (Fig. 3).

Table 1 includes data of CSF 5HIAA, HVA, and MHPG, the metabolites of serotonin (5HT), dopamine (DA) and noradrena- line (NA) respectively. Comparison of changes between treat- ment groups for 5HIAA was just outside the 5% level of significance. HVA increased in both treatment groups. MHPG showed no significant changes. Correlations of pretreatment blood and CSF SAM levels in all patients versus the various monoamine metabolites were not significant (table 2). However a highly significant correlation was found between CSF SAM levels and CSF HVA after SAM treatment. The changes in SAM and HVA pre and post-treatment were related. This was not seen in placebo treated patients. There was a

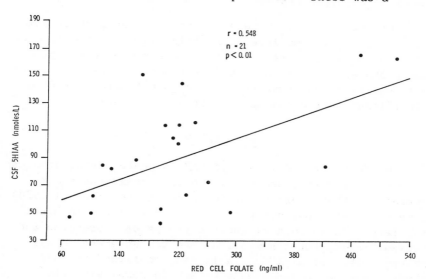

Fig. 3. Correlation between red cell folate and CSF 5HIAA in depressed patients.

	CORRELATION COEFFICIENT					
	Pre-treatment			Post–SAM–Treatment		
	r	n	p	r	n	p
Blood SAM vs CSF MHPG	0.327	20	n.s.	0.328	10	n.s.
CSF SAM vs CSF MHPG	0.246	20	n.s.	0.224	10	n.s.
Blood SAM vs CSF HVA	0.318	20	n.s.	0.166	12	n.s.
CSF SAM vs CSF HVA	0.323	20	n.s.	0.830	12	<0.001
Blood SAM vs CSF 5HIAA	0.112	20	n.s.	0.111	12	n.s.
CSF SAM vs CSF 5HIAA	0.017	20	n.s.	0.529	12	<0.10

Table 2.   Correlation coefficients between blood and CSF
SAM and various neurotransmitter metabolites.

strong trend for a correlation of CSF SAM and CSF 5HIAA
post–SAM treatment ($r = 0.529$) but this was outside the 5%
level of significance.

Plasma prolactin were estimated pre and post treatment
in 20 patients. The levels of prolactin decreased in each
case in the same treated group whereas those in the placebo
group showed changes in both directions. Comparison of the
mean values of the changes pre and post treatment showed a
significant decrease after SAM treatment (table 1).

DISCUSSION

Decreased blood levels of SAM in acute schizophrenics
have been reported, whereas in chronic schizophrenia and
depression there were no differences (Andreoli et al 1978).
A more recent study did not show any difference in blood
SAM levels in various diagnostic groups of depression and
schizophrenia, but a sex difference was apparent in all
groups (Cohen et al 1982), a finding confirmed in this
study. The decreased levels of SAM in females may be
related to substrate concentrations of methionine which, as
is true of all the other amino acids, is lower in females.

Physiologically methionine adenosyl-transferase (MAT) is
unsaturated and increasing methionine can increase SAM
concentrations. The extent to which CSF SAM may reflect
brain tissue concentrations is uncertain as we are unaware
of any studies to demonstrate this. However we did not
find any sex differences in CSF SAM content as we did for
erythrocytes. It has been shown that systemic administration of SAM to rats can increase brain levels of SAM
(Stramentinoli et al 1977). We have demonstrated increases
in CSF SAM after drug treatment indicating that in man SAM
can cross the blood brain barrier where it may act on the
central nervous system.

A close relationship between SAM and folate exists
with SAM influencing enzymes involved in the folate one
carbon cycle. Folate deficiency is common in dementia as
it is also in depression. Our findings of low CSF SAM in a
group of dementias may be influenced by the low folate
status also observed. Decreased levels of SAM in liver but
not brain tissue have been reported in mice fed folate
deficient diets (Middaugh et al 1979) and it appears that a
rather severe reduction in folic acid is required to
noticeably influence SAM. Low CSF SAM in dementia may be
related to other pathways i.e. synthesis of choline or
incorporation of phospholipids into membranes both of which
have been shown to be defective in this condition and in
which SAM is involved. Further investigations of SAM in
dementia are warranted.

We have confirmed previous studies of folate deficiency
in depression. It was also interesting that red cell folate
correlated with CSF 5HIAA. In previous studies one in
psychiatric patients (Bowers and Reynolds 1972) and one in
senile dementia (Shaw et al 1971) folate deficiency was not
found to be associated with CSF 5HIAA. These studies were
based on serum folate, whereas red cell folate may be more
indicative of tissue levels and may represent a more stable
pool. Animal studies have shown that rats fed folate deficient diets had decreased brain 5HT content (Botez et al
1979), and that treatment with folate in folate deficient
depressed patients increased CSF 5HIAA (Botez et al 1982).

The anatomical distribution of 5-methyl-tetrahydrofolate
(THF) in rat brain shown to correlate with indolamine
neurones, and that it makes up approximately 50% of
synaptosomal folate. Considered together it tends to
suggest a role for folates in the synaptic region more
specifically within the serotonergic synapse. Methyl-THF
is the transport form of folate across the blood brain
barrier (Chanarin et al 1974). Given in this form it may
increase brain levels more rapidly. Methyl-THF given to a
child with 5,10, methylene-THF reductase deficiency with
associated neuropsychiatric complications was shown to
increase CSF acid metabolites (I. Smith et al personal
communication). CSF SAM in this patient examined by our
laboratory was extremely low, 5.0 ng/ml (unpublished
observations).

SAM has been shown to influence neurotransmitters in
particular the serotonergic (Curcio et al 1978) and also
the nor-adrenergic (Algeri et al 1979) system in rats.
Increases in CSF 5HIAA have also been reported after
treatment with SAM in man (Angoli et al 1977) using the
probenecid technique to prevent egress of acid metabolites.
We observed a strong tendency for CSF SAM to correlate with
CSF 5HIAA after SAM treatment which is consistent with previous reports of SAM affecting the 5HT system. The correlated
changes after SAM treatment with HVA suggest more than just
a casual role for SAM in its effect on neurotransmitter
systems in man. In rats brain SAM levels can be decreased
by administration of methyl group acceptors notably L-DOPA
(Wurtman and Ordenz 1979) with parallel increases in
S-adenosylhomocysteine (SAH) (Wagner et al 1984) and
therefore they could modulate brain synthesis of methyl
groups. This opens the possibility for some kind of servo
control linking methyl group synthesis and utilization with
neuronal activity.

Our observations of decreased prolactin levels after
SAM treatment tend to suggest an influence on the dopamine
system. Prolactin secretion is under the influence of
inhibitory and releasing factors. Dopamine secreted by the
tubero-infundibular system is the main inhibitory factor

involved in the control of prolactin secretion. Neuroleptics
can greatly increase plasma prolactin by blockade of DA
receptors and drugs such as L-DOPA and bromocryptine which
can elevate DA cause a decrease. SAM may be exerting a DA
agonist like action or alternatively be acting in other ways
which leads to decreases in prolactin. Protein carboxymethylation of neurohormones have been demonstrated in vitro with
luteinizing hormone showing the greatest substrate
specificity followed by follicle-stimulatrng hormone, adreno-
corticotropic hormone growth hormone and then prolactin
(Diliberto and Axlerod, 1974). Studies are in progress to
determine the time course of the decrease in prolactin.

Perhaps it is not surprising that SAM may affect a
variety of processes as it is involved in methylation of
neurotransmitters, proteins, phospholipids as well as
participating in the metabolism of folates and polyamines
and that the metabolites of SAM particularly SAH and
methyl-thioadenosine (MTA) are themselves active compounds.
From our studies we can only attempt to demonstrate obvious
effects of SAM that can be monitored and relate these to
clinical improvement, but it is a first step in a human
study approach. Certainly the effects of SAM will not be
confined to any one clinical condition.

REFERENCES

1. Agnoli, A., Ruggieri, S. and Cerone, G. (1977) in
   Depressive Disorders (Garattini, G., Ed) pp 447-458,
   Stuttgart : Schattauer-Verlag.
2. Algeri, S., Catto, E. and Curcio, M. (1979) in
   Biochemical and Pharmacological roles of adrenosyl
   methionine and the central nervous system. (Zappia,
   V., Usdin, E., Salvatore, F. Ed) pp. 81-87, Oxford,
   Pergamon Press.
3. Andreoli, V., Maffei, F., Tonon, G. (1978) in
   Transmethylations and the central nervous system.
   (Andreoli, V., Agnoli, A., Fazio, C. Ed) pp. 147-150,
   Springler-Verlag.

4. Botez, M.I., Young, S.N. and Bacheralier, J. (1979) Nature 278, 182–183.

5. Botez, M.I., Young, S.N. and Bachevalier, J. (1982) Annals of Neurology 12, 479–485.

6. Bottiglieri, T., Lim, C.K. and Peters, T.J. (1984) J Chromatog. 311, 354–360.

7. Bowers, M.B. and Reynolds E.H. (1972) Lancet ii, 1376.

8. Carney, M. W. P. and Sheffield, B. F. (1970) J. Nerv. Ment. Dis. 150, 404–412.

9. Cohen, B., Lipinski, J. F., Vuckovic, A. (1982) Am. J. Psychiat. 139, 229–231.

10. Chanarin, I., Perry, J. and Reynolds, E. H. (1974) Clin. Sci. Mol. Med 46, 369–373.

11. Curico, M., Catto, E. and Stramentinoli, G. (1978) Progress in Neuropsychopharmacology 2, 65–71.

12. Diliberto, E.J. Jr., Axelrod, J. (1974) Proc. Nat. Acad. Sci. USA 71, 1701–1704.

13. Fazio, C., Andreoli, V., Agnoli, A. (1974) IRCS Medical Science-Nervous System 2, 1015.

14. Ghadrian, A. M., Anarth, J. and Engelsmann, F. (1980) Psychomatics 21, 926–929.

15. Giulidori, P. and Stramentinoli, G. (1984) Anal. Biochem. 137, 217–220.

16. Joseph, M. H. and Davies, P. (1983) J. Chromatog. 277, 125–136.

17. Middaugh, L. A., Grover, T. A. and Zemp, J.W. (1979) in Folic acid in Neurology, Psychiatry and Internal Medicine (Botez, M. I., Reynolds, E. H. Ed) pp. 213–228. Raven Press.

18. Reynolds, E. H., Toone, B. K. and Carney, M. W. P. (1984) The Lancet ii, 196–198.

19. Shaw, D. M., MacSweeney, D. A. and Johnson, A. L. (1971) Psychol. Med. 1, 166–171.

20. Stramentinoli, G., Catto, E., Algeri, S. (1977) Communications in Psychopharmacology 1, 89–97.

21. Wurtman, R. S. and Ordonez, L. A. (1979) in Biochemical and Pharmacological roles of adenosylmethionine and the central nervous system (Zappia, V., Usdin, E., Salvatore, F. eds) pp. 132–143, Oxford Pergamon Press.

22. Wagner, J., Danzin, C. and Huot-Oliver, S. (1984) J. Chromatog. 290, 247–262.

NORADRENERGIC AND CARDIOVASCULAR EFFECTS OF CHRONIC S-ADENYOSYL-METHIONINE IN HEALTHY VOLUNTEERS

Michael A. Sherer, M.D., Matthew V. Rudorfer, M.D.,

Giulio L. Cantoni, M.D.*, Robert N. Golden, M.D.,

William Z. Potter, M.D., Ph.D.

Section on Clinical Pharmacology, Laboratory of
Clinical Science and
*Laboratory of General and Comparative Biochemistry
National Institute of Mental Health
Bethesda, Maryland 20205 U.S.A.

INTRODUCTION

S-Adenosyl-Methionine (SAMe), the universal methyl donor in methylation reactions, has been extensively studied over the past twenty years in a variety of neuropsychiatric conditions (Agnoli et al., 1976; Fazio et al., 1974; Carney et al., 1983). Following early case reports indicating that SAMe might have a mood-elevating effect, studies were conducted in Italy (Agnoli et al., 1976; Del Vecchio et al., 1978; Miccoli et al., 1978; Muscettola et al., 1982; Salvadorini et al., 1980), Germany (Kufferle et al., 1982) and in the United States (Lipinski et al., 1984); these provide evidence that parenterally administered SAMe can produce clinical improvement in depressed patients. In comparison to standard antidepressants, SAMe is claimed to be as effective as the tricyclics while producing fewer side effects.

The mechanism by which SAMe exerts its possible anti-depressant action has not been studied in man. As the two neurotransmitters most frequently considered to be involved in the affective illness are norepinephrine (NE) and serotonin, we decided to explore the possibly relevant pharmacology of SAMe on the NE system in young healthy volunteers.

339

SUBJECTS AND METHODS

Subjects were eight healthy men aged 18 to 25, housed
in a clinical research unit at the National Institute of
Mental Health. There was no history of psychiatric illness
in the subjects or their first-degree relatives. They were
in good physical health, as confirmed by physical exam,
EKG, blood chemistries, hematology, urinalysis and thyroid
testing. Subjects were all free from any medications in
the three weeks prior to testing and avoided alcohol or
drugs. The study consisted of a 12-day stay in the in-
patient unit and required that subjects adhere to a
standard low monoamine diet.

Following a 24-hour acclimatization, patients were
studied on days 2 and 3 with either a single 400 mg dose
of SAMe or placebo (saline) infusion. The order of
administration was randomized and both the subjects and
unit staff (but not the administering physician) were blind
to the treatment condition. At 7 AM, following an overnight fast, subjects were allowed to void and then rest in
bed for an additional 120 minutes. An intravenous
butterfly needle was then inserted into an antecubital
vein and kept open throughout the study with a slow normal
saline drip. The SAMe or saline placebo was given by slow
bolus injection at 9:30 AM and 20 minutes later blood
samples were drawn for measurement of plasma NE and its
major metabolite, 3-methoxy-4-hydroxyphenylglycol (MHPG).

Blood pressure (BP) and heart rate (HR) were monitored
every five minutes. Ten minutes after the initial blood
drawing, the subjects were instructed to assume a standing
position. BP and HR were monitored every one to two
minutes and a second blood sample was drawn after the
subject had been standing for five minutes.

On days 5 through 11 of the study, subjects received
a daily (9 AM) 400 mg dose of SAMe administered by slow
bolus infusion. Subjects were not blind to these administrations. On day 12 the physiologic challenge described
above was repeated.

Plasma NE concentrations were measured after alumina
gel extraction with electrochemical detection high
performance liquid chromatography (HPLC), using N-methyl

dopamine as an internal standard. Reverse phase HPLC with electrochemical detection was also used to assay plasma MHPG concentration, with 3-ethoxy-4-hydroxyphenylglycol as the internal standard. Data were analyzed with repeated measures analysis of variance (ANOVA), paired Student's t test, and Spearman's correlation coefficient.

Twenty-four hour urine samples (7 AM to 7 AM) were collected daily into plastic containers, preserved with 3% sodium bisulfite and kept frozen at -20°C until analyzed for the norepinephrine metabolites MHPG and vanillylmandelic acid (VMA) using gas chromatography/mass spectrometry. All urine samples were analyzed for a given substance within a single run. A urine sample of at least 900 ml was collected during the placebo period and during each of the ten study days. Adequate collections were available and were analyzed for four of the eight subjects.

RESULTS

Data on the subjects' supine and upright HR are presented in Table 1, as is delta HR, the change following the physiologic challenge. No differences were noted in supine HR between placebo and chronic conditions. In the acute condition supine HR was slightly, but insignificantly, higher. Upright HR, however, was lower on the chronic condition compared to either placebo (p<.02), or acute (p<.02) conditions, reflecting a decrease in 6 of 8 subjects, with unchanged values for another. Delta HR was significantly higher in the placebo condition, compared to either the acute (p<.02) or chronic (p<.02) conditions, although blood pressure continued to rise following the physiologic challenge under all conditions.

Supine diastolic BPs did not vary over the three treatment conditions (Table 1). Upright diastolic BPs were higher than corresponding supine values in all conditions. The rise in diastolic BP was significant for the placebo (p<.02) and chronic conditions (p<.02). The rise for the acute condition did not reach statistical significance.

Supine systolic BP did not differ among the three conditions. However, in 6 of 8 subjects, upright systolic BP was lower in the chronic condition compared to placebo.

Table 1.   CARDIOVASCULAR EFFECTS OF SAMe   ($\overline{X} \pm$ SEM)

	Placebo	Acute	Chronic
Supine BP (mmHg)	$\dfrac{120.3 + 1.7}{66.0 \pm 1.7}$	$\dfrac{121.3 + 3.8}{65.3 + 3.2}$	$\dfrac{120.0 + 3.0}{63.5 + 3.1}$
Upright BP (mmHg)	$\dfrac{125.9 + 3.2}{76.0 \pm 4.1}$	$\dfrac{124.6 + 4.4}{71.7 \pm 2.9}$	$\dfrac{118.6 + 4.5}{73.1 + 3.6}$
Supine Pulse (bpm)	60.0 ± 3.5	64.0 ± 4.2	58.6 ± 3.7
Upright Pulse (bpm)	86.2 ± 2.1[a]	85.4 ± 2.3[a]	80.1 ± 3.0[b]
Delta Pulse (bpm)	26.2 ± 3.0[c]	21.4 ± 3.6[d]	21.5 ± 1.5[d]

a vs b, p <.02
c vs d, p <.02

Supine plasma MHPG, supine and upright plasma NE and delta NE, the NE rise following the physiologic challenge, are presented in Table 2. Upright NE was lower on the chronic condition vs. placebo (p<.05), reflecting a decrease in the upright NE for five of the eight subjects in the chronic compared to the placebo condition. No subjects had higher upright NE values in the chronic condition compared to placebo; in three subjects the values were unchanged. Supine MHPG and supine NE values were not affected by either acute or chronic SAMe, with an equal number of subjects showing mild increases or decreases in supine NE. The NE increment was reduced on chronic drug. However, with the small number of subjects, this did not reach statistical significance.

Results for the 24 hour urinary MHPG and VMA collections are presented in Table 3 and Figure 1. In one of the four subjects, a gradual decrease was noted over the treatment days for both metabolites. A trend can be noted for lower catecholamine excretion during the mid-phase of treatment (day four). Overall ANOVA was not significant for the treatment effect, however. As we had seen in unmedicated depressed patients (Linnoila et al., 1982a) there was a high (r>0.9) correlation between the urinary NE metabolites both before and during SAMe administration.

Table 2.   SAMe EFFECTS ON PLASMA CATECHOLAMINES

                              (pmol/ml, $\overline{X}$ ± SEM)

	Placebo	Acute	Chronic
Supine NE	1.04 ± 0.18	0.86 ± 0.17	0.86 ± 0.15
Upright NE	2.91 ± 0.49[a]	2.66 ± 0.50	2.22 ± 0.20[b]
Delta NE	1.87 ± 0.36	1.80 ± 0.39	1.37 ± 0.15
MHPG (supine)	13.90 ± 0.95	14.95 ± 0.40	14.97 ± 0.25

a vs b, p<.05

Throughout the treatment conditions, no subjects complained of dizziness following the physiologic challenge, although it is important to note that we were evaluating healthy young volunteers with considerable cardiac reserve. Daily mood and anxiety rating scales showed no change over the 12 days of this study. Subjects were unable to accurately distinguish between the placebo and acute administration days (four subjects guessed correctly; four did not). Overall, subjects uniformly reported an inability to detect any effect of the SAMe administration, except for local erythema at the site of the I.V. administrations in several of the subjects.

Table 3.

URINARY CONCENTRATIONS OF NOREPINEPHRINE METABOLITES

                              (g/l, $\overline{X}$ ± SEM)

	MHPG	VMA
Placebo	2.69 ± 0.15	4.70 ± 0.31
SAMe Day 1	2.51 ± 0.19	4.22 ± 0.29
SAMe Day 4	2.06 ± 0.12	3.67 ± 0.17
SAMe Day 7	2.43 ± 0.22	4.15 ± 0.26

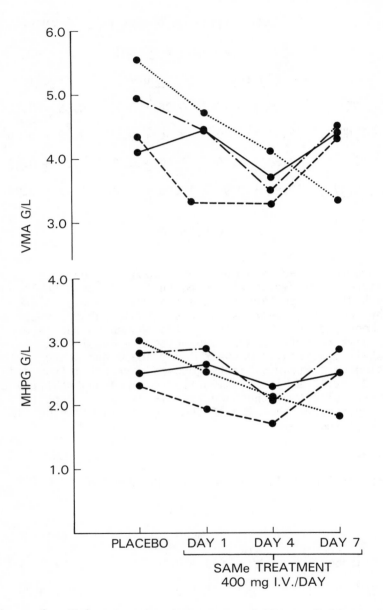

Figure 1. Urinary excretion rates of NE metabolites VMA
(top panel) and MHPG (bottom panel) before and during week
of SAMe administration in four volunteers.

DISCUSSION

The main finding of our study is that SAMe, in healthy male volunteers, affects peripheral cardiovascular measures of adrenergic function in the challenged, but not resting, state. We also confirm previous reports on the lack of behavioral effects of SAMe in volunteers (Baldessarini et al., 1979); self-rating scores showed no changes in mood or anxiety, and the subjects were unable to distinguish SAMe administration from placebo. Ours is the first study in man to specifically address the relationship of SAMe to adrenergic function, following either acute or chronic treatment. Acute biochemical effects have been studied in rat, following SAMe and probenecid, with evidence of increased synthesis and levels of NE in the brainstem and hypothalamus (Algeri et al., 1979). Thus, it is reasonable to look for longer term effects on the noradrenergic system.

As reviewed elsewhere (McDevitt et al., 1979) the normal physiologic response to the challenge of assuming a standing posture from a supine position includes clear increases in diastolic blood pressure and heart rate. Since selective beta blockers reduce the HR response to orthostasis or exercise by 15-20% (Frishman et al., 1980; Carruthers et al., 1974; Kofi-Ekue et al., 1974), the increase in heart rate on standing is considered to be an indicator of beta receptor function. Interestingly, chronic SAMe reduces the mean HR response to orthostasis from 26.2 to 21.5 bpm (Table 1), a decrease similar in magnitude to that seen after beta blockers.

SAMe does not appear to affect the diastolic BP rise seen on standing. The upright systolic BP shows a trend toward reduction which, while not significant, is reminiscent of the BP response to various antidepressant treatments, particularly the monoamine oxidase inhibitors (MAOIs). In our study, the alterations of heart rate in response to the physiologic challenge are paralleled by changes in plasma NE levels. Thus, the upright NE values are significantly lower following chronic administration compared to placebo, with only a nonsignificant decline in supine plasma NE.

The regulation of cardiovascular parameters, and their relationship to quantitative (and often indirect)

measures of synaptic transmission, are obviously complex.
Nonetheless, under well-controlled conditions with young
healthy volunteers, pulse increases on standing can be
related to increases in plasma NE (Rudorfer et al., in
press; Goldstein et al., 1983; Ross et al., 1983). The
associations found in this study between plasma measures of
adrenergic function and measures of cardiovascular function
are consistent with these earlier findings. Available
evidence indicates that in young healthy adults cardiovascular response is proportional to sympathetic nervous
system activation. Thus, the most apparent explanation for
our data is that SAMe treatment produces a modest depression of sympathetic nervous system release of NE in
response to standing, reflected most clearly in the blunted
cardiovascular response. Evidence favoring a specific
pharmacological effect rather than an overall reduction in
noradrenergic responsivity related to time or adaptation
to testing includes data derived in an earlier study of
similar volunteers, in which 8 days of lithium treatment
failed to alter plasma NE change to the same orthostatic
challenge (Rudorfer et al., 1985).

All effective antidepressant agents studied thus far
reduce whole-body NE turnover in depressed patients
(Linnoila et al., 1982a; 1983). Healthy volunteers showed
this effect when treated with the serotonin reuptake
inhibitor zimelidine (Rudorfer et al., 1984) but not with
lithium (Rudorfer et al., 1985).

In the current study, despite an intriguing decrease
for one subject of both urinary MHPG and VMA, the overall
excretion of these metabolites was unchanged in the group
of subjects in whom these measures were obtained.
Similarly, plasma MHPG was unchanged under any of the
three conditions. Taken together, these results can be
seen as further evidence for an unaltered baseline of the
adrenergic system following SAMe treatment. To the extent
that SAMe affected the noradrenergic system, this was
evident only in the challenged state. No data are available at this time on the effect of SAMe on urinary
noradrenergic measures in depressed patients.

The significant attenuation of the pulse and plasma
NE responses to the physiologic challenge, with no significant changes in urinary NE measures may offer a clue to
the putative antidepressant action of SAMe. In a recent

study with the same cardiovascular challenge used here, untreated unipolar and bipolar depressed patients showed an elevated noradrenergic response to the orthostatic challenge, compared to normal volunteers, while showing no elevation of supine NE (Rudorfer et al., in press). The increased response of untreated patients to the physiologic challenge can be seen as evidence of an "inefficient" noradrenergic system, as can the greater urinary turnover in the untreated vs. the treated state (Potter et al., in press).

Recent studies provide increasing evidence on the interaction of central and peripheral adrenergic measures. Locus coeruleus stimulation appears to cause peripheral NE release (Crawley et al., 1978) and, conversely, alterations of the sympathetic nervous system may produce parallel changes in the central nervous system (Maas et al., 1983). The α_2 agonist clonidine reduces peripheral release of NE and MHPG, presumably due to the central effects on locus coeruleus and without effect on the presynaptic α_2-receptors (Kobinger et al., 1978; Fitzgerald et al., 1981).

It therefore is possible that peripheral measures obtained in blood and urine may reflect central adrenergic function. This is particularly important if we compare the cardiovascular effects of SAMe to MAOIs. The mechanism of the orthostatic effect following MAOIs remains obscure. Most recently, central mechanisms have been invoked: using a pithed rat as a model of a noradrenergic system isolated from CNS influences, no decrement was noted in effective noradrenergic function as a result of treatment with clorgyline, an MAO type A inhibitor (Cohen et al., 1982). This finding suggests either central regulation or, alternatively, peripheral regulation with a centrally mediated reflex component. A central mechanism for the peripheral noradrenergic functional changes we observed after SAMe could, by analogy, be present since qualitatively the changes are the same as observed following administration of clorgyline to patients (Ross et al., 1985).

In summary, we find a blunted noradrenergic responsivity in volunteers following chronic SAMe administration, consistent with what we might expect from an antidepressant.

No changes were noted in the measures of the unchallenged
adrenergic system, as measured by urinary turnover of MHPG
and VMA and plasma NE and MHPG. It is important to note,
however, that we do not always find identical drug effects
in patients and volunteers. Particularly interesting in
comparison is lithium, which appears to have little effect
on adrenergic measures in volunteers but decreases NE
turnover in patients. Studies in patients on the effects
of SAMe on urine, plasma, and cerebrospinal fluid adrenergic
measures will be helpful in clarifying its mechanism of
antidepressant action.

REFERENCES

Agnoli, A., Andreoli, V., Casacchia, M. and Cerbo, R.
    (1976) Effect of S-adenosyl-L-methionine (SAMe) upon
    depressive symptoms. J. Psychiatr. Res. 13, 43.
Agnoli, A., Andreoli, V., Casacchia, M., Maffei, F. and
    Fazio, C. (1978) in Transmethylations and the Central
    Nervous System (Andreoli, V., Agnoli, A. and Fazio, C.,
    Eds.) p. 170. Springer-Verlag, New York.
Algeri, S., Catto, E. and Curcio, M. (1979) in Biochemical
    and Pharmacological Roles of Adenosylmethionine in
    the Central Nervous System, (Zappia, V. and Usdin, E.,
    Eds.) Pergamon Press, London.
Baldessarini, R.J., Stramentinoli, G. and Lipinski, J.F.
    (1979) Methylation hypothesis. Arch. Gen. Psychiatry,
    36, 303.
Carney, M.W.P., Martin, R., Bottigheny, T., Reynolds, E.H.,
    Nissenbaum, H., Toone, B.K. and Sheffield, B.F. (1983)
    Switch mechanism in affective illness and S-adenosyl-
    methionine. Lancet, 1, 820.
Carruthers, S.G., Ghosal, A., McDevitt, D.G., Nelson, J.K.
    and Shanks, R.G. (1974) The assessment of beta-
    adrenoceptor blocking drugs in hyperthyroidism. Br.
    J. Clin. Pharmacol. 1, 93.
Cohen, R.M., Campbell, I.C. and Yamaguchi, I. (1982)
    Cardiovascular changes in response to selective
    monoamine oxidase inhibition in the rat. Eur. J.
    Pharmacol. 80, 155.
Crawley, J.N., Hattox, S.E., Maas, J.W. and Roth, R.H.
    (1978) 3-methoxy-4-hydroxyphenethyleneglycol increase
    in plasma after stimulation of the nuclear locus
    coeruleus. Brain Res. 141, 380.

Del Vecchio, M., Iorio, G., Cocorullo, M., Vacca, L. and
    Amati, A. (1978) Has SAMe (AdoMet) an antidepressant
    effect A preliminary trial versus chlorimipramine.
    Rivista Sperimentale di Freniatria, 102, 344.
Fazio, C., Andreoli, V., Agnoli, A., Casacchia, M., Cerbo,
    R. and Pinzello, A. (1974) Therapy of schizophrenia
    and depressive disorders with S-adenosyl-L-methionine.
    IRCS (Research on: Clinical Pharmacology and
    Therapeutics; Human Metabolism and Nutrition;
    Psychiatry and Clinical Psychology; Psychology),
    2, 1015.
Fitzgerald, G.A., Watkins, J. and Dolby, C.T. (1981)
    Regulation of norepinephrine release by peripheral
    alpha-2 receptor stimulation. Clin. Pharmacol. Ther.
    29, 160.
Frishman, W.A. (ed.) (1980) Comparison of Tindolol and
    Propanolol Treatment, p. 145, Appleton-Century-Crofts,
    New York.
Goldstein, D.S., McCarty, R., Polinsky, R.J. and Kopin, I.J.
    (1983) Relationship between plasma norepinephrine and
    sympathetic neural activity. Hypertension, 5, 552.
Karoum, F. and Neff, N.H. (1982) in Modern Methods in
    Pharmacology (Spector, S. and Beck, N., Eds.)
    pp. 39-54, Alan R. Liss, New York.
Kobinger, W. (1978) Central alpha-adrenergic systems as
    targets for hypotensive drugs. Rev. Physiol. Biochem.
    Pharmacol. 8, 39.
Kofi-Ekue, J.M., Shanks, R.G. and Walsh, M.J. (1974)
    Observations on the effects of beta-adrenoceptor
    blocking drugs on glyceryl trinitrate tachycardia.
    Br. J. Clin. Pharmacol. 1, 19.
Kufferle, B. and Grinberger, J. (1982) in Typical and
    Atypical Antidepressants: Clinical Practice (Costa, E.
    and Racagni, G., Eds.) p. 175, Raven Press, New York.
Linnoila, M., Karoum, F., Calil, H.M., Kopin, I.J. and
    Potter, W.Z. (1982a) Alteration of norepinephrine
    metabolism with desipramine and zimelidine in depressed
    patients. Arch. Gen. Psychiatry 39, 1025.
Linnoila, M., Karoum, F. and Potter, W.Z. (1982b) High
    correlation of norepinephrine and its major metabolite
    excretion rates. Arch. Gen. Psychiatry 39, 521.
Linnoila, M., Karoum, F., Rosenthal, N. and Potter, W.Z.
    (1983) Electroconvulsive treatment and lithium
    carbonate. Arch. Gen. Psychiatry 40, 677.
Lipinski, J.F., Cohen, B.M., Frankenburg, M.D., Tohen, M.,
    Waternaux, C., Altesman, R., Jones, B. and Harris, P.
    (1984) Open trial of S-adenosyl-methionine for treat-
    ment of depression. Am. J. Psychiatry 141, 448.

Maas, J.W. (ed.) (1983) MHPG: Basic Mechanism and Psychopathology, p. 33. Academic Press, New York.

McDevitt, D.G. (1979) in Advances in Pharmacology and Therapeutics, Proceedings of the Seventh International Congress of Pharmacology. (Tillement, J.P., Ed.) p.77, Pergamon Press, Oxford.

Miccoli, L., Porro, V. and Bertolina, A. (1978) Comparison between the antidepressant activity of S-adenosyl-methionine (SAMe) and that of some tricyclic drugs. Acta Neurologica 33, 243.

Muscettola, G., Galzenati, M. and Balbi, A. (1982) in Typical and Atypical Antidepressants: Clinical Practice, (Costa, E. and Racagni, G., Eds.) p. 151, Raven Press, New York.

Potter, W.Z., Rudorfer, M.V. and Linnoila, M. (in press) New clinical studies support a role of norepinephrine in antidepressant action. Proceedings of the Earl Usdin Memorial Symposium.

Ross, R.J., Scheinin, M., Lesieur, P., Rudorfer, M.V., Hauger, R.L., Siever, L.J., Linnoila, M. and Potter, W.Z. (1985) The effects of clorgyline on noradrenergic function. Psychopharmacology 85, 227.

Ross, R.J., Zavadil, A.P. III, Calil, H.M., Linnoila, M., Kitanaka, I., Blombery, P., Kopin, I.J. and Potter, W.Z (1983) Effects of desmethylimipramine on plasma norepinephrine, pulse and blood pressure. Clin. Pharmacol. Ther. 33, 429.

Rudorfer, M.V., Karoum, F., Ross, R.J., Potter, W.Z. and Linnoila, M. (1985) Differences in lithium effects in depressed and healthy subjects. Clin. Pharmacol. Ther. 37, 66.

Rudorfer, M.V., Ross, R.J., Linnoila, M., Sherer, M.A. and Potter, W.Z. (in press) Exaggerated orthostatic responsivity of plasma norepinephrine in depression. Arch. Gen. Psychiatry.

Salvadorini, F., Mariani, G., Galeone, F. and Saba, P. (1980) Evaluation of S-adenosyl-methionine (SAMe) effectivenes on depression. Cur. Ther. Res. 27, 908.

Spector, S. and Beck N. (eds.) (1982) Modern Methods in Pharmacology, pp. 39-54. Alan R. Liss, New York.

Zavadil, A.P. III, Ross, R.J., Calil, H.M., Linnoila, M., Blombery, P., Jimerson, D.C., Kopin, I.J. and Potter, W.Z. (1984) The effect of desmethylimipramine on the metabolism of norepinephrine. Life Sci. 35, 1061.

ROLE OF THE ONE-CARBON CYCLE IN NEUROPSYCHIATRY

J.R. Smythies, R.D. Alarcon, A.J. Bancroft, J.A. Monti, D.A. Morere, L.C. Tolbert, and W.G. Walter-Ryan

Neurosciences Program & Clinical Studies Unit, Department of Psychiatry, University of Alabama at Birmingham, Birmingham, Alabama 35294

ABSTRACT

This paper reviews the work available to date suggesting that elements of the one-carbon cycle may be involved in psychiatric illnesses. Two enzymes of the one-carbon cycle (in erythrocytes) - methionine adenosyltransferase (MAT) and serine hydroxymethyltransferase (SHMT) - have been reported by our group to be underactive in schizophrenia and depression and overactive in mania. This correlates with the reported anti-depressant effects of S-adenosylmethionine in humans. SHMT has also been found by another group to be underactive in serum of schizophrenics. This defect appears to be linked to abnormalities in the distribution of phospholipids in the membrane, with a relative deficiency of phosphatidylcholine and a relative excess of phosphatidylserine. Evidence showing that medications do not appear to be responsible for these findings will be presented. A review is then made of the role of transmethylation systems for lipids and proteins in cellular control systems. Lipid transmethylation is related in many systems to receptor-final messenger coupling and so to information transfer across the membrane. Protein methylation is involved in many cellular systems including chemotaxis in bacteria and leucocytes, neurotransmitter release, sperm motility and calmodulin function.

351

     This paper reviews evidence suggesting that transmethylation reactions (using S-adenosylmethionine (SAM) as a methyl donor) play a significant role in neuropsychiatric disorders. Historically, the first hypothesis relating transmethylation reactions and neuropsychiatry was made by Osmond, Smythies, Harley-Mason and Redmill in 1952, who suggested that a fault in the transmethylation of catecholamines could lead to the production in the brain of abnormal psychotoxic metabolites related to mescaline. Later this hypothesis was extended to cover the production of psychotomimetic derivatives of tryptamine such as dimethyltryptamine (DMT) and O-methylbufotenin (OMB). Although we were able to identify DMT and OMB in human cerebrospinal fluid by definitive GC/MS methodology, there were no important correlations between levels of these compounds and the clinical situation (Smythies et al., 1979).

     In 1963 a second "transmethylation" hypothesis was presented (Smythies, 1963). This suggested that there was some defect in the mechanism of transmethylation itself rather than in any psychotoxic products. Carl et al. (1978) showed that the levels of activity of two enzymes of the one-carbon cycle (Fig. 1) were low in schizophrenia (Fig. 2). These two enzymes were methionine adenosyltransferase (MAT) and serine hydroxymethyltransferase (SHMT). Using a kinetic assay, Kelsoe et al. (1982) confirmed that MAT activity in erythrocytes from schizophrenics was significantly lower than normal. Recently, Tolbert et al. (1983) found in addition that MAT activity in depressed patients is also low, whereas it is above normal in

RELEVANT PARTS OF THE ONE CARBON CYCLE

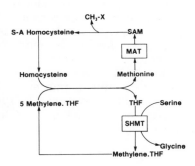

Fig. 1 – Elements of the one-carbon cycle.

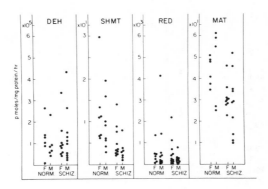

Fig. 2 – Activity of four enzymes of the one-carbon cycle
in male and female schizophrenic patients and normal controls.

mania (Fig. 3). This is in harmony with the many reports over
the last ten years (see review by Carney et al., 1983) that SAM
has antidepressant properties when given by intravenous infusion
in humans. It is claimed that SAM is as effective as standard
tricyclic antidepressants, works faster and has fewer side effects.
However, patients who do not respond to TCAs do not respond
to SAM.

A further link between transmethylation and psychiatric
disorders is the report, first made in 1961 by Pollin, Cardon and
Kety (1961) and confirmed many times since (see Cohen et al.
(1974) for a review), that some 40 per cent of chronic
schizophrenics react to 20 G/day L-methionine (plus or minus
a MAOI) with an acute florid psychosis. Normal subjects do
not show this response. This effect was at one time explained
by the supposition that the methionine load increased
transmethylation reactions and so the production of the
hypothetical methylated psychotoxic compounds. However,
it has since been shown that methionine loading does not increase
urinary levels of methylated metabolites of catecholamines (Antun
et al., 1971), does not increase SAM levels in human blood or
methylation of L-dopa in rat tissues, and actually decreases

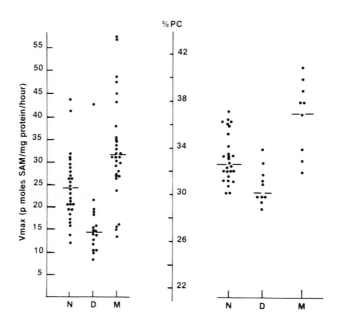

Fig. 3 – MAT kinetics (Vmax) in erythrocytes in depression, mania and schizophrenia.

the production of DMT by rabbit lung (Stramentinoli and Baldessarini, 1978). The latter effect may be due to the production of homocysteine (Fig. 1) which is a powerful inhibitor of transmethylation reactions (Schatz et al., 1981; Baudry et al., 1973). Another hypothesis to explain the "methionine" effect in chronic schizophrenia is that this represents, not an exacerbation of the schizophrenia, but rather a manic-type reaction superimposed on the chronic schizophrenia.

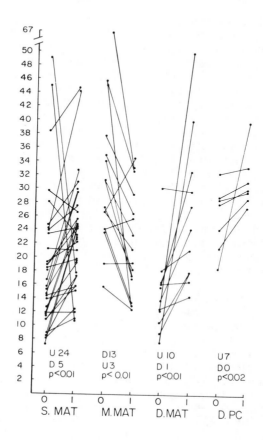

Fig. 4 - Changes in MAT kinetics (Vmax) in schizophrenia (S), mania (M) and depression (D), drug-free and after two weeks of medication (S - neuroleptics; M - neuroleptics ± lithium; D - anti-depressants). PC - % changes in membrane phosphatidylcholine in depression before and after treatment.

Another system that may be relevant in this context is the role that the methylation of phospholipids is thought to play in transferring information across cell membranes (Loh and Law, 1980). Hirata and Axelrod (1980) have suggested that the biochemical basis of this reaction is the successive methylation of phosphatidylethanolamine (PE) to form phosphatidylcholine (PC). Previous reports (Stevens, 1972; Henn and Henn, 1983) have found that RBCs from schizophrenic patients have lower PC and higher phosphatidylserine (PS) -(the immediate precursor of PE) levels - than normal. The most recent study in this area was by Hitzemann et al. (1985). These workers report that schizophrenic patients, but not manics, have a significant deficit in RBC phosphatidylcholine and patients with the most severe deficiency show a marked decrease in Na^+-Li^+ counter flow activity. The phospholipid methylation activity was measured in ghost RBC membranes by the Axelrod method. The patient group was composed of 20 DSM-III schizophrenics, 13 DSM III schizophreniform disorder patients and 11 DSM III manics. All three groups had decreased phospholipid methylation activity, although manics, especially drug-free patients, showed the least deviation from normal. However, there was no significant correlation between methylation and PC levels. They did not find that drug exposure significantly altered phospholipid methylation activity.

One problem to be examined is the possible role of medications (i.e. neuroleptics and lithium) in patients, in that the reported changes in MAT activity and phospholipid levels could be due to the previous medication rather than the disease process. To answer this question we have studied a group of 57 patients (Morere et al., 1985) with DSM III diagnoses of schizophrenia (29), mania (16) and major depression (12) in the Clinical Studies Unit of the University Hospital. Vmax was significantly increased (p < 0.01) after two weeks of neuroleptic therapy in schizophrenics and of antidepressant treatment in depressives, and was significantly decreased in manics (from a pre-drug high level) following lithium/neuroleptic therapy. Since these changes concomitant with medication are opposite in direction to those seen in the particular illnesses before medication, it seems unlikely that the levels found in the illness could be due to drug effects. Figure 4 shows the significant changes in MAT activity values after medication in schizophrenics (S), depressed (D) and manic (M) patients, as well as changes in per cent PC in the depressed population. In the case of per cent PC changes in schizophrenic and manic patients, the trends did not reach statistical significance. To confirm this point in vitro, studies were carried out adding neuroleptics to RBC preparations from three control subjects and comparing Vmax for MAT with and without preincubation with the neuroleptics. Table 1 shows that these drugs had no effect in vitro. Thus

TABLE 1

IN VITRO NEUROLEPTICS

SUBJECT	Control		CPZ		Hal		Flu		Thio	
	Vmax	Km	Vmax	Km	Vmax	Km	Vmax	Km	Vmax	Km
H.O.	25.01	1.99	24.87	2.59	25.36	2.87	24.92	3.49	25.42	4.96
J.K.	21.04	3.68	21.23	3.97	20.86	4.08	21.03	4.36	20.95	4.25
L.T.	23.40	5.44	23.61	5.86	24.12	5.73	23.51	6.02	23.46	6.54

CPZ = chlorpromazine, 500 ng/ml; Hal = haloperidol, 30 ng/ml; Flu = fluphenazine, 5 ng/ml; Thio = thioridazine, 500 ng/ml.

The preincubation with neuroleptics resulted in no consistent effect on Vmax. An increase in the Km was observed.

it is possible that the normalization in MAT activity and PC levels seen in the patient population are due to the changes in the clinical condition of the patients rather than to a direct drug effect on the enzyme. Further studies to elucidate this point are underway.

Transmethylation reactions are now known to play an important role in a number of cellular control processes. The Axelrod mechanism of lipid methylation has been implicated in the coupling of the receptor to second messenger mechanisms in a number of systems. For example, vasopressin, Ca^{++} transport, lymphocyte mitogenesis, histamine secretion (Prasad and Edwards, 1981), bradykinin (Dave et al., 1981), nerve growth factor (Pfenninger and Johnson, 1981), beta-adrenergic agonists in some tissues (Hirata et al., 1979), (but not all – see Koch et al., 1983), and others.

Another area of growing importance is protein carboxymethylation. This reaction methylates carboxyl groups in protein and so reduces the negative charge on the molecule. One enzyme, which is found only in bacteria, methylates glutamic acid residues (McFadden et al., 1983) and has been shown to control bacterial chemotaxis in E. coli (Kehry et al., 1983). Chemoattractants inhibit demethylation and chemorepellants have the opposite effects (Toews et al., 1979; Kleene et al., 1979). These demethylation mechanisms in turn control the movement of the bacterium's flagella which determines its mode of locomotion. In other systems carboxymethylation is effected by a second enzyme which methylates specifically d-aspartate, an amino acid found in aged proteins. The methylated residue then may racemate back to the normal L-isomer. Carboxymethylation also controls neurotransmitter release (e.g. beta-adrenergic stimulation of amylase secretion by the parotid) (Strittmatter et al., 1979). The methylation may reduce the mutually repelling negative charges on the protein of the external surface of the synaptic vesicle and the interior surface of the cell so that these membranes may fuse prior to exocytosis. Dopamine agonists stimulate carboxymethylation in striatal synaptosomes (Billingsley and Roth, 1982). This effect is blocked by (+) butaclamol, but not by its inactive (-) isomer. Pretreatment with 6OH dopamine abolishes the effect, which must therefore be limited to dopamine autoreceptors. Other loci where carboxymethylation is important are sperm motility, leucocyte chemotaxis and calmodulin function (Campillo and Ashcroft, 1982).

Other evidence indicating some disturbance of the one-carbon cycle in schizophrenia has been presented. Wilcox et al. (1985) reported that plasma serine hydroxymethyltransferase activity is low in schizophrenic patients (51 ($\pm$ 42 S.D.) nmol/mg protein v. 110 ($\pm$56) (p < 0.01) in normals (which we had found to be the case also for erythrocytes (Carl et al. (1978)). This coexisted with abnormally high plasma serine levels (202.6 ($\pm$ 385 S.D.) ug/ml v. 130.7 ($\pm$18.5) (p < 0.0001). However, administration of serine (4 mM/kg) to the psychotic patients produced no observable clinical effects. They observed that TCAs, lithium and neuroleptics did not affect plasma levels of serine or SHMT activity. Using another patient population of episodic psychotic patients with psychedelic symptoms, Bruinvels and Pepplinkhuizen, 1985, found that in ten such cases who were symptom free at the time, seven developed their characteristic symptoms to serine loading and three to glycine loading (2 mmol/kg). Administration of methionine to these patients was without effect. Administration of glycine and serine to eleven normal controls and three recovered manic depressives had no effect.

Patients who had a psychotic exacerbation of symptoms after administration of serine showed increased blood taurine levels and decreased blood serine levels.

Other data suggested some weakness in receptor-coupling in schizophrenia due in turn to defective methylation of phospholipids. In white blood cells from schizophrenics, less cyclic AMP is released by PGE_1 than normal (Rotrosen et al., 1980), but the cyclic AMP released by sodium fluoride activation is normal (Garver et al., 1982). This has been confirmed in platelets from male (but not female) schizophrenics (Kafka and van Kammen, 1983). The faulty link in the causal chain connecting the PGE_1 receptor and adenylate cyclase may be provided by lipid methylation.

SAM has been shown in normal volunteers to reduce the heart rate and to decrease blood levels of norepinephrine (NE) in the standing posture (Sherer et al., 1985). This is similar to the effects of MAOIs. Increased standing blood NE levels are found in depression. This effect of SAM may be related to its antidepressant effect.

REFERENCES

Antun, F., Eccleston, D. and Smythies, J.R. (1971) in Brain Chemistry and Mental Disease (B.T. Ho and W.M. McIsaac, Eds.), pp. 61–71, Plenum Press, New York.

Baudry, M., Chast, F. and Schwartz, J.C. (1973) J. Neurochem. 20, 13–21.

Billingsley, M.L. and Roth, R.H. (1982) J. Pharm. Exp. Therap. 223, 681–688.

Bruinvels, J. and Pepplinkhuizen, L. (1984) J. Psychiat. Res. 18, 307–318.

Campillo, J.E. and Ashcroft, S.J.H. (1982) FEBS Letts. 238, 71–75.

Carl, G.F., Crews, E.L., Carmichael, S.M., Benesh, F.C. and Smythies, J.R. (1978) Biol. Psychiat. 13, 773–776.

Carney, M.V.P., Martin, R., Bottiglieri, T., Reynolds, F.H., Nussenbaum, H., Toone, B.K. and Sheffield, B.F. (1983) Lancet(i), 820–821.

Cohen, S., Nichols, A. and Wyatt, R. (1974) Biol. Psychiat. 8, 109–221.

Dave, J.R., Knazek, R.A. and Liu, S.C. (1981) Biochem. Biophys. Res. Comm. 103, 727–738.

Garver, D.L., Johnson, C. and Kanter, D.R. (1982) Life Sci. 31, 1987–1992.

Henn, F.A. and Henn, S.W. (1982) in Biological Markers in Psychiatry and Neurology (E. Usdin and I. Hanin, Eds.), pp. 183–185, Pergamon Press, New York.

Hirata, F., Strittmatter, W.J. and Axelrod, J. (1979) Proc. Nat. Acad. Sci. 76, 368–372.

Hirata, F. and Axelrod, J. (1980) Science 209, 1082–1090.

Hitzemann, R., Mark, C., Hirschowitz, J. and Garner, D. (1985) Biol. Psychiat. 20, 397–407.

Kalka, M.S., and van Kammen, D.P. (1983) Arch. Gen. Psychiat. 40, 264-270.

Kehry, M.R., Bond, M.W., Hunkapiller, M.W. and Dahlquist, F.W. (1983) Proc. Nat. Acad. Sci. 80, 3599-3603.

Kelsoe, J.R., Tolbert, L.C., Crews, E.L. and Smythies, J.R. (1982) J. Neurosci. Res. 8, 88-103.

Kleene, S.J., Hobson, C. and Adler, J. (1979) Proc. Nat. Acad. Sci. USA 76, 6309-6313.

Koch, T.K., Gordon, A.S. and Diamond, I. (1983) Biochem. Biophys. Res. Comm. 114, 339-347.

Loh, H.H. and Law, P.Y. (1980) Ann. Rev. Pharmacol. Toxicol. 20, 201-231.

McFadden, P.N., Horwitz, J. and Clarke, S. (1983) Biochem. Biophys. Res. Comm. 113, 418-424.

Morere, D.A., Alarcon, R.D., Monti, J.A., Walter-Ryan, W.G., Bancroft, A.J., Smythies, J.R. and Tolbert, L.C. Submitted for publication, J. Clin. Psychopharmacology.

Osmond, H., Smythies, J.R., Harley-Mason, J. and Redmill, J. (1952) J. Ment. Sci. 98, 309-315.

Prasad, C. and Edwards, R.M. (1981) Biochem. Biophys. Res. Comm., 103, 559-564.

Pfenninger, K.H. and Johnson, M.P. (1981) Proc. Nat. Acad. Sci. 78, 7797-7800.

Rotrosen, J., Miller, A.D., Mandeo, D., Traficanto, C.J., and Gershon, S. (1980) Arch. Gen. Psychiat. 37, 1047-1054.

Schatz, R.A., Wilens, T.E. and Sellinger, O.Z. (1981) J. Neurochem. 36, 1739-1748.

Sherer, M.A., Golden, R.N. and Potter, W.F. (1985) Proc. Soc. Biol. Psychiat., 40th Annual Convention, p. 83.

Smythies, J.R. (1963) Postgrad. Med. J. 39, 26-33.

Smythies, J.R., Morin, R.D. and Brown, G.B. (1979) Biol. Psychiat. 14, 549-556.

Stevens, J.D. (1972) Schizophrenia Bull. 6, 60-61.

Stramentinoli, G. and Baldessarini, R.J. (1978) J. Neurochem. 31, 1015-1020.

Strittmatter, W.J., Gaynor, C. and Axelrod, J. (1979) J. Pharm. Exp. Therap., 207, 419-424.

Toews, M.L., Goy, M.F., Springer, M.S. and Adler, J. (1979) Proc. Nat. Acad. Sci. USA, 76, 6309-6313.

Tolbert, L., Monti, J.A., O'Shields, H., Walter-Ryan, W., Meadows, D., and Smythies, J.R. Psychopharm. Bull. 19, 594-599.

Wilcox, J., Wazivi, R., Sherman, A. and Mott, J. (1985) Biol. Psychiat., 20, 41-49.

DOUBLE-BLIND STUDY OF S-ADENOSYL-METHIONINE VERSUS PLACEBO

IN HIP AND KNEE ARTHROSIS

Caruso I.,Montrone F.,Fumagalli M.,Sarzi P.,Boc-
cassini L.,Santandrea S.,Locati M.,Volpato R.
Rheumatology Service, L. Sacco Hospital.

via G.B. Grassi, 74 - 20157 Milan (Italy)

ABSTRACT

A double-blind study comparing the efficacy and tolerabili-
ty of S-Adenosyl-Methionine (SAMe) (39 patients,400 mg t.i.
d.) versus placebo (37 patients) in the treatment of osteoarthrosis of hip and or knee was carried out. A significant
improvement in all 5 clinical parameters of SAMe group and
in 3 out of 5 of placebo group was obtained. The comparison
between the two groups showed a noticeable change in favour
of SAMe in all clinical parameters, a statistical significance being obtained only in 2. Side effects were experienced in 3 patients receiving SAMe and in 6 of placebo group.
They were mainly gastro-intestinal. All 3 patients of SAMe
group and 2 of those receiving placebo withdrew the treatment. Both groups (39 patients on SAMe and 37 on placebo)
were homogenous as far as age, sex, weight, duration of disease, functional class and baseline status of arthrosis are
concerned.

INTRODUCTION

S-Adenosyl-Methionine (SAMe)is a physiological substance
which is involved in a great number of metabolic processes
(Usdin et al.,1979).

In particular, SAMe has proved to be a metyl-donor and a
precursor of endogenous sulfurated products, like glutathione (Jacoby & Habig, 1980). Owing to these caracteristics,
SAMe was suggested for use in various forms of liver diseases as an antisteatosic and detoxicating agent (Micali et
al.,1983) as well as in the management of psychiatric disorders as an antidepressant (Agnoli et al.,1976) (Caruso et
al.,1984). Open clinical studies conducted with SAMe, administered parenterally in patients affected by degenerative
joint disease, have shown that this drug is effective and
excellently tolerated (Ballabio & Caruso, 1978)(Ceccato et
al.,1979)(Polli et al.,1975).
Pharmacological studies performed by analyzing prostaglandin activity in inflammatory exudates of laboratory animals
demonstrated an anti-inflammatory action of SAMe. This drug
has been reported to have also an analgesic activity (Stramentinoli, 1975)(Gualano et al., 1983).
The aim of the present study was to verify in a double-blind
trial versus placebo for a 21 days period the therapeutic
effectiveness and tolerance of SAMe administered orally in
a group of patients with hip or knee arthrosis.

PATIENTS & METHODS

Seventy-six outpatients aged 40-75, with osteoarthrosis of
hip or knee lasting more than one year, were eligible for
the study (Table I). Arthrosis, diagnosed on the basis of
clinical and X-ray signs, was classified according to ARA
functional classes.
Only patients belonging to II and III classes were included
(Table I). The following patients were excluded from the
trial:
-marked alterations to liver, cardiocirculatory apparatus
 and kidney;
- acute gastritis or peptic ulcer;
- other rheumatic diseases;
- pregnancy.
The two groups appear to be homogenous with respect to all
parameters considered.

TABLE I

GENERAL DATA ON PATIENTS

		SAMe (39)	Placebo (37)	
Age	Mean	56.5	57.4	n.s.
(in years)	(range)	(42-73)	(44-75)	
Sex (F/M)		23/16	22/15	n.s.
Duration of OA.	Mean	4.7	5.1	
(years)	(range)	(1.5-8.0)	(1.5-7.6)	n.s.
Functional class*				
	II	24	22	n.s.
	III	15	15	n.s.

(*) No patient has grades I or IV.

n.s. = Not significant between groups.

The distribution of 76 patients by affected joint is reported in Table II.
Upon entering the study, previous therapy was discontinued
for a wash-out period of one week, after which the patients
began the double-blind treatment that lasted 21 days.
Physical therapy, including kinesitherapy, was excluded during the trial. Concomitant medications for conditions other
than osteoarthrosis were permitted, with every effort to minimize changes.
SAMe and placebo were issued in 200 mg tablets identical as
to colour, shape and taste. The daily dose was 1200 mg divided into three administrations of 400 mg each, after meals.
The therapeutic activity of SAMe and placebo was assessed by
evaluating the following clinical and physical parameters :
 night pain, weight-bearing pain and pain associated on per-
 forming a group of specific activities (going upstairs and
 downstairs, getting out of bed, standing up from a chair),
 was rated on a scale from 0 to 3.
Knee flexion angles and hip abduction measured as intermal-
leolar distance in centimeters were assessed.
Recordings were made in baseline conditions and at the end
of the trial. At the end of the treatment in double-blind
conditions, both the physician and patients expressed a judgement on the overall effectiveness of the therapy according to an arbitrary scale graded from 0 to 3.
To monitor for toxicity a complete blood count (including

TABLE II

DISTRIBUTION OF 76 PATIENTS BY
JOINTS OF MAJOR INVOLVEMENT

	SAMe	Placebo	Tot.
HIP	12	13	25
KNEE	27	24	51
TOTAL	39	37	

hematocrit, red blood cell count, hemoglobin, white blood
cell count, differential WBC and platelet counts), a urinalysis, a chemical blood survey (including liver function
tests, blood urea nitrogen, creatinine, total protein and
albumin, electrolytes) and ESR were performed on admission
and conclusion.
Patients were interviewed at completion about new symptoms
or possible side effects.

STATISTICAL ANALYSIS

The omogeneity of both groups in baseline conditions was
verified using the following tests: unpaired t test for
the "quantitative variables" age, weight , height and duration of the disease; X^2 test for impaired joints, functional and X-ray alterations and subjective symptoms. In addition, Sign test was used to evaluate improvement of symptoms
within the groups.
Mann-Whitney and X^2 tests were used to compare improvements
between the two groups (considering the frequency of improvements of subjective symptoms).
The physician's and patients' overall judgement on the therapeutic response were compared by X^2 test.
Changes in laboratory parameters were evaluated by t Student's test.

RESULTS and CONCLUSIONS

Table IIIa reports the evaluation results of subjective individual symptoms.

TABLE IIIa

CLINICAL RESPONSE TO SAMe OR PLACEBO

	SAMe (32)	Placebo (34)
loading pain	p < 0.01	p < 0.05
Night pain	"	n.s.
Pain pool	"	n.s.
Going upstairs and downstairs	"	p < 0.01
Standing up from a chair	"	n.s.
Getting out of bed	"	p < 0.05
"Difficulty in specific activity" pool.	"	p < 0.01

(comparison within groups made by sign test)

TABLE IIIb

CLINICAL RESPONSE TO SAMe OR PLACEBO
COMPARISON BETWEEN GROUPS

Loading pain	p < 0.03
Night pain	n.s.
Pain pool	p < 0.03
Going upstairs and downstairs	n.s.
Standing up from a chair	p < 0.03
Getting out of bed	n.s.
"Difficulty in specific activity" pool.	p < 0.03

(comparison made by Mann-Whitney test)

The comparison of baseline and final conditions in each of
the two treatment groups yielded significant results in all
5 symptoms for SAMe while placebo showed significant results
as far as loading pain ($p < 0.03$) and 2 out of 3 of the specific activities considered (going upstairs and downstairs
and getting out of bed, $p < 0.01$ and $p < 0.05$ respectively)
are concerned.

The comparison between the two groups showed noticeably
change in favour of SAMe in all 5 variables taken in account,
but it was statistically significant in 2 (loading pain and
standing up from a chair).(TABLE IIIb)

TABLE IV
EVALUATION ON THE TREATMENT EFFECTIVENESS
Physician

	No change	Improvement	
SAMe (32)	13	19	$p < 0.025$
Placebo (34)	25	9	

Patient

	No change	Improvement	
SAMe (32)	13	19	$p < 0.05$
Placebo (34)	22	12	

TABLE V
TOLERABILITY DATA

	SAMe(39)	Placebo(37)
Side effects	3*	6**
Withdrawals	3	2
Lost to follow-up	4	1

* Epigastralgia, biliary colic
** Epigastralgia, nausea, vomiting, diarrhea, headhache.

Knee flexion angles, as well as hip abduction did not change significantly at the end of the trial.
Concerning the physician's and patients' final judgement, favourable evaluation were considerably prevailing for SAMe group, $p < 0.05$ and $p < 0.025$ respectively (TABLE IV).
Mainly gastrointestinal side effects were experienced in 3 patients receiving SAMe and in 6 of placebo group (Table V). All 3 patients of SAMe group (2 epigastralgia, 1 biliary colic) and 2 out of 6 belonging to placebo group (1 diarrhea, 1 nausea) withdrew treatment (TABLE V) during the first week of the trial and were consequently excluded from the statistical evaluation.
Five of 76 patients are not included because they were lost

to follow up (TABLE V).

The exact mechanism of action of SAMe is still unknown. However, some preliminary data suggest that SAMe may inhibit, at some level, prostaglandin synthesis.

If this would be confirmed, it would be more clear why, in this trial, unlike previous studies, a greater number of side effects appeared.

It must be considered, however, that also the placebo group exhibited gastrointestinal intolerance and, therefore,such an untoward effect may be related rather to an inadeguate preparation of the tablets (our study was carried out with tablets ; now blisters are available) than to a SAMe induced pharmacological action.

The above data are preliminary and no definite conclusions can be drawn.

Aa a matter of fact, other clinical trials comparing SAMe vs commonly used NSADs are needed in a larger number of patients with osteoarthrosis to clear up the effect of SAMe.

REFERENCES

Agnoli A. et al., 1976: Effects of S-adenosyl-L-methionine (SAMe) upon depressive symptoms. J. Psychiat. Res., 13, 43-54.

Ballabio & Caruso, 1978: Le traitement medical de la coxartrose. J. Med. Strasbourg (Europa Medica), 9, 313-319.

Caruso et al., 1984: Antidepressant activity of S-adenosyl-methionine. Lancet, i, 904.

Ceccato et al., 1979: Indagine clinica aperta e comparativa sull'impiego della SAMe e del Ketoprofen nella osteoartrosi. Progresso Medico, 35, 177-191.

Gualano et al., 1983: Anti-inflammatory activity of S-adenosyl-L-methionine: interference with eicosanoid system. Pharmacol. Res. Commun., 15, 683-696.

Jacoby & Habig, 1980: Glutathione Transferase. In: Enzymatic basis of detoxicating (Jacoby, W. B., Ed.) pp. 63-94, Academic Press.

Micali et al., 1983: Double-blind controlled clinical trial of SAMe administered orally in chronic liver diseases. Curr. Therap. Res., 33, 1004-1013.

Polli et al., 1975: Aspetti farmacologici e clinici della Solfo-adenosyl-L-metionina (SAMe) nell'artropatia degenerativa primaria (osteoartrosi). Min. Med., 66, 4443-4449.

Stramentinoli G., 1975: Azione antiflogistica ed analgesica della S-adenosyl-L-metionina (SAMe) in prove sperimentali su animali da laboratorio. Min. Med., 66, 4434-4442.

Usdin et al., 1978: Transmethylation. Proceedings of the Conference on Transmethylation. Bethesda, Maryland, U.S.A., October 16-19. Elsevier North Holland, New York, 1979.

E. Design, Synthesis, and Biological Evaluation of Transmethylation and Inhibitors

Methionine Analog Inhibitors of S-Adenosylmethionine

Biosynthesis as Potential Antitumor Agents

Janice R. Sufrin[1,2], J.B. Lombardini[3],
Debora L. Kramer[2], Vitauts Alks[2], Ralph J.
Bernacki[2] and Carl W. Porter[2]

[1]Department of Surgical Oncology and [2]Grace
Cancer Drug Center, Roswell Park Memorial
Institute, Buffalo, New York 14263; [3]Depart-
ment of Pharmacology, Texas Tech University,
Health Sciences Center, Lubbock, Texas 79430

INTRODUCTION

The essentiality of S-adenosylmethionine (AdoMet) in
transmethylation reactions and polyamine biosynthesis
provides a rationale for the development of methionine
(Met) analog inhibitors of AdoMet synthesis as potential
antitumor agents. Recent studies indicating that "Met
dependent" tumors have defects in Met and AdoMet metabolism suggest that certain tumors may be particularly susceptible to growth inhibition by Met analogs (Hoffman,
1985). Systematic approaches to the design of such
analogs have been facilitated by the earlier studies on
Met analog inhibitors of microbial and mammalian iso-
functional methionine adenosyltransferases (MAT; EC
2.5.1.6) reported by Talalay and coworkers (Chou et al.,
1977), in which certain critical features of the enzyme
bound conformation of L-Met and of the complementary
topography at its L-Met binding site were defined.

One of the more interesting Met analogs to emerge
from these studies was 1-aminocyclopentane-1-carboxylic
acid, more commonly known as cycloleucine. The ready
availability of cycloleucine has made it quite valuable

for examining the effects of inhibition of AdoMet biosynthesis and transmethylation pathways in isolated biological systems (Caboche and Bachellerie, 1977; Dimock
and Stoltzfus, 1978). Moreover, the metabolic disposition and antitumor activity of cycloleucine have been
extensively evaluated (Sterling and Henderson, 1963;
Sterling et al., 1962). In clinical trials, cycloleucine showed specific therapeutic effects towards
patients with leiomyosarcoma (Aust et al., 1970). However, it is important to note that the in vivo biological
effects of cycloleucine are not restricted to its inhibitory activity towards AdoMet biosynthesis, but relate
also to its activity as an amino acid antagonist of
valine and leucine (Sterling et al., 1962), its resistance to metabolism and its slow excretion rate
(Sterling and Henderson, 1963). It is these latter
effects which may have been responsible for the associated nonspecific toxicity that ultimately made cycloleucine unsuitable for clinical regimens.

Our more recent studies have focused on detecting
possible exploitable differences in the L-Met binding
site of tumor versus normal MAT forms (Sufrin and
Lombardini, 1982a; Lombardini and Sufrin, 1983). In the
course of these studies, a novel and potent Met analog
inhibitor, L-2-amino-4-methoxy-cis-but-3-enoic acid (L-
cis-AMB), was identified which shows greater specificity
for the inhibition of AdoMet biosynthesis than cycloleucine (Sufrin et al., 1982). It is presumed that the
presence of a strategic conformational restraint in
L-cis-AMB (Fig. 1) provides an excellent correlation
between its enzyme bound conformation and that of L-Met,
and appears to be the basis for its observed specificity.

At the previous Transmethylation Conference in Lake
of the Ozarks (1981) we reported our observations relat-
ing to the differing substrate activities of several Met
analogs towards tumor versus normal MAT forms (Sufrin and
Lombardini, 1982b). These data suggested an additional
chemotherapeutic strategy, the design of Met analog substrates of MAT that might selectively interfere with Ado-
Met biosynthesis in tumor cells; and, as is apparent from
the metabolism of AdoMet, each AdoMet analog formed in
this manner, in vivo, would have unique biological
effects, related to its specific metabolic disposition
within both transmethylation and polyamine pathways.

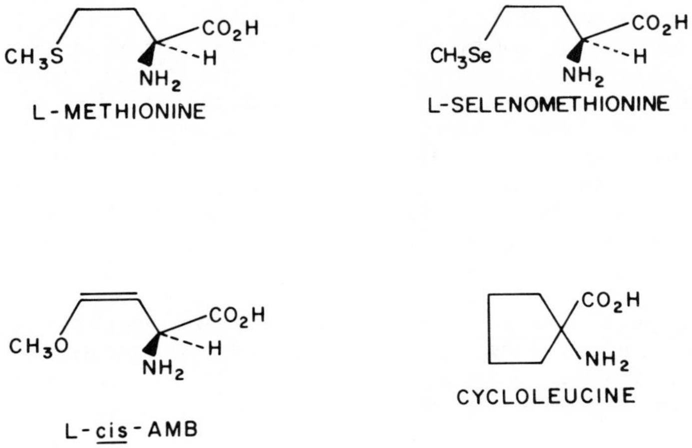

Figure 1:   Structures of Methionine Analogs

    The present study compares biological and antitumor
effects of the Met analogs, L-cis-AMB, cycloleucine and
selenomethionine (SeMet) in L1210 murine leukemia cells,
in culture, as well as their inhibitory or substrate
activity towards L1210 MAT preparations, and examines a
possible approach to enhancing the growth inhibitory
effects of these Met analogs by restricting cellular
access of exogenous Met in tumor cells.

MATERIALS AND METHODS

Materials. L-cis-AMB was synthesized with minor modifi-
cations in the published procedure (Sufrin et al., 1982).
Cycloleucine and DL-SeMet were obtained from Sigma
Chemical Co., St. Louis, MO.

MAT from L1210 Cells: Partial Purification and Fractionation. All operations were conducted at 0-4°C. Ascites
L1210 cells (3g) obtained from DBA-2 Jackson mice, were
suspended in 10 ml of 20 mM Tris-HCl buffer, pH 8.0 and
the mixture homogenized with a ground glass homogenizer

and pestle. The homogenate was centrifuged for 20 minutes at 16,000 x g and the pellet was discarded. Solid ammonium sulfate was added with stirring to the supernatant to a final concentration of 0.6 M. The supernatant was centrifuged for 20 minutes at 16,000 x g to remove any precipitate. The supernatant fraction was then chromatographed on a phenyl Sepharose column, using gradient elution (1.5 x 13 cm) as described previously (Sullivan and Hoffman, 1983; Lombardini and Sufrin, 1983). Two forms, designated L1210 MAT-I and L1210 MAT-II according to their order of elution, were obtained (Fig. 2).

MAT Enzymatic Assays. MAT activity was measured as described (Chou and Lombardini, 1972; Lombardini and Sufrin, 1983). Substrate activity of SeMet was determined as described (Sufrin and Lombardini, 1982a).

Cell Culture. Murine leukemia cells were maintained in logarithmic growth as a suspension culture and were treated with Met analogs using conditions as described previously (Porter et al., 1984).

AdoMet and Polyamine Determinations. AdoMet pools and polyamine pools were determined according to our described procedures (Porter et al., 1984) on cells treated for 48 hr in the presence or absence of the Met analogs and at media Met levels of 30 μM or 100 μM.

AdoMet Decarboxylase Activity. The methods used for determination of AdoMet decarboxylase activity have been described elsewhere (Porter et al., 1984).

In Vivo Experiments. DBA/2 mice weighing approximately 20 gm were implanted (i.p.) with 10^6 L1210 cells on day 0. Animals were then treated (i.p.) with an aqueous solution of L-cis-AMB, at appropriate concentrations, on days 1, 3 and 5. Increase in life span of treated animals is reported as the mean percent increase over the mean survival time of untreated controls as described previously (Bernacki et al., 1985).

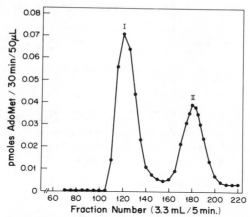

Figure 2:   Phenyl Sepharose Chromatography of L1210
            MAT Forms

RESULTS AND DISCUSSION

      The separation, by phenyl Sepharose chromatography of
two MAT forms from L1210 cells (L1210 MAT-I and L1210
MAT-II) in relative amounts of 2:1, is shown in Fig. 2.
The apparent K_m (L-Met) and V_{max} values were determined (Table 1).   The low K_m (Met) values for these
L1210 forms are of interest because they indicate that
measurements of growth inhibitory activities of Met
analog inhibitors (and substrates) of MAT towards L1210
cells grown in standard culture medium (100 µM Met)
appear to present unfavorable conditions, not correspond-
ingly found in vivo, for examination of competitive inhibition by these analogs.

      The K_i values of L-cis-AMB and cycloleucine towards
L1210 MAT forms were determined (Table 2) and, used as a
measure of their inhibitory activity, it is seen that
L-cis-AMB is 3-10 fold more potent than cycloleucine.
The potency of these two analogs as inhibitors of L1210
cell growth was assessed by measuring the inhibitory concentration required to reduce growth by 50% after 48 hr
(IC_{50}).   The respective IC_{50} values of L-cis-AMB (0.8
mM) and cycloleucine (4.0 mM) (Table 2) show L-cis-AMB to
be 5-fold more potent than cycloleucine; these data
correlate well with their observed K_i values towards
L1210 MAT preparations.

TABLE 1: Kinetic Constants for L1210 MAT Forms I and II[a]

Form	K_m (L-Met) (μM)	V_{max} (pmoles/μg/30/min)
L1210 MAT-I	2.03 ± 0.43	4.11 ± 1.19
L1210 MAT-II	1.34 ± 0.52	0.88 ± 0.05

[a]Data are expressed as means ± S.E.M. The number of experiments was 4 for K_m determinations and 2, for V_{max} determinations. L-Met concentrations varied from 0.2 to 10 μM. ATP concentration was 5 mM.

SeMet was chosen for study as a model substrate analog of MAT. The relative substrate activity of SeMet, (compared to Met at the same concentration) towards L1210 MAT-I was found to be 45% (data not shown), and is indicative of the expected formation of Se-adenosyl-selenomethionine (AdoSeMet) in L1210 cells treated with SeMet. It has been established by others that AdoSeMet can serve very effectively as a methyl donor and as a substrate of AdoMet decarboxylase, thus allowing maintenance of transmethylation reactions and polyamine biosynthesis (Mudd and Cantoni, 1957; Pegg, 1969). In L1210 cells, the IC_{50} value of SeMet is approximately 0.13 mM (Table 3) and demonstrates the greater effectiveness, compared to L-cis-AMB and cycloleucine, of this substrate analog as an inhibitor of growth.

TABLE 2: Comparison of Inhibition of L1210 MAT Forms with L1210 Cell Growth Inhibition by L-cis-AMB and Cycloleucine

Analog	Ki MAT-I	MAT-II (μM)	IC_{50} (48 hr) (mM)
L-cis-AMB	5.0	15.8	0.8
Cycloleucine	48.3	48.4	4.0

TABLE 3: Effects of Exogenous L-Met Levels on L1210 Cell
          Growth Inhibition and Depletion of AdoMet Pools
          by L-cis-AMB, Cycloleucine and SeMet

Inhibitor[a] (48 hr)	Growth (% Control)		AdoMet Pools (% Control)	
	Exogenous Met			
	30 μM	100 μM	30 μM	100 μM
None	98	100	85	100[b]
1.0 mM L-cis-AMB	20	34	36	63
4.0 mM Cycloleucine	32	41	56	63
0.13 mM SeMet	9	45	83[c]	79[c]

[a]The media was replenished at 24 hr to maintain
exogenous Met levels at 30 μM.
[b]Control AdoMet levels were 2.7 nmoles/10^7 cells.
[c]AdoMet plus AdoSeMet (relative amounts not determined)

    We have shown previously that L-cis-AMB, cycloleucine
and SeMet at their IC_{50} concentrations, lowered AdoMet
pools by ~ 50% (Porter et al., 1984). Since growth inhibition was found to precede effects on protein
synthesis (leucine incorporation) by 24 hr, a causal
relationship between AdoMet depletion and growth inhibition was inferred. Furthermore, since the intracellular
polyamine pools of spermidine and spermine were not
affected by treatment with the Met analogs (at IC_{50}
values), alterations in transmethylation pathways, via
reductions in AdoMet pools, may be responsible for the
observed growth inhibition.

    The growth inhibitory effects of these same three Met
analogs were also studied at different media Met concentrations* to determine: 1) the possible enhancement of
their growth inhibitory activity in the presence of lower
media concentrations of Met, and 2) a possible correlation between any observed enhancement of growth inhibition and increased interference with AdoMet biosynthesis.

*The concentration of Met in human and mouse serum is
 36 μM (Drewes and McKee, 1967) and in standard RPMI
 culture medium is 100 μM.

The ability of L1210 cells to grow in varying concentrations of Met restricted media was examined and it was
determined that 30 μM Met is the minimum concentration
which sustains their normal growth rate during a 48 hr
incubation (Fig. 3). When the growth inhibitory effects
of L-cisAMB, cycloleucine and SeMet on L1210 cells were
compared at 100 μM Met and 30 μM Met (Table 3) enhancements in activity of 40% and 73% were seen for L-cis-AMB
and SeMet, respectively, at the lower Met concentration.
This increased activity for L-cis-AMB was accompanied by
a significant depletion in AdoMet levels. For SeMet, the
observed enhancement does not immediately appear to be
associated with changes in AdoMet levels. However, since
our recorded HPLC measurements did not distinguish between AdoMet and its closely related analog, AdoSeMet, it
is presumed that the enhanced growth inhibitory activity
is an initial consequence of the increased formation of
AdoSeMet at the expense of AdoMet. In contrast, a more
modest enhancement of growth inhibition (21%) and AdoMet
depletion is seen for cycloleucine at the lower Met
concentration, suggesting that other biochemical
mechanisms might also contribute to the observed growth

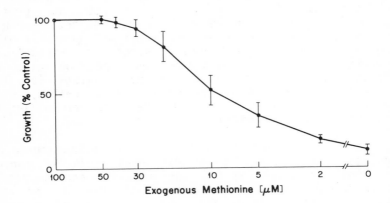

Figure 3:   Effects of Methionine Restriction on L1210
            Cell Growth at 48 hr.

inhibitory activity of cycloleucine. This is not surprising, in view of its known activity as an inhibitor of amino acid transport (Sterling and Henderson, 1963).

Our previous observations that polyamine pools remain virtually unchanged in L1210 cells treated with IC_{50} concentrations of L-cis-AMB, cycloleucine and SeMet (Porter et al., 1984) made it of further interest to determine whether the maintenance of polyamine levels occurs under more extreme conditions of growth inhibition and AdoMet depletion, as were seen when L1210 cells were treated with 1.0 mM L-cis-AMB at 30 μM Met (Table 4). Despite an observed depletion in AdoMet of >90%, spermine and spermidine levels remain unchanged. The resultant increases in AdoMet decarboxylase activity and putrescine levels, are apparent compensatory responses by the pathway to the highly reduced AdoMet levels. These data provide further indications that polyamine biosynthesis is exceedingly well regulated and conserved, even under conditions which might be expected to induce substantial alterations in their pools.

We have initiated in vivo pharmacological evaluation of the antitumor activity of L-cis-AMB and have found that treatment of mice bearing L1210 leukemia with 10, 25 50 or 100 mg/kg L-cis-AMB x 3, i.p., on days 1, 3, 5 produces increases in lifespan of 30, 53, 23 and 7%, respectively (Table 5). In these studies, it is seen that with administration of 25 mg/kg of L-cis-AMB, an optimum and significant therapeutic effect was achieved.

CONCLUSION

This study has provided substantial evidence for the greater specificity of L-cis-AMB, compared to cyclo-leucine, as an inhibitor of L1210 MAT preparations and consequently of AdoMet formation and growth inhibition in cultured L1210 cells. Furthermore, it has been shown that the growth inhibitory effects of SeMet, a model sub-strate analog of MAT and of L-cis-AMB, but not of cyclo-leucine, are significantly enhanced in culture when the supply of exogenous Met is restricted. Preliminary in vivo evaluation of the antitumor activity of L-cis-AMB in L1210 leukemic mice is encouraging. Overall, the data support the continuing development of L-cis-AMB and

TABLE 4: Effects of Exogenous Met Levels on Growth Inhibition, AdoMet Levels and Polyamine Synthesis in L1210 Cells Treated with L-cis-AMB

Conditions[a]	Growth (% Control)	AdoMet (% Control)	AdoMet DC[b] (nmol/hr/mg Protein)	Put	Spd	Spm[c]
				(nmol/10[6]cells)		
100 μM Met	100	100	1.03	0.25	3.68	1.15
100μM Met, 1 mM L-cis-AMB	34	63	2.39	0.69	3.88	1.36
30 μM Met[d]	89	85	N.D.[e]	2.14	3.65	1.08
30 μM Met, 1 mM L-cis-AMB[d]	20	36	N.D.	2.11	3.89	1.29
30 μM Met, 1 mM L-cis-AMB	35	<10%	4.90	3.10	3.94	1.13

a Cells were treated for 48 hr in media containing the indicated concentration of Met at 0 hr.
b AdoMet DC, AdoMet decarboxylase.
c Polyamines: Put, putrescine; Spd, spermidine; Spm, spermine.
d Exogenous Met in media replenished at 24 hr.
e N.D., not determined.

TABLE 5: Life Span of L1210 Leukemic Mice Treated with L-cis-AMB

Group No.[a] (No. Animals)	Dose[b] (mg/kg)	Survival Range (Days)	Median Survival (Days)	Lifespan (% Increase)	Significance[c] (P)
1 (20)	None	6-8	6.5	0	---
2 (10)	10	7-13	8.5	30	<0.01
3 (10)	25	8-12	10	53	<0.01
4 (15)	50	7-12	8	23	<0.01
5 (10)	100	7-8	7	7	0.076

[a]Mice were implanted with 10^6 tumor cells, i.p. on day 0.

[b]Route and schedule of administration: i.p. on days 1, 3, 5.

[c]Significance determined by Cox-Mantel and Dunn procedures.

related Met analogs which interfere with AdoMet biosynthesis as potential antineoplastic agents and as
experimental probes in cellular physiology and
pharmacology.

References

Aust, J.B., Andrews, N.C., Schroeder, J.M. and Lawton,
    R.L. (1970). Cancer Chemo. Rep. 54, 237-241.
Bernacki, R.J., Wilson, G.L., Mossman, B.T., Angelino, N.,
    Kanter, P.M. and Korytnyk, W. (1985). Cancer Res.
    45, 695-702.
Caboche, M. and Bachellerie, J.-P. (1977). Eur. J. Bio-
    chem., 74, 19-29.
Chou, T.-C. and Lombardini, J.B. (1972). Biochim.
    Biophys. Acta 267, 399-406.
Chou, T.-C., Coulter, A.W., Lombardini, J.B., Sufrin
    J.R. and Talalay, P.T. (1977). In The Biochemistry
    of Adenosylmethionine (Salvatore, F., Borek, E.,
    Zappia, Z., Williams-Ashman, H.G. and Schlenk, F.,
    eds.), pp. 18-36, Columbia University Press, New York.
Dimock, K. and Stoltzfus, C.M. (1978). Biochemistry, 17,
    3627-3632.
Drewes, P.A. and McKee, R.W. (1967). Nature 213, 411-412.
Hoffman, R.M. (1985). Anticancer Res. 5, 1-30.
Lombardini, J.B. and Sufrin, J.R. (1983). Biochem.
    Pharmacol. 32, 489-495.
Mudd, S.H. and Cantoni, G.L. (1957). Nature 180, 1052.
Pegg, A.E. (1969). Biochim. Biophys. Acta 177, 361-364.
Porter, C.W., Sufrin, J.R. and Keith, D.D. (1984). Bio-
    chem. Biophys. Res. Commun. 122, 350-357.
Sterling, W.R., Henderson, J.F., Mandal, H.G. and Smith,
    P.K. (1962). Biochem. Pharmacol. 11, 135-145.
Sterling, W.R. and Henderson, J.F. (1963). Biochem.
    Pharmacol. 12, 303-316.
Sufrin, J.R., Lombardini, J.B. and Keith, D.D. (1982).
    Biochem. Biophys. Res. Commun. 106, 551-552.
Sufrin, J.R. and Lombardini, J.B. (1982a). Molec.
    Pharmacol. 22, 752-759.
Sufrin, J.R. and Lombardini, J.B. (1982b). In
    Biochemistry of S-Adenosylmethionine and Related
    Compounds (Usdin, E., Borchardt, R.T. and Creveling,
    C.R., eds.), pp. 687-690, MacMillan Press, London.
Sullivan, D.M. and Hoffman, J.L. (1983). Biochemistry
    22, 1636-1641.

Metabolism and Mechanism of Action of Neplanocin A - A Potent Inhibitor of S-Adenosylhomocysteine Hydrolase.

Bradley T. Keller and Ronald T. Borchardt

Departments of Biochemistry and Pharmaceutical Chemistry

University of Kansas, Lawrence, KS 66045

Neplanocin A [(-)-9-[trans-2, trans-3-dihydroxy-4-(hydroxy-methyl)cyclopent-4-enyl] adenine] (Figure 1) is a cyclopentenyl analog of adenosine which has been isolated from the culture filtrate of the microorganism *Ampullariella regularis* (Yaginuma et al., 1980, 1981; Hayashi et al., 1981). Despite having minimal antibacterial and antifungal activity, this novel antibiotic was initially observed to be cytotoxic at 0.2 µg/ml against cultured L5178Y lymphoma cells (Yaginuma et al., 1981). It also exhibited significant antitumor activity in mice bearing L1210 leukemia, increasing the life span by 120% at 5 mg/kg/day (Tsujino et al., 1980; Yaginuma et al., 1981).

Based on the structural similarity to adenosine, our laboratory investigated the possibility that some of the pharmacological activity of neplanocin A involves an alteration in cellular transmethylation mediated through an effect on S-adenosylhomocysteine (AdoHcy) hydrolase (EC 3.3.1.1.). This enzyme, by catalyzing the reversible hydrolysis of AdoHcy to adenosine and homocysteine, plays a pivital role in regulating cellular levels of AdoHcy, a potent product inhibitor of S-adenosylmethionine (AdoMet)-dependent methylation reactions. We observed that neplanocin A produced both concentration-dependent and time-dependent inhibition of purified bovine liver AdoHcy hydrolase, having a Ki of 8.39 nM (Borchardt et al., 1984). Analysis of the apparent irreversible inactivation of the enzyme demonstrated that the analog is a tight-binding inhibitor, exhibiting a stoichiometry of one molecule of inhibitor to one molecule (tetramer) of enzyme. Thus, it is not surprising that neplanocin A was not observed to serve as a substrate in the reverse reaction to form the corresponding S-neplanocyhomocys-

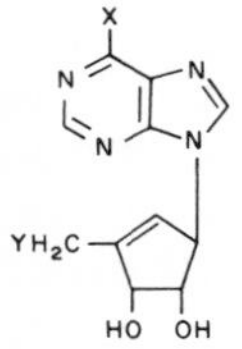

	X	Y
Neplanocin A	$-NH_2$	$-OH$
Neplanocin D	$-OH$	$-OH$
Neplanocin Triphosphate	$-NH_2$	$-O(PO_3)_3^{-4}$
S−Neplanocylmethionine	$-NH_2$	$\overset{\oplus}{-}S(CH_2)_2CHCOOH$ with CH_3 and NH_2
decarboxylated S−Neplanocylmethionine	$-NH_2$	$\overset{\oplus}{-}S(CH_2)_2CH_2NH_2$ with CH_3
S−Neplanocylhomocysteine	$-NH_2$	$-S(CH_2)_2CHCOOH$ with NH_2

Fig. 1. **Structures of potential neplanocin A metabolites.**

teine derivative (Figure 1). Fluorescence studies on the inactivated bovine enzyme have further shown that the mechanism of inhibition by neplanocin A involves a reduction of the enzyme-bound NAD^+ to NADH (Matuszewska and Borchardt, unpublished data). This inhibition was found to be completely reversible in a time-dependent manner by incubation with excess NAD^+. However, in contrast to the release of enzyme-bound NAD^+ during the cAMP-induced inhibition of AdoHcy hydrolase (Hohman et al., 1985), no dissociation of the bound coenzyme was detected following treatment with neplanocin A.

Inhibition of AdoHcy hydrolase by neplanocin A has also been demonstrated in a number of cultured cell lines. We have shown that addition of 1 μM neplanocin A to the cell culture medium of both mouse L929 fibroblasts and N2a neuroblastoma cells results in a rapid, time-dependent inhibition with loss of more than 95% of the enzymatic activity within 30 minutes (Borchardt et al., 1984; Ramakrishnan and Borchardt, 1984). Moreover, prolonged exposure to the analog maintains the hydrolase activity at this negligible level through 24 hours, after which it slowly begins to recover (Figure 2). Coinciding with the inhibition of cellular AdoHcy hydrolase activity is an intracellular accumulation of AdoHcy leading to a 10- to 12-fold increase in the cellular ratio of AdoHcy/AdoMet. A major consequence of this increase, as demonstrated with N2a neuroblastoma cells, is an inhibition of cellular AdoMet-dependent methylation, including a 40-50% decrease in both lipid methylation and protein carboxymethylation (Ramakrishnan and Borchardt, 1984). Inhibition of RNA methylation has also been observed in virus-infected L929 cells (see below).

Like the purified bovine AdoHcy hydrolase, inhibition of the L929 cell enzyme by neplanocin A (K_i = 0.2 nM) was similarly observed to be stoichiometric in a 1:1 ratio of inhibitor to enzyme (Bartel and Borchardt, 1985). Consequently, titration of the enzyme with this inhibitor was used to determine the concentration of the enzyme in intact L929 cells, which was calculated to be 0.8 μM. It was also established that the 27% increase in the specific activity of AdoHcy hydrolase observed in these cells within 12 hours of providing fresh culture medium was not due to an increase in enzyme concentration. Instead, it appears as though an endogenous inhibitor or readily reversible type of enzyme modification is regulating the enzyme *in vivo*.

Corroborating our findings in the murine cell lines, Chiang and coworkers have reported the inhibition of AdoHcy hydrolase by neplanocin A in human red blood cells, K_i = 3 nM (Whaun et al., 1985)

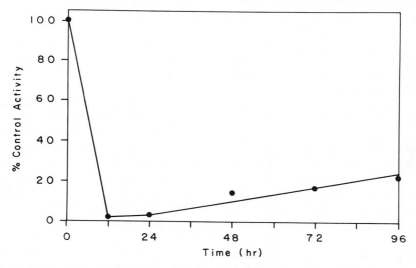

*Fig. 2. **Time course of L929 cell AdoHcy hydrolase activity following treatment with 1 μM neplanocin A.** Monolayers of mouse L929 cells were refed with culture medium containing or lacking 1 μM neplanocin A and incubated for the indicated time. The cells were then harvested by trypsinization and assayed for AdoHcy hydrolase activity as previously described (Borchardt et al., 1984).*

and HL-60 promyelocytic leukemia cells, K_i =2 nM (Aarbakke et al., 1985). In the former cell line, the antimalarial action of the drug against two strains of *Plasmodium falciparum* was suggested to be related to an inhibition of AdoMet-dependent transmethylation reactions as a result of the increase in cellular AdoHcy levels. The induction of differentiation observed in the latter cell line following neplanocin A treatment was similarly associated with an increase in AdoHcy and appeared to be correlated with a decrease in methylation of 5-methylcytosine in the cellular DNA.

Although the effects of neplanocin A on these cell lines are closely related to changes in the intracellular levels of AdoHcy (and presumably to AdoMet-dependent methylation reactions), the identification of cellular metabolites of this analog pose the possibility of additional or alternative mechanisms for its action. Tsujino and colleagues (1980), in their initial studies on the biological activity of neplanocin A, showed that it was a substrate for adenosine deaminase and, consequently, was rapidly deaminated to biologically inactive neplanocin D (Figure 1). While we observed this conversion in lysates of L929 cells, the co-addition of an adenosine deaminase inhibitor, e.g. deoxycoformycin; erythro-9-(2-hydroxy-3-nonyl)adenine (EHNA), to the culture medium did not potentiate the effects of the compound either in our cell system or in those of other investigators (Glazer and Knode, 1984; Saunders et al., 1985). Thus, catabolism of neplanocin A via adenosine deaminase appears to be of little significance in the effects observed in these cell culture systems.

Based on the HPLC analyses of extracts from neplanocin A-treated cells, our laboratory subsequently reported the metabolic conversion of neplanocin A to its corresponding AdoMet derivative, S-neplanocyl-methionine (NpcMet; Figure 1), in both mouse L929 fibroblasts and N2a neuroblastoma cells (Keller and Borchardt, 1984; Ramakrishnan and Borchardt, 1984). Identification of this metabolite was particularly important considering the proposed effects of neplanocin A on AdoMet-dependent methylation reactions. Similar metabolism has also been reported by Glazer and Knode (1984) in HT-29 human colon carcinoma cells, Whaun et al. (1985) in red blood cells and Aarbakke et al. (1985) in the HL-60 promyelocytic leukemia cell line. Of interest, however, is the finding that the HT-29 carcinoma cells, unlike the others mentioned here, exhibited no inhibition of AdoHcy hydrolase and consequently, no accumulation of AdoHcy. The reported cytocidal activity of neplanocin A on this cell line has instead been directly attributed to the formation of NpcMet and its apparent specificity for inhibiting RNA methylation in this system. In addition to red blood cells and HT-29 carcinoma cells, di- and trinucleotide metabolites of neoplanocin A (Figure 1) which are required for NpcMet formation have also been reported in Chinese hamster ovary (CHO) cells (Saunders et al., 1985). In contrast to the carcinoma cells, though, the high cytotoxicity of neoplanocin A to CHO cells did not appear to be related to the formation of these metabolites, as an adenosine kinase deficient mutant (which did not produce the nucleotides) was only slightly more resistant than the wild type cell line.

In mouse L929 cells treated with 1 µM neoplanocin A, NpcMet can accumulate to levels equal to or slightly greatly than AdoMet itself (approximately 500 pmoles/10^6 cells) within 12-24 hours (Keller and Borchardt, 1984). As a result of this accumulation, it was important to evaluate the effects of this metabolite on the two major pathways requiring AdoMet i.e., transmethylation and polyamine biosynthesis. Analysis of the turnover rates of NpcMet and AdoMet in the presence of 20 mM cycloleucine (an inhibitor of AdoMet synthetase) indicated that, during the first two hours, the utilization of NpcMet was much slower than AdoMet itself ($t_{1/2}$ = 13 hours vs. 1 hour; Keller et al., 1985). Moreover, the turnover of AdoMet in the neoplanocin-treated cells was unaffected by the accumulated NpcMet, suggesting that the neoplanocin derivative had little metabolic activity.

A more specific assessment of the activity of this metabolite was performed using unlabeled NpcMet, [^{3}H-methyl]NpcMet and [^{14}C-carboxyl]NpcMet which were purified by reverse phase HPLC from extracts of neoplanocin A-treated L929 cells incubated with the appropriately radiolabeled methionine compound (Keller et al., 1985). Of interest was the finding that this purification could be significantly improved by utilizing the inherent stability of the carbocyclic structure of NpcMet to moderately alkaline conditions (pH 10) under which AdoMet has been shown to be readily degraded (Borchardt, 1979). Using the unlabeled compound, we observed NpcMet to be a poor inhibitor of both [^{3}H-methyl]AdoMet-dependent lipid methylation and protein carboxymethylation in lysates of L929 cells. An IC_{50} value of 205 µM was determined for both reactions. The [^{3}H-methyl]-labeled analog was similarly found to be a poor substrate (i.e., methyl donor) for these reactions, exhibiting K_m values 25-30 fold higher than [^{3}H-methyl]-AdoMet under the same conditions, while less than 40% difference in the corresponding V_{max} values was observed. The lack of activity by NpcMet in AdoMet-dependent methylation reactions was also supported by our ability to detect the appearance of little, if any , NpcHcy in extracts of neoplanocin A-treated cells by HPLC. Thus, NpcMet appears to be a weak competitive inhibitor of these L cell methylation reactions.

As an initial approach to assessing the effects of the AdoMet derivative on polyamine biosynthesis via AdoMet decarboxylase, polyamine levels were measured in L929 cells treated with 1 µM neplanocin A for 12, 24 or 36 hours to induce the maximal accumulation of NpcMet. The largest effects, observed after 24 hours, were a 3.8-fold decrease in putrescine and a 1.7-fold decrease in spermidine while spermine levels were relatively unaffected. These results are in sharp contrast to the elevation of putrescine and depletion of spermidine that would be expected if NpcMet were an inhibitor of AdoMet decarboxylase, and are more consistent with the transient cytostatic effect of neplanocin A on L929 cells which we reported previously (Borchardt et al., 1984). The lack of inhibition of AdoMet decarboxylase by NpcMet was also confirmed by *in vitro* studies using purified enzyme from either *E. coli* or rat prostate, with less than 10% loss of activity observed at concentrations of the AdoMet analog as high as 100 µM. In addition, virtually no substrate activity with either enzyme was detected using [^{14}C-carboxyl]NpcMet under conditions in which [^{14}C-carboxyl]AdoMet was observed to be extensively decarboxylated. The change in polyamine levels in L929 cells following neplanocin A treatment, therefore, does

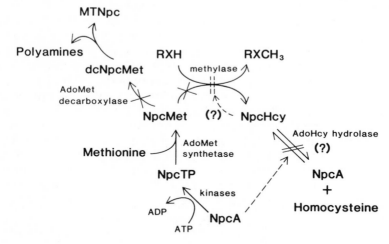

*Fig. 3. **Metabolic scheme for neplanocin A in mouse L929 cells.** dcNpcMet, decarboxylated S-neplanocylmethionine; MTNpc, 5'-methylthioneplanocin; Npc A, neplanocin A; NpcTP, neplanocin A triphosphate; NpcMet, S-neplanocylmethionine; NpcHcy, S-neplanocyl-homocysteine; RXH, unmethylated acceptor molecule; RXCH$_3$, methylated acceptor molecule.*

not appear to be related to a direct effect of NpcMet on AdoMet decarboxylase.

The metabolism of neplanocin A in mouse L929 cells, as discussed above, is summarized in Figure 3. At present, it appears as though many of the biological effects of the analog are mediated through its inhibition of AdoHcy hydrolase and subsequently, AdoMet-dependent methylation reactions. Although the formation of NpcHcy does not seem to occur *in vivo*, it is important to determine the effect of this compound on AdoHcy hydrolase and AdoMet-dependent methyltransferases in future studies.

In addition to the metabolic effects of neplanocin A on L929 cells, our laboratory has demonstrated that the compound is also a potent inhibitor of vaccinia virus multiplication in this host cell line (Borchardt et al., 1984). The analog exhibited greater than 90% inhibition of viral plaque formation when 1 μM neplanocin A was added to the culture medium. As previously mentioned, this concentration of the drug produces a transient cytostatic effect on the cells (i.e., inhibition of cellular DNA synthesis and cell division) although it is not observed to be cytotoxic. The antiviral action of neplanocin A is consistent with that reported for other adenosine analog inhibitors of AdoHcy hydrolase such as (S)-9-(2,3-dihydroxypropyl)adenine (De Clercq et al., 1978), 3-deazaaristeromycin (De Clercq and Montgomery, 1983) and adenosine dialdehyde (Keller and Borchardt, 1983). Moreover, De Clercq and Cools (1985) have demonstrated that there is a close correlation between the antiviral potency and the inhibition of AdoHcy hydrolase for several adenosine analogs, including neplanocin A. The presumable mechanism of action of these compounds involves an inhibition of methylation of the 5'-cap structure on the viral messenger RNA due to the increase in intracellular AdoHcy/AdoMet following hydrolase inhibition. The viral methyltransferases responsible for these AdoMet-dependent methylations have previously been shown to be sensitive to inhibition by AdoHcy and a number of its analogs (Borchardt and Pugh, 1979). As a result of this inhibition of RNA methylation the efficiency of ribosome attachment to the mRNA is decreased and the translation of viral proteins (required for virus replication) would be significantly impaired. In support of this mechanism, Figure 4 illustrates that the synthesis of [^{35}S]methionine-labelled viral proteins is dramatically reduced in neplanocin A-treated cells during early stages of infection. Although it appears as though host synthesis is also inhibited in this study, it should be noted that the cells were infected with a very high titer of virus (15 plaque-forming-units/cell) and that vaccinia virus infection has been shown to induce degradation of host mRNA, thereby inhibiting host protein synthesis (Rice and Roberts, 1983).

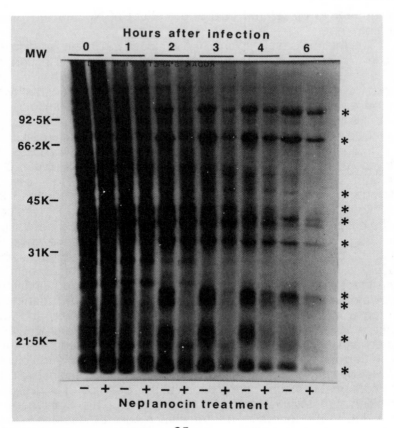

Fig. 4. **Autoradiogram of [35S]methionine-labelled proteins from vaccinia virus-infected L cells.** *Monolayers of mouse L929 cells were pretreated for 12 hours with or without 1 μM neplanocin A then infected for 1 hour with vaccinia virus at 15 pfu/ cell. At the indicated times after infection the cultures were labelled for 15 minutes with 25 μCi/dish [35S]methionine. The cells were solublized in Laemmli sample buffer and the protiens analyzed by SDS-PAGE using a gel of 10% acrylamide concentration. * = virus proteins.*

To further confirm this mechanism of action, we have initiated studies to compare the methylation of mRNA from neplanocin A-treated and untreated, virus-infected L cells. Preliminary results presented in Table I show that there is a 51% decrease in the ratio of [3H-methyl]-methionine/[14C]uridine incorporation into total cytoplasmic RNA from treated cells. When the poly A+-RNA was isolated from these samples by

Table I. Effect of Neplanocin A on RNA Methylation in Vaccinia Virus-Infected Mouse L929 Cells.[a]

1 µM Neplanocin A	sample	dpm [³H]methionine	dpm [¹⁴C]uridine	$\frac{[^3H]}{[^{14}C]}$
–	total cRNA	2.39×10^6	4.06×10^5	5.89
+	total cRNA	1.70×10^6	5.93×10^5	2.87
–	poly A⁺RNA	7.14×10^4	3.77×10^4	1.89
+	poly A⁺RNA	1.03×10^5	6.37×10^4	1.62

[a]*Monolayer cultures of L929 cells were treated with 1 µM neplanocin A for 12 hours, after which vaccinia virus was added (10 pfu/cell) and the incubation continued for another 5 hours. The infected cells were then labelled for 2·5 hours with medium containing 15 µCi/ml [³H-methyl]methionine and 0·4 µCi/ml [¹⁴C]uridine. Total cytoplasmic RNA (cRNA) was extracted from the cells and the poly A⁺RNA isolated by poly U-sepharose chromatography.*

poly U-sepharose chromatography, 14% inhibition of the $[^3H]/[^{14}C]$ ratio was observed in the neplanocin A-treated cells. Ongoing studies are being carried out to hybridize this poly A⁺-RNA to viral DNA in order to obtain the virus-specific poly A⁺-RNA as further confirmation of the mechanism of antiviral action of neplanocin A.

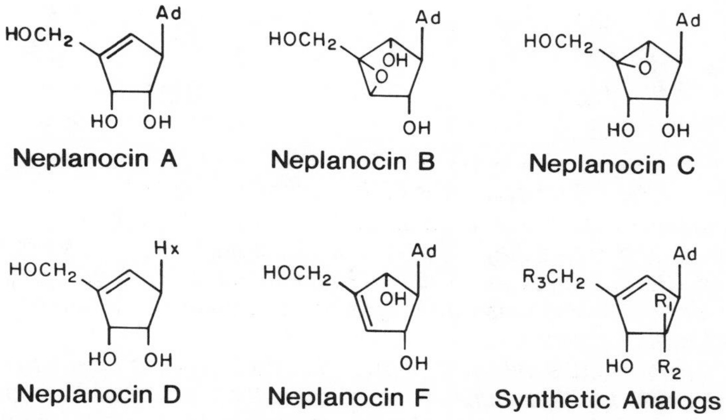

Fig. 5. Structures of Naturally Occurring and Synthetic Neplanocin Analogs.

In addition to neplanocin A, we have also obtained a number of other natural and synthetic analogs of the neplanocins (Figure 5) which were screened for their inhibition of L cell AdoHcy hydrolase as well as their antiviral activity against vaccinia virus in this host cell line.   The results, shown in Table II, indicate that in comparison to neplanocin A, none of these analogs were found to exhibit significant inhibition against either the hydrolase or the virus. These findings, which are consistent

Table II. **Effect of Naturally Occurring and Synthetic Analogs of Neplanocin on L929 Cell AdoHcy Hydrolase Activity and Vaccinia Virus Plaque Formation.**

Analog[a]			Percent Inhibition of [b] AdoHcy Hydrolase	Percent Inhibition of [c] Plaque Formation
Natural Analogs				
Neplanocin A			91	87.5
Neplanocin B			4	5.4
Neplanocin C			18	25.9
Neplanocin D			15	0.9
Neplanocin F			12	2.7
Synthetic Analogs				
R_1	R_2	R_3		
I	H	OH	24	42.0
Br	H	OH	19	8.9
Cl	H	OH	24	15.2
OH	H	OH	24	0
N_3	H	OH	5	9.8
OAc	H	OH	10	0
H	OH	N_3	24	0
H	OH	iBuS	20	4.2

[a] *Refer to Figure 5 for structures of the potential inhibitors.*

[b] *Monolayers of L929 cells were treated with 1 μM of the potential inhibitor for 24 hours and then assayed for AdoHcy hydrolase activity as previously described (Borchardt et al., 1984).   Each result is the average of two independent determinations and values are expressed as a percent of the untreated control cultures.*

[c] *Monolayers of L929 cells were exposed to vaccinia virus inoculum for one hour, then refed with culture medium containing 1 μM of the potential inhibitor. After 72 hours plaques were quantitated as previously described (Borchardt et al., 1984).   Each result is the average of at least four independent determinations and the values are expressed as a percent of the untreated controls which had between120-200 plaques in these studies.*

with those of De Clercq (1985), also support the premise that the antiviral activity of adenosine analogs is closely related to the inhibition of AdoMet-dependent methylation reactions mediated by AdoHcy hydrolase activity.

Acknowledgements - This work was supported by United States Public Health Service Grant GM-29332. Neplanocin A and its natural and synthetic analogs were kindly provided by the Toyo Jozo Co., Ltd., Japan.

References

Aarbakke, J., Gordon, R.K., Cross, A.S., Miura, G.A. and Chiang, P.K. (1985) Fed. Proc. 44, 464, abst.#313.

Bartel, R.L. and Borchardt, R.T. (1985) Anal. Biochem. 149, 191-196.

Borchardt, R.T. (1979) J. Amer. Chem. Soc. 101,458-463.

Borchardt, R.T. and Pugh, C.S.G. (1979) in Transmethylation (Usdin, E., Borchardt, R.T. and Creveling, C.R., eds.) pp. 197-206, Elsevier/North-Holland, New York.

Borchardt, R.T., Keller, B.T. and Patel-Thombre, U. (1984) J. Biol. Chem. 259, 4353-4358.

De Clercq, E. (1985) Antimicrob. Agents Chemother. 28, 84-89.

De Clercq, E. and Cools, M. (1985) Biochem. Biophys. Res. Commun. 129, 306-311.

De Clercq, E. and Montgomery, J.A. (1983) Antiviral Res. 3, 17-24.

De Clercq, E., Descamps, J., De Somer, P. and Holy, A. (1978) Science 200, 563-565.

Glazer, R.I. and Knode, M.C. (1984) J. Biol. Chem. 259, 12964-12969.

Hayashi, M., Yaginuma, S., Yishioka, H. and Nakatsu, K. (1981) J. Antibiot. (Tokyo) 34, 675-680.

Hohman, R.J., Guitton, M.C. and Vernon, M. (1985) Proc. Natl. Acad. Sci. USA, 82, 4578-4581.

Keller, B.T. and Borchardt, R.T. (1983) Fed. Proc. 42, 2139, abst.#2230.

Keller, B.T. and Borchardt, R.T. (1984) Biochem. Biophys. Res. Commun. 120, 131-137.

Keller, B.T., Clark, R.S., Pegg, A.E. and Borchardt, R.T. (1985) Mol. Pharmacol. 28, 364-370.

Ramakrishnan, V. and Borchardt, R.T. (1984) Fed. Proc. 43, 1556, abst. #814.

Rice, A.P. and Roberts, B.E. (1983) J. Virology 47, 529-539.

Saunders, P.P., Tan, M.T. and Robins, R.K. (1985) Biochem. Pharmacol., 34, 2749-2754.

Tsujino, M., Yaginuma, S., Fujii, T., Hayano, K., Matsudo, T., Watanabe, T. and Abe, J. (1980) in Current Chemotherapy and Infectious Disease, Proceedings of the 11th International Congress of Chemotherapy (Nelson, J.D. and Grassi, C., eds.) Vol. 2, pp. 1559-1561, The American Society for Microbiology, Washington, DC.

Whaun, J.M., Miura, G.A., Brown, N.D., Gordon, R.K. and Chiang, P.K.. (1985) Fed. Proc. 44, 499, abst.#516.

Yaginuma, S., Tsujino, M., Muto, N., Otani, M., Hayashi, M., Ishimura, F., Fujii, T., Watanabe, S., Matsuda, T., Watanabe, T. and Abe, J. (1980) in Current Chemotherapy and Infectious Disease, Proceedings of the 11th International Congress of Chemotherapy (Nelson, J.D. and Grassi, C., eds.) Vol. 2, pp. 1558-1559, The American Society for Microbiology, Washington, DC.

Yaginuma, S., Muto, N., Tsujino, M., Sudate, Y., Hayashi, M. and Otani, M. (1981) J. Antibiot. (Tokyo) 34, 359-366.

BIOLOGICAL CONSEQUENCES OF S-ADENOSYL-L-HOMOCYS-
TEINASE INHIBITION BY ACYCLIC ADENOSINE ANALOGS

A.Holý[a], I.Votruba[a], A.Merta[a], E.DeClercq[e],
R.Jelínek[b], K.Sláma[c], K.Beneš[d], O.Melichar[a],

[a]Inst.Org.Chem.Biochem.; [b]Inst.Exp.Med.;
[c]Inst.Entomol.; [d]Inst.Exp.Botany, Praha
(Czechoslovakia); [e]Rega Instituut, Leuven
(Belgium)

S-Adenosyl-L-homocyteinase (SAH-hydrolase)
is recognized as an important enzyme in the regulation of biological transmethylations mediated
by methyl transferases. Thus, the inhibitors of
this enzyme can be expected to evoke a multitude
of biological effects. The numerous examples of
such activities have been reviewed recently
(Ueland,1982).

In the past few years we have been examining
the biological aspects of a newly developed type
of SAH-hydrolase inhibitors which should not undergo any appreciable catabolic changes in vivo.
Our investigation encircles three spheres of problems: (a) Search for active compounds, (b) effective isolation and purification of SAH-hydrolases from the target cells or organs and (c) correlation of enzyme inhibitory properties with the
biological effects of the inhibitors.

ISOLATION OF SAH-HYDROLASES

The majority of SAH-hydrolases are not abun-
dantly stable and their activity (interpreted in
kinetic parameters) may well differ in dependence
upon the isolation techniques. We have therefore
developed affinity chromatography procedures

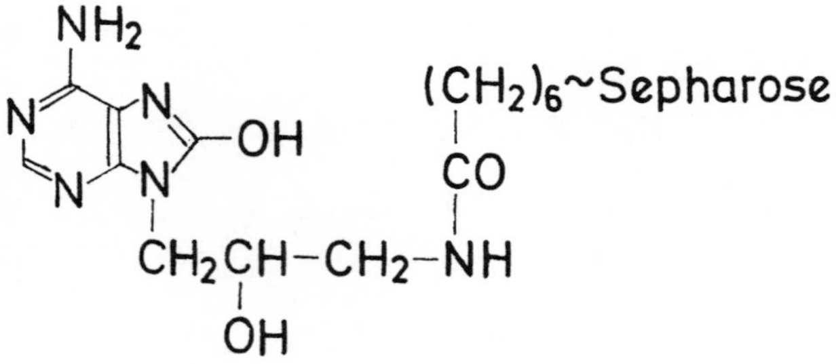

I

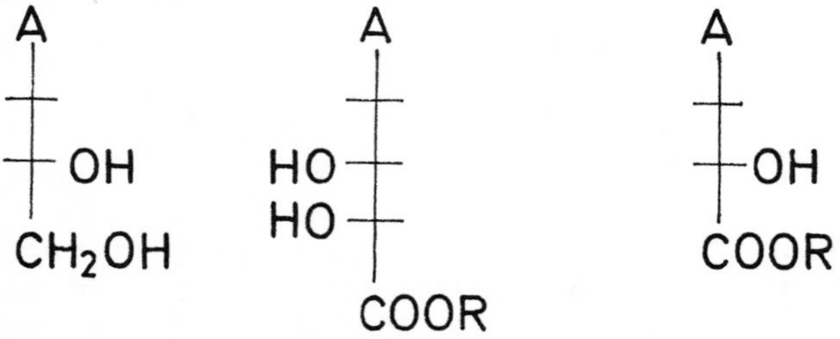

II

III R=H
IV R=alkyl

V R=H
VI R=alkyl

A = adenin-9-yl residue

which simplify and accelerate isolation (Votruba et al.,1983a). Now, this method has been substantially improved by an introduction of a novel affinity support represented by Formula I. This material consists of a ligand, 9-(3-amino-2-hydroxypropyl)-8-hydroxyadenine, which is linked to the 6-carboxyhexyl-Sepharose matrix. The unique specific affinity of this material (Holý et al., 1985c) toward SAH-hydrolases is in a striking contrast to the lack of inhibitory activity of the ligand toward the enzyme under in vitro conditions.

This new principle of affinity chromatography has been verified by applications which comprize the purification of SAH-hydrolases from leukemic

Table 1 Some properties of SAH-hydrolases purified by affinity chromatography

Enzyme source	MW	Subunit MW	pI	K_M^{Ado} $\mu mol.l^{-1}$	K_M^{SAH} $\mu mol.l^{-1}$	Specific activity[d] $nkat.mg^{-1}$	Purif. factor
L1210 cells	230000[a] 183000[b]	43000[a]	5.6-5.7	3.8	4.4	113.2	590.0
Mouse liver	230000[a] 172000[b]	43000[a]	5.6-5.7	–	–	–	–
Nicotiana tabacum cells	220000[a]	55000[a]	5.15[c] 5.25[c]	5.15	11.0	73.0	40.7
Pyrrhocoris apterus ovaries	–	–	–	1.0	3.5	–	–

a Determined by PAGE electrophoresis; b determined by ultracentrifugation;
c two components; d in the direction of synthesis.

cells, mouse liver, plant tissue cells and insect ovaries. The properties of thus-obtained enzymes are comprized in Table 1.

The affinity support can be used for rapid isolation of electrophoretically homogeneous enzyme from partially purified material(Votruba et al.,1983a; Merta et al.,1983) or, alternatively, for a one-step isolation from the supernatant fraction of the crude cell homogeneate (Šebestová et al.,1984). The latter alternative permits an isolation of the pure enzyme from minute samples of tissue (Votruba et al.,1985). Contaminating materials are removed by an increasing salt concentration; finally, the enzyme is liberated by elution with a dilute solution of adenosine.

The SAH-hydrolase which has been isolated from murine leukemia (L1210) cells by this procedure (Merta et al.,1983) was compared with an enzyme obtained from mouse liver by affinity chromatography. The amino acid composition of both enzymes (Table 2) is very similar; however, in contrast to the liver enzyme which is reported to contain a substituted N-terminal amino acid (Ueland et al.,1978), the L1210 enzyme contains L--glutamic acid as the only N-terminal group.

The isoelectric focusing of the two enzymes is depicted in Fig.1. The pI values of the two enzymes are in the range of pH 5.6-5.7. The enzymes are evidently microheterogeneous; a similar microheterogeneity was also encountered in the polyacrylamide gradient gel (5-15%) electrophoresis in which the L1210 enzyme dissociates into three bands (result not shown). The SAH-hydrolase isolated by the same affinity chromatography technique from Nicotiana tabacum (Šebestová et al., 1984) separates on isoelectric focusing into two zones (pI 5.15 and 5.25, resp., cf. Table 1) in the ratio 1:1.

Thus, the novel affinity chromatography method enables the rapid isolation of SAH-hydrolases which exhibit a high specific activity (witnessing the native character of the enzyme). It can be recommended for use owing to the easy accessibility of the affinity ligand, reproducibility of the affinity carrier, reproducibility and rapidity of the isolation procedure; it also makes

Table 2   Amino acid composition of SAH-hydrolase

Amino acid	N(L1210)[a]	N(mouse liver)[a,b]
Lys	27.15	27.75
His	10.73	11.30
Arg	15.61	12.72
Asp	45.19	44.98
Thr	21.32	21.16
Ser	12.33	14.47
Glu	37.54	39.08
Pro	19.06	17.89
Gly	34.77	36.53
Ala	36.25	37.76
Cys	8.00	5.94
Val	28.40	30.15
Met	15.50	16.14
Ile	25.52	28.99
Leu	35.85	37.83
Tyr	11.70	12.92
Phe	10.95	11.69
Try	(10.77)[c]	10.77

[a]Number of amino acid residues calculated for one subunit; [b] taken from (Ueland et al.,1978); [c] calculated from the value estimated for mouse liver enzyme (Ueland et al.,1978).

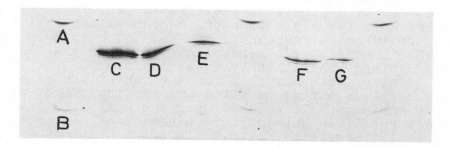

Fig.1. IEF of SAH-hydrolases in PAGE. (A) Bovine carbonic anhydrase B (pI 5.85); (B) β-lactoglobuline A (pI 5.2), (C)(D)(E) mouse liver SAH-hydrolase, (F)(G) L1210 SAH-hydrolase.

possible to concentrate and purify the enzyme
from very small amounts of biological material
(Votruba et al.,1985). Nevertheless, the electro-
migration properties of the enzyme proteins isolated by this technique do differ from those of
enzymes purified by other procedures. It remains
to be established whether the above findings are
consistent with the reported subunit homogeneity
of SAH-hydrolases isolated by other procedures
(Gomi et al.,1985).

OPEN-CHAIN ADENOSINE ANALOGS AS INHIBITORS
OF SAH-HYDROLASE

Since the discovery of (S)-9-(2,3-dihydroxy-
propyl)adenine (DHPA, II) inhibition of rat liver
SAH-hydrolase (Votruba & Holý,1980), an exhausti-
ve study of structure-activity relationship in the
series of open-chain adenosine analogs revealed
many additional reversible and irreversible inhibitors of SAH-hydrolase (Holý et al.,1985a,1985b).
Three types of compounds are particularly interesting: DHPA (II) as a representative of reversible
competitive inhibitors, D-eritadenine (III) and
3-(adenin-9-yl)-2-hydroxypropanoic acids (V) as
example of powerful irreversible inactivators
(Votruba & Holý,1982; Holý et al.,1985b) and esters of the latter acids (IV,VI) as non-inhibito-
ry prodrugs of inhibitors III and V.

The SAH-hydrolases purified from different
sources by affinity chromatography (cf. Table 1)
were used for evaluation of the inhibitory activity of selected compounds. The data comprized in
Table 3 confirm the general character of the SAH-
-hydrolase inhibition by these analogs.

The effects observed for the inhibition of
mouse liver enzyme in vitro and for the effect of
the inhibitors II and III upon the enzyme in intact rat liver hepatocytes (Schanche et al.,1984)
are also consistent with the above inhibitory
activities.

Table 3   Inhibition of SAH-hydrolases by open-
          -chain analogs of adenosine

Enzyme source	IC_{50} $(nmol.l^{-1})$[a]		
	II	III	V
Rat liver	–	7.0	20.0
L1210 cells	900	3.0	12.0
Nicotiana tabacum	1500	1.5	12.5
Insect ovaries	600	2.0	14.0

a For hydrolytic reaction.

BIOLOGICAL EFFECTS OF SAH-HYDROLASE INHIBITORS

1. Antiviral Activity

Neutral open-chain adenosine analogs which
act as reversible SAH-hydrolase inhibitors generally display a non-specific broad-spectrum antiviral activity (Holý et al.,1985a; DeClercq & Holý,1979). There is a correlation between the enzyme inhibitory effect and antiviral activity
(Holý et al.,1985a). However, the irreversible
inactivators (e.g. III,V) do not exhibit stronger
effects than the reversible inhibitors. In order
to circumvent polarity as the obvious cause of
hindered cell penetration the alkyl esters of the
above compounds (IV,VI) were developed as potential prodrugs; these compounds really exhibit
markedly increased antiviral effect (DeClercq &
Holý,1985). The antiviral spectra of both reversible and irreversible inhibitors are identical.
    The open-chain analogs possess an undisputab-
le advantage: their inertia toward cellular metabolic processes practically excludes target enzymes which are affected by phosphorylated metabolites of other nucleoside analogs (araA, acyclo-
guanosine, etc.). Thus, SAH-hydrolase and related
enzymes of the regulatory pathway connected with
transmethylations might be regarded as the only
target available. However, it is not easy to find
a general explanation of the antiviral effects
observed on one side and low cytotoxicity on the
other. The direct connection with viral multipli-

cation is feasible only with (-)stranded RNA viruses which are dependent on capping of viral mRNA.

The characteristic features of SAH-hydrolase inhibitors as antivirals can be summarized as follows: (a) Typical antiviral spectrum with profound preference for (-)stranded RNA viruses (rhabdo-, paramyxo-, reoviridae). However, also DNA viruses are sensitive (poxviridae, plant viruses). This spectrum is also similar for other SAH-hydrolase inhibitors (carbocyclic nucleosides) (DeClercq et al.,1984). (b) Antiviral effect of the reversible and irreversible SAH-hydrolase inhibitors depends upon the host cell used (DeClercq & Holý,1985); in those cells in which the drug displays an antiviral effect the intracellular level of DHPA significantly increases after virus infection whereas the opposite is true for the cells in which the virus multiplication is drug-insensitive (Votruba et al.,1983b). Since the drug transport is not affected by the viral infection (Dragún et al.,1983), this finding suggests an involvement of intracellular factors which actively captivate the drug.

The obvious importance of transmethylation reactions in rapidly proliferating systems implicates the role of SAH-hydrolase inhibitors in non--pathological processes occurring in living systems:

2. Embryotoxicity and Teratogenicity

DHPA (30-100 µg) administered subgerminally (day 2) or intraamniotically (day 3) to embryonic chick produces a wide array of malformations accompanied with significant embryonic mortality. The distribution analysis confirmed that for expression of the embryotoxic properties no metabolic activation of the drug is needed (Jelínek et al.,1981). Microscopic-anatomical examination of drug-treated chick-embryo revealed a serious damage to the spinal cord, optic cup and limb buds, resulting in the development of hydromyely, microphtalmia and reduction limb deformities (Jelínek et al.,1985).

Teratological analysis of additional SAH-hydrolase inhibitors performed in the chick embryo disclosed compounds exceeding DHPA in both seve-

Table 4 Teratogenic doses of SAH-hydrolase inhi-
         bitors in 2-day-old chick embryo

Compound	Teratogenic dose (μg)
II	30-100
III	3-100
(S)-IV	30-100
(R)-IV	10-100
(RS)-V	3-100[a], 10-100[b]
3-Deaza-($\pm$)aristeromycin	30-100
3-Deazaadenosine	30-100

[a] R = ethyl, isopropyl, n-butyl, sec-butyl, iso-
butyl;   [b] R = methyl, isopentyl.

Table 5 Aspermatogenic effect of SAH-hydrolase
         inhibitors (administered intratesticularly)

Compound	Decrease of testes weight, %
II	30
III	50
(S)-V	68
(R)-V	80

Table 6 Inhibition of larval hatching (Pyrrho-
         coris apterus)[a]

Compound	IC_{50}[b] ($mg.ml^{-1}$)	IC_{100} ($mg.ml^{-1}$)
II	0.12	1.0
III	0.007	0.05
(S)-V	0.01	0.1
(R)-V	0.15	1.0
VI (R=CH$_3$)	0.05	1.0

[a]Drug administered in drinking water: 1 $mg.ml^{-1}$
corresponds to a consumption of 1$g.kg^{-1}.day^{-1}$;
[b]drug concentration which causes 50% or 100% inhibition of larval hatching.

rity of the embryotoxic action and duration of
sensitivity period which extended, in the extreme, up to day 5 of incubation (Table 4). The
effect concerned, above all the central nervous
system, **eye** anlage, facial outgrowths and anlages
of the limbs. These four embryonic morphogenetic
systems may be considered specific for the SAH-
-hydrolase inhibitors. It seems plausible that
the primary target cell population may be the neural crest elements of the organ anlages affected.

Teratogenicity was absent at 100 µg per embryo
for 15 additional open-chain analogs tested which
do not inhibit SAH-hydrolase.

3. Aspermatogenic Activity

Prolonged oral administration of DHPA to male
mice results in testicular germinal aplasia and
sterility; this effect is fully reversible (De
Clercq et al.,1981). Additional SAH-hydrolase inhibitors also induce severe aspermatogenic effects:
on intratesticular application (3x0.1 mg daily for
three following days) of irreversible inhibitors
to male mice, the weight of testes dramatically decreases (Table 5). No data are available whether
these affects can also be stimulated by different
routes of administration, neither on reversibility of the effects. (These experiments were performed by Dr J.Matoušek, Institute of Animal Physiology and Genetics, Liběchov, Czechoslovakia).

4. Insect Chemosterilant Activity

DHPA administered orally to females of hemi-
pteran insects induces egg-sterility and a dose-
-dependent suppression of fecundity (Sláma et al.,
1984). The connection of this effect with the inhibition of ovarian enzyme was proved by enzyme
determination and isolation, as well as by estimating the drug level in ovaries (Votruba et al.,
1985). Similar sterilizing effect was observed with
viviparous apterous females Aphis fabae which received the drug via the host plant. Additional experiments with irreversible inhibitors confirm the
link between the inhibition of the enzyme and the
chemosterilizing effect (Table 6), (Gelbič et al.,
1984).

Table 7   The effect of SAH-hydrolase inhibitors
on seedling root development (Vicia faba L.)[a]

Compound	Conc. mg. l^{-1}	Suppression (%)[b] of (A)	(B)	(C)
II	10	39.5	69.0	90.0
III	10	55.5	17.5	80.0
IV (R=CH$_3$)	10	3.0	20.0	20.0
(RS)-V	10	61.5	88.0	98.0
VI (R=CH$_3$)	1	53.5	58.5	73.5

[a] 3-Day-old seedlings kept for 7 days at 25°C in
the drug solution; [b] (A) main root length; (B)
side roots number; (C) total side roots length.

5. Plant Root Inhibition

Shoot and root development of the seedlings
of Vicia faba L. planted in a diluted Knop's solution is substantially suppressed in presence of
DHPA. The microscopic examination revealed the
block of mitosis and/or cytokinesis accompanied
by the formation of binucleate cells (Beneš et al.,
1984). Similar effects were encountered with additional SAH-hydrolase inhibitors (Table 7). In
particular, compounds V and VI proved to be much
more powerful inhibitors than DHPA. No connection
is evident between effects of SAH-hydrolase inhibition and metabolism or effects of cytokinins.

The therapeutic application of SAH-hydrolase
inhibitors can be accompanied by serious side-
-effects; the compounds can serve for studying
the consequences of disturbances in transmethylations and/or the adenine nucleotide pool.

REFERENCES

Beneš,K., Holý,A. and Melichar,O. (1984) Biol.
    plant. 26, 144-150.
DeClercq,E. and Holý,A. (1979) J.Med.Chem.,22,510.
DeClercq,E., Leyten,R., Sobis,H., Matoušek,J.,
    Holý,A. and DeSomer,P. (1981) Toxic.Appl.Phar-
    macol. 59, 441-451.

DeClercq,E., Bergstrom,D.E., Holý,A. and Montgo-
  mery,J.A. (1984) Antiviral Res. 4, 119-133.
DeClercq,E. and Holý,A. (1985) J.Med.Chem.28,
  282-287.
Dragúň,M., Rada,B. and Holý,A.(1983) Acta Virol.
  27, 119-129.
Gelbič,I., Tonner,M. and Holý,A. (1984) Acta ent.
  bohemoslov. 81, 46-53.
Gomi,T., Ishiguro,Y. and Fujioka,M. (1985) J.
  Biol.Chem. 260, 2789-2793.
Holý,A., Votruba,I. and DeClercq,E. (1985a)
  Collect.Czech.Chem.Commun. 50, 245-261.
Holý,A., Votruba,I. and DeClercq,E. (1985b)
  Collect.Czech.Chem.Commun. 50, 262-279.
Holý,A., Kohoutová, J., Merta,A. and Votruba,I.
  (1985c) Collect.Czech.Chem.Commun., in press.
Jelínek,R., Holý,A. and Votruba,I. (1981) Tera-
  tology 24, 267-275.
Jelínek,R., Doskočil,M. and Holý,A. (1985) Tera-
  togenesis, Carcinogenesis, Mutagenesis, in press
Merta,A. Votruba,I., Veselý,J. and Holý,A. (1983)
  Collect.Czech.Chem.Commun. 48, 2701.
Schanche,J.S., Schanche,T., Ueland,P.M., Holý,A.
  and Votruba,I. (1984) Molec.Pharmacol. 26,
  553-558.
Sláma,K., Holý,A. and Votruba,I.(1983) Ent.exp.
  appl. 33, 9-14.
Šebestová,L., Votruba,I. and Holý,A. (1984)
  Collect.Czech.Chem.Commun. 49, 1543-1551.
Ueland,P.M., Skotland,T., Døskeland,S.O. and Flat-
  mark,T. (1978) Biochim.Biophys.Acta 553, 57-65.
Ueland,P.M. (1982) Pharmacol.Revs. 34, 223-253.
Votruba,I. and Holý,A. (1980) Collect.Czech.Chem.
  Commun. 45, 3039-3044.
Votruba,I. and Holý,A. (1982) Collect.Czech.Chem.
  Commun. 47, 167-172.
Votruba, I., Holý,A. and Rosenberg,I.(1983a)
  Collect.Czech.Chem.Commun. 48, 2549-2557.
Votruba,I., Holý,A. and DeClercq,E. (1983b) Acta
  Virol. 27, 273-276.
Votruba,I., Holý,A., Rosenberg,I. and Sláma,K.
  (1985) Insect Biochem., in press.

NUCLEOSIDE ANALOGS AS ANTIVIRAL AGENTS

John A. Montgomery and John A. Secrist III

Southern Research Institute

P. O. Box 55305, Birmingham, Alabama   35255

INTRODUCTION

Neither 3-deaza- (**7**) nor 7-deazaadenosine (**13**) is very selective in its antiviral activity. 3-Deaza-adenosine (c^3-Ado) is moderately active against some viruses, vaccinia, vesicular stomatitis, parainfluenza type 3, and reo type 1 but at concentrations only 5- to 20-fold lower than the cytotoxic concentration (150 µM) (see Table 1). 7-Deazaadenosine (c^7-Ado) is much more cytotoxic than the 3-deaza compound, causing disruption of cells at 1.5 µM. 7-Deazaadenosine inhibits some viruses, e.g., vesicular stomatitis and polio type 1 at concentrations (0.03 µM) that are 50-fold lower than its cytotoxic concentration, but for other viruses it is inhibitory only at concentrations approaching cytotoxicity. Certain substitutions at C-7 of c^7-Ado reduce its cytotoxicity and increase its potency (see Table 1).

The carbocyclic analogs of adenosine (C-Ado, **1**) and 7-deazaadenosine (C-c^7-Ado, **13**) are both cytotoxic at about 38 µM and inhibit the replication of some viruses at slightly lower concentrations (5- to 10-fold at most). On the other hand, a dramatic improvement in both potency and selectivity is demonstrated by the carbocyclic analog (C-c^3-Ado) of 3-deazaadenosine. While not cytotoxic to PRK, HeLa, or Vero cells at 1500 µM, C-c^3-Ado inhibits the replication of vaccinia,

Table 1. Antiviral Activity of 3- and
7-Deazaadenosine and Related Compounds[a]

Virus	Cell Culture	Therapeutic Index[b]				
		c^3-Ado	c^7-Ado	C-c^3-Ado	C-c^7-Ado	7-MeCHOH-c^7-Ado
Vaccinia	PRK	5.6	20.0	>500.0	5.0	14.0
HSV-1	PRK	$\leq$1.0	5.6	$\leq$2.0	$\leq$1.0	5.0
HSV-2	PRK	$\leq$1.0	20.0	$\leq$1.3	1.4	1.4
VSV	PRK	5.6	56.0	>2000.0	$\leq$1.0	25.0
Polio 1	HeLa	$\leq$1.0	56.0	1.0	$\leq$1.0	200.0
Coxsackie B4	HeLa	$\leq$1.0	20.0	1.0	1.4	57.0
Sindbis	Vero	$\leq$1.0	20.0	>20.0	$\leq$1.0	5.7
Measles	Vero	$\leq$1.0	20.0	>1000.0	2.5	<1.0
Parainfluenza 3	Vero	20.0	5.6	>2000.0	5.0	57.0
Reo 1	Vero	4.0	5.6	>400.0	2.5	100.0

[a]Based on data in DeClercq et al., 1984. [b]Cytotoxic concentration/minimum
concentration required to inhibit viral cytopathogenicity by 50%.

vesicular stomatitis, measles, parainfluenza, and reo
type 1 viruses at 0.75-3.8 μM, giving a selectivity
index of 400-2000. The activity spectrum is similar
to that of c^3-Ado, but C-c^3-Ado is 10-100 times more
potent and at least 10 times less cytotoxic (see Table
1) (DeClercq et al., 1984).

Neither c^3-Ado nor C-c^3-Ado is deaminated or phosphorylated to any extent in cells (Chiang et al., 1977;
Montgomery et al., 1982). They are both alternative
substrates for, and consequently competitive inhibitors
of, adenosylhomocysteinase (Chiang et al., 1977;
Montgomery et al., 1982). Both compounds and the corresponding adenosylhomocysteine analogs are inhibitors
of adenosylmethionine decarboxylase (Gordon et al.,
1983). Further, C-c^3-Ado has no effect on DNA, RNA,
or protein synthesis in L1210 cells at 200 μM concentration, significantly above the cytotoxic concentration
for these murine leukemia cells in culture. A mutant

1 (C-Ado): X=CH$_2$, R=HOCH$_2$
2: X=O, R=H$_2$NCO
3: X=CH$_2$, R=H$_2$NCO
4: X=O, R=HO$_2$CCH(NH$_2$)(CH$_2$)$_2$CHNH$_2$CH$_2$
5: X=O, H$_2$N(CH$_2$)$_2$CH(NH$_2$)CH$_2$
6: X=O, H$_2$N(CH$_2$)$_3$CH(NH$_2$)CH$_2$

7 (c^3-Ado): X=O, R-HOCH$_2$
8: X=O, R=MeSCH$_2$
9: X=O, R=i-BuSCH$_2$
10 (C-c^3-Ado): X=CH$_2$, R=HOCH$_2$
11: X=CH$_2$, R=ClCH$_2$
12: X=CH$_2$, R=CH$_3$

13 (c^7-Ado): X=O, R$_1$=HOCH$_2$, R$_2$=H
14: X=O, R$_1$=R$_2$=HOCH$_2$
15 (C-c^7-Ado): X=CH$_2$, R$_1$=HOCH$_2$, R$_2$=H

16 (c^3-Ino): X=O
17 (C-c^3-Ino): X=CH$_2$

subline (AKR-4) of adenosine kinase deficient Rl.1 murine T lymphoma cells is 50-fold resistant to these compounds. These AKR-4 cells are characterized by elevated levels of methionine adenosyltransferase activity (Kajander et al., 1985). Thus, although the exact mechanism of the antiviral activity of these compounds is uncertain, it seems to be related to perturbations in adenosylmethionine metabolism.

c^7-Ado (tubercidin) is not deaminated but is rapidly phosphorylated to the triphosphate in cells (Suhadolnik, 1970). Cells lacking adenosine kinase cannot phosphorylate c^7-Ado and are highly resistant to it (Bennett et al., 1966). Although there is not a clear picture of its cytotoxic mechanism, its primary effect appears

18 (c[7]-Ino): X=O, R=H
19: X=O, R=Br
20: X=O, R=NO$_2$
21: X=O, R=NH$_2$
22: X=O, R=CN
23: X=O, R=CH$_2$OH
24: X=O, R=CH$_2$NH$_2$
25 (C-c[7]-Ino): X=CH$_2$, R=H

to be on macromolecular synthesis (Suhadolnik, 1970). As mentioned above, only certain 7-substituted derivatives of c[7]-Ado have significant antiviral activity in vitro (Bergstrom et al., 1984), but there is no information on their metabolism or mechanism of action. Both these compounds and C-c[3]-Ado have in vivo activity in mouse models also (DeClercq et al., 1984).

Sinefungin (**4**), a potent inhibitor of viral methyl-transferases, inhibits plaque formation by vaccinia virus in L-cells (Pugh et al., 1978; Borchardt, 1980) and has shown in vivo activity against Herpes simplex (Nagarajan, 1979).

As part of our ongoing program on antiviral agents, we have prepared a number of derivatives and congeners of these lead structures and evaluated them for their antiviral activity, with interesting results.

CHEMISTRY

The carboxamide derivatives **2** and **3** of adenosine (Chiang et al., 1981) and C-Ado were prepared from their isopropylidene derivatives by basic permanganate oxidation followed by conversion of the acid to the acid chloride with thionyl chloride, reaction with alcoholic ammonia, and acidic removal of the isopropyl-idene group. The sinefungin analog **5** was prepared from 2',3'-O-isopropylidene-5'-C-(2-oxotetrahydro-3-furanyl)-5'-deoxyadenosine (Lyga and Secrist, 1983) by a complex eleven-step sequence. The homolog **6** was prepared from sinefungin by protection of the amino groups, photolytic decarboxylation, and deprotection. The 5'-chloro derivative of c^3-Ado (Chiang et al., 1978) was converted to the methylthio compound **8** by reaction with sodium methylmercaptide. The 5'-chloro derivative of C-c^3-Ado (**11**) was prepared similarly (Montgomery et al., 1982) and catalytically reduced to the 5'-deoxy compound **12**. The 7-hydroxymethyl derivative (**14**) of c^7-Ado was prepared by a literature procedure (Bergstrom et al., 1981). Compound **14** and other 7-substituted derivatives of c^7-Ado, also prepared by literature procedures (Watanabe and Ueda, 1983; Bergstrom and Brattesani, 1980), were deaminated to the c^7-Ino analogs **19-23** by treatment overnight with sodium nitrite, in three additions to a solution of the compound in dilute acetic acid. Compounds **16-18** and **25** were prepared in a similar manner from the c^3-Ado, C-c^3-Ado, c^7-Ado, and C-c^7-Ado. Compound **24** was prepared from the reduction of **22**.

BIOLOGIC EVALUATIONS

The 5'-carboxamide derivative of adenosine (**2**), which inactivates adenosylhomocysteinase (Chiang et al., 1981), showed minimal activity against vaccinia (Lederle CA) in L-929 cells, but its carbocyclic analog **3** was a potent inhibitor of this virus replication with a virus rating (VR) of 3.4 and an MIC_{50} of 6.5 μg/mL (for the definition of VR and MIC_{50}, see Montgomery et al., 1982). Compound **3** also showed activity against HSV-1(377) in Vero cells (VR=1.3, MIC_{50}=90 μg/mL) but only marginal activity against HSV-2 (MS) in Vero cells or vesicular stomatitis in L-929 cells. The sinefungin analogs **5** and **6** were less active than sinefungin itself against HSV-1 or vaccinia, but **5** is the most potent known inhibitor of spermine synthase, with an I_{50} of 12 μM, and also inhibits E. coli adenosylmethionine decarboxylase (I_{50}=1 mM) (Pegg, personal communication). The 5'-isobutylthio derivative (**9**) of c^3-Ado (Chiang et al., 1978; Bodner et al., 1981) showed significant activity against influenza Ao/PR/8/34 in MDCK cells (VR=1.6; MIC_{50}=7 μg/mL). The 5'-chloro derivative of C-c^3-Ado (**11**) has a VR against vaccinia of 1.5 (MIC_{50}=32 μg/mL), whereas the 5'-deoxy compound **12** is much better (VR=3.2, MIC_{50}=2.7 μg/mL). The values for C-c^3-Ado itself are VR=3.6 (MIC_{50}=2.8 μg/mL).

Montgomery and Secrist

Table 2. Antiviral Activity

Compound	Vaccinia		HSV-1		HSV-2		Influenza				Rhino 1A	
							Ao		A_2			
	VR	C[a]	VR	C	VR	C	VR	C	VR	C	VR	C
AraA	2.0	11.0	2.0	15	2.0	3						
Ribavirin							4.0	9.0	1.5	32.0	0.6	>300
2	0.8	~90.0										
3	3.4	6.5	1.3	~90	0.5	90						
8	0.5	70.0										
9							1.6	~7.0				
11	1.9	32.0										
12	3.2	2.7										
14	~7.0	~0.2	0.0				0.5	~300.0			0.0	
16	1.2	160.0										
17	1.5	160.0										
18	0.2		0.0				1.4	2.5	0.7	5.1	3.8	1.4
19	3.4	~100.0	0.0				0.4				0.2	

[a]Minimum concentration (µg/mL) of drug required for 50% inhibition of virus-induced cytopathogenic effects in infected cell cultures.

The 7-hydroxymethyl derivative of c[7]-Ado was the only one of five 7-substituted c[7]-Ado derivatives that showed significant antiviral activity, having a VR of 5.7 (MIC_{50} ca 0.2 µg/mL) against vaccinia (Lederle CA) and a VR of 0.5 (MIC_{50} ca 300 µg/mL) against influenza Ao/PR/8/34. These results are in agreement with previous work on related compounds (DeClercq et al., 1984; Bergstrom et al., 1984). Deamination of c[7]-Ado to the inosine analog c[7]-Ino (18) caused a dramatic change in antiviral activity. c[7]-Ino is a potent inhibitor of Rhino 1A(2060) in MRC_5 cells (VR=3.8, MIC_{50}=1.4 µg/mL) and a good inhibitor of influenza Ao/PR/8/34 (VR=1.4, MIC_{50}=2.5 µg/mL). It was less effective against influenza A_2/Aichi/2/68 (VR=0.7, MIC_{50}=5.1 µg/mL) and inactive against vaccinia as was C-c[7]-Ino.. Substitution at the 7 position of c[7]-Ino again produced a marked change in antiviral activity. Although compounds 20-24

showed at best marginal activity, the 7-bromo derivative
19 had a VR of 3.4 against vaccinia (MIC_{50} ca 100 µg/mL),
marginal activity against influenza Ao/PR/8/34, and
little activity against Rhino 1A. The significant
antiviral activity of these new nucleoside analogs
is summarized in Table 2.

   Acknowledgment. The authors wish to thank
Dr. W. M. Shannon and his associates for the antiviral
data reported herein. This work was supported in part
by the National Institutes of Health, P01 CA-34200.

REFERENCES

Bennett, Jr., L. L., Schnebli, H. P., Vail, M. H.,
Allan, P. W., and Montgomery, J. A. (1966) Mol.
Pharmacol. 2, 432.

Bergstrom, D. E. and Brattesani, A. J. (1980) Nucleic
Acids Res. 8, 6231.

Bergstrom, D. E., Brattesani, A. J., Ogawa, M. K.,
and Schweickert, M. J. (1981) J. Org. Chem. 46, 1423.

Bergstrom, D. E., Brattesani, A. J., Ogawa, M. K.,
Reddy, P. A., Schweickert, M. J., Balzarini, J., and
De Clercq, E. (1984) J. Med. Chem. 27, 285.

Bodner, A. J., Cantoni, G. L., and Chiang, P. K. (1981)
Biochem. Biophys. Res. Commun. 98, 476.

Borchardt, R. T. (1980) J. Med. Chem. 23, 347.

Chiang, P. K., Richards, H. H., and Cantoni, G. L.
(1977) Mol. Pharmacol. 13, 939.

Chiang, P. K., Guranowski, A., and Segall, J. E. (1981)
Arch. Biochem. Biophys. 207, 175.

Chiang, P. K., Cantoni, G. L., and Bader, J. P. (1978)
Biochem. Biophys. Res. Commun. 82, 417.

De Clercq, E., Bergstrom, D. E., Holy, A., and
Montgomery, J. A. (1984) Antiviral Res. 4, 119.

Gordon, R. K., Brown, N. D., and Chiang, P. K. (1983) Biochem. Biophys. Res. Commun. 114, 505.

Kajander, E., Kubota, M., Yamanaka, H., Montgomery, J., and Carson, D. (1985) The Biochemistry of S-Adenosylmethionine as a Basis for Drug Design, An International Symposium (Borchardt, R. T., Creveling, C. R., and Ueland, P. M., Eds.), Humana Press, Inc., Clifton, New Jersey.

Lyga, J. W. and Secrist III, J. A. (1983) J. Org. Chem. 48, 1982.

Montgomery, J. A., Clayton, S. J., Thomas, H. J., Shannon, W. M., Arnett, G., Bodner, A. J., Kim, I.-K., Cantoni, G. L., and Chiang, P. K. (1982) J. Med. Chem. 25, 626.

Nagarajan, R. (1979) U. S. Patent No. 4,158,056.

Pugh, C. S. G., Borchardt, R. T., and Stone, H. O. (1978) J. Biol. Chem. 253, 4075.

Suhadolnik, R. J. (1970) Nucleoside Antibiotics, John Wiley & Sons, Inc., New York.

Watanabe, S.-I., Ueda, T. (1983) Nucleosides Nucleotides 2, 113.

STUDIES CONCERNING THE MECHANISM OF ACTION

OF 3-DEAZAADENOSINE IN LEUKOCYTES

Thomas P. Zimmerman, Gerald Wolberg, Carolyn R. Stopford, Karen L. Prus and Marie A. Iannone

Wellcome Research Laboratories, Burroughs Wellcome Co., Research Triangle Park, North Carolina 27709

INTRODUCTION

3-Deazaadenosine (c^3Ado) is a fascinating compound that exhibits interesting biological activities but whose mechanism of action remains an enigma. Although the synthesis of c^3Ado was first reported in 1966 (Rousseau et al., 1966), during the subsequent eleven years little was reported concerning biological activities of this adenosine analogue. During this interval, c^3Ado was shown to be resistant to deamination by adenosine deaminase (Ikehara & Fukui, 1974) and to be nontoxic to tumor cells (Kitano et al., 1975; May & Townsend, 1975). In 1977, however, widespread interest in c^3Ado was awakened by the discovery that c^3Ado is both a substrate and a potent inhibitor of S-adenosylhomocysteine (AdoHcy) hydrolase (Chiang et al., 1977); in this same report it was shown that c^3Ado caused a buildup of AdoHcy and was metabolized to S-3-deazaadenosylhomocysteine (c^3AdoHcy) in rat hepato-cytes. Following this landmark publication, numerous reports began to appear describing diverse biological effects of c^3Ado, particularly with respect to leukocyte functions (reviewed by Ueland, 1982, and by Chiang, 1985). In many of these experimental systems, exogenously supplied L-homocysteine (Hcy) has been found to enhance the biolog-ical activity of c^3Ado.

The biochemical mechanism(s) by which c^3Ado affects these various cellular functions is understood poorly.

417

Because c^3Ado has been shown to cause a buildup of AdoHcy and to be metabolized to c^3AdoHcy in many tissues, as well as to cause inhibition of cellular transmethylation reactions (Ueland, 1982; Chiang, 1985), it has become widely accepted that most, if not all, of the biological effects of c^3Ado result ultimately from the inhibition of some critical methylation reaction(s) within the affected cells. The potentiation of many of the biological effects of c^3Ado by Hcy, a co-substrate with c^3Ado for AdoHcy hydrolase (Chiang et al., 1977), is consistent with this view. Moreover, this methylation hypothesis of c^3Ado action has received indirect support from reports that: (i) c^3Ado is not metabolized detectably to 5'-nucleotides (Bader et al., 1978; Zimmerman et al., 1978, 1979; Miller et al., 1979); (ii) c^3Ado is not incorporated detectably into cellular nucleic acids (Bader et al., 1978); (iii) c^3Ado does not affect basal levels of leukocyte cAMP (Zimmerman et al., 1978, 1979); and (iv) c^3Ado does not decrease leukocyte ribonucleoside 5'-triphosphate pools (Zimmerman et al., 1978, 1979).

Nevertheless, recent studies concerning the effects of c^3Ado on neutrophil chemotaxis (Garcia-Castro et al., 1983) and on lymphocyte-mediated cytolysis (LMC) (Zimmerman et al., 1984) have begun to cast doubt upon the universality of the methylation hypothesis of c^3Ado action. This report summarizes the current efforts in our laboratory to elucidate the biochemical mechanism(s) by which c^3Ado inhibits LMC and macrophage phagocytosis.

MATERIALS AND METHODS

[G-^{3}H]3-Deazaadenosine (22 Ci/mmol) was custom synthesized by Moravek Biochemicals, Inc. Quin-2, tetraacetoxymethyl ester, was obtained from Amersham International, and ionomycin was from Calbiochem. Other materials were from sources identified elsewhere (Stopford et al., 1985; Wolberg et al., 1984; Zimmerman et al., 1976, 1978, 1979, 1980, 1984).

Cytolytic lymphocytes were obtained from CD-1 mice 10 or 11 days after intraperitoneal injection of 3 x 10^7 EL4 cells, while C57BL leukemia EL4 cells were maintained, harvested and labeled with $Na_2{}^{51}CrO_4$ as described (Zimmerman et al., 1976). Resident peritoneal macrophages were prepared from CD-1 mice (Stopford et al., 1985). Lymphocyte

experiments were conducted with Dulbecco's phosphate-
buffered saline supplemented with 5% fetal calf serum
(heat-inactivated) as the medium. Macrophage experiments
were conducted with RPMI-1640 medium containing 10% fetal
calf serum (heat-inactivated), penicillin (100 units/ml),
streptomycin (100 µg/ml) and 25 mM Hepes as the medium.

The in vitro assay of LMC determines the amount of ^{51}Cr
released during a 70-min incubation at 37° of ^{51}Cr-labeled
EL4 cells and specifically sensitized cytolytic lymphocytes
(Wolberg et al., 1973). With a 1:1 ratio of cytolytic
lymphocytes to EL4 target cells, 24% lysis occurred in the
control assays. Macrophage antibody-dependent phagocytosis
was measured at 37° during 30-min incubations of adherent
macrophages and antibody-coated sheep red blood cells
(Stopford et al., 1985).

The effect of various agents on the relative levels of
$[^{35}S]$AdoHcy and $[^{35}S]c^3$AdoHcy in leukocytes was assessed
in L-$[^{35}S]$methionine-prelabeled cells (Zimmerman et al.,
1984; Stopford et al., 1985). Acid-soluble extracts of
cells were analyzed for cAMP by radioimmunoassay and for
ribonucleoside 5'-triphosphates by anion-exchange HPLC
(Zimmerman et al., 1976).

Intracellular levels of free Ca^{2+} were determined with
the Ca^{2+}-sensitive fluorescent probe Quin-2 (Tsien et al.,
1982). Macrophages (4 x 10^6 cells/ml of medium) were
incubated for 60 min at 37° with 48 µM Quin-2, tetraacetoxymethyl ester. These Quin-2-loaded cells were harvested
by a brief centrifugation (1000 x g for 5 min) and resuspended in fresh medium. Prior to use, cells were collected
by brief centrifugation and resuspended to a density of
2 x 10^6 cells per ml in a medium consisting of 145 mM NaCl,
5.0 mM KCl, 1.0 mM sodium phosphate, 1.0 mM $CaCl_2$, 0.5 mM
$MgSO_4$, 5.0 mM glucose, 10 mM Hepes, pH 7.4, for fluorescence measurements (Tsien et al., 1982).

Macrophage microfilaments were visualized either by
staining with rhodamine-labeled phalloin (Faulstich et al.,
1983) or by indirect immunofluorescent staining (Stopford
et al., 1985).

RESULTS AND DISCUSSION

In view of the above-mentioned evidence that c^3Ado inhibits some leukocyte functions by a mechanism that appears to be independent of the drug's effects upon cellular levels of AdoHcy and c^3AdoHcy (Garcia-Castro et al., 1983; Zimmerman et al., 1984), recent experimentation in our laboratory has been directed towards two alternative aspects of c^3Ado pharmacology: (i) effects of c^3Ado on the leukocyte cytoskeleton; and (ii) leukocyte metabolism of radiolabeled c^3Ado to 5'-nucleotides.

Cytoskeleton Effects of c^3Ado

Interest in the possible effect of c^3Ado on the leukocyte cytoskeleton was stimulated by certain similarities in the ways in which c^3Ado and cytoskeleton-modifying agents affect mouse cytolytic lymphocytes. For example, c^3Ado and cytochalasin B, a microfilament-disrupting agent (Wessells et al., 1971), inhibited LMC by 50% at concentrations of 5.0 and 1.25 μM, respectively, when the cytolytic lymphocytes were pretreated for 60 min with each drug (Fig. 1). Of particular interest, pretreatment (60 min) of cytolytic lymphocytes with either c^3Ado (Fig. 2A) or cytochalasin B (Fig. 2B) resulted in an augmented cAMP accumulation when these cells were subsequently stimulated with prostaglandin E_1 (PGE_1, 2.0 μM). However, neither agent alone caused a significant increase in the basal level of lymphocyte cAMP (Fig. 2). Although microtubule-disrupting agents also inhibited LMC and caused enhancement in the lymphocyte cAMP response to PGE_1, both of these effects of the microtubule-directed agents were antagonized by taxol (Wolberg et al., 1984). By contrast, taxol had no effect upon the inhibition of LMC caused by either c^3Ado or cytochalasin B and actually increased slightly the enhancement of the PGE_1-stimulated cAMP accumulation caused by both c^3Ado and cytochalasin B (Wolberg et al., 1984). Collectively, these observations led us to speculate that c^3Ado might, in some manner, be altering the microfilament system present in the cytolytic lymphocytes.

Attempts were made to study drug effects on the microfilaments of these cytolytic lymphocytes by staining filamentous actin with a fluorescent ligand (Faulstich et al., 1983) and then visualizing the microfilaments microscopically. However, this endeavor was unsuccessful

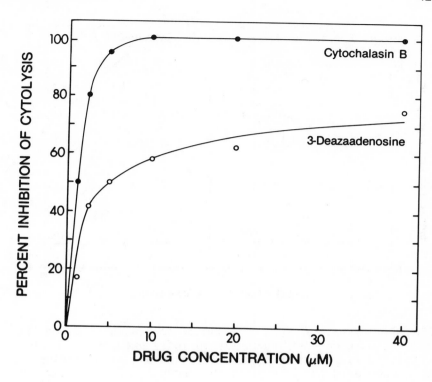

Fig. 1. Effect of c³Ado and cytochalasin B on LMC. The
cytolytic lymphocytes were incubated for 60 min with the
indicated concentration of each drug prior to the start of
the LMC assays.

due to the round configuration and small size of these
lymphocytes.

These developments led us to examine mouse macrophages
as an alternative experimental system with which to investigate the mechanism of action of c³Ado. The principal
advantage offered by macrophages over lymphocytes is that
the former cells adhere and spread well upon surfaces and
are thus highly suitable for fluorescence microscopy
studies. Moreover, of equal importance, it was known that

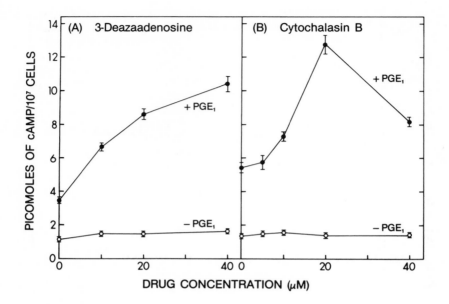

Fig. 2. Effect of c³Ado (A) and cytochalasin B (B) on the PGE₁-stimulated cAMP accumulation in lymphocytes. Mouse cytolytic lymphocytes (1.0 x 10⁷ cells/5.0 ml of medium) were incubated for 60 min in the presence of the indicated concentration of c³Ado or cytochalasin B. Ethanol (O) or PGE₁ (2.0 µM) (●) was then added and the cells were acid-extracted for cAMP determinations after an additional 30-min incubation. This experiment was performed in duplicate and each column-purified extract was radioimmuno-assayed in duplicate for cAMP. Each point represents the mean ± SEM for four determinations.

c³Ado is inhibitory to macrophage phagocytosis (Leonard et al., 1978).

Many of the experimental results obtained with macro-phages have been the subject of a separate report (Stopford et al., 1985) and are only summarized here. Inhibition of macrophage phagocytosis by c³Ado (IC₅₀ = 10 µM) was confirmed. Concentrations of c³Ado ≥ 5 µM were observed to alter markedly both the morphology and, as assessed by fluorescence microscopy, the microfilament pattern of adherent cells. All of these effects of c^3Ado on macrophages were readily reversible after drug washout. Two other potent inhibitors of AdoHcy hydrolase, periodate-oxidized adenosine (Adox) (Hoffman, 1979) and 3-deaza($\pm$)-aristeromycin (c^3Ari) (Montgomery et al., 1982), were even more effective than c^3Ado in increasing the relative macrophage content of AdoHcy. However, since neither Adox nor c^3Ari inhibited phagocytosis or altered macrophage morphology or microfilaments, c^3Ado is presumed to be producing these effects on macrophages by a mechanism independent of AdoHcy levels. Moreover, since Adox prevented the metabolism of c^3Ado to c^3AdoHcy in macrophages but did not alter these different cellular effects of c^3Ado, the latter do not appear to depend upon the cellular buildup of c^3AdoHcy.

In spite of the dramatic changes in both morphology and microfilament patterns caused by c^3Ado and cytochalasin B in adherent macrophages, neither of these two drugs affected the PGE_1-stimulated cAMP accumulation of these cells (data not shown). These results confirm that macrophages (Grunspan-Swirsky & Pick, 1978), unlike lymphocytes (Insel & Koachman, 1982), do not exhibit a cytochalasin B enhancement in their response to stimulators of adenylate cyclase.

Current efforts are being directed towards an elucidation of the molecular mechanism by which c^3Ado causes disorganization of macrophage microfilaments. We have investigated the possibility that this might be an indirect effect of c^3Ado, due to a drug-induced alteration of intracellular Ca^{2+} levels. However, measurement of cell associated Quin-2 fluorescence has shown that 20 μM c^3Ado did not change the concentration of cytoplasmic free Ca^{2+} in these macrophages (139 $\pm$ 35 nM in control cells versus 144 $\pm$ 39 nM in c^3Ado-treated cells). Under these same experimental conditions, 50 nM ionomycin caused a 4.2-fold increase in the concentration of macrophage free Ca^{2+}.

Metabolism of c^3Ado to 5'-Nucleotides

The recent acquisition of [^{3}H]c^3Ado has allowed us to reinvestigate, with greater sensitivity than previously available (Zimmerman et al., 1978, 1979), the possible metabolism of c^3Ado to 5'-nucleotides in leukocytes. Acid-

soluble extracts of mouse cytolytic lymphocytes were
prepared and analyzed by anion-exchange HPLC after the
cells had been incubated for 60 min with 10-40 μM [^{3}H]-
c^{3}Ado. The column effluent was monitored both for UV
absorbance (254 and 280 nm) and for radioactivity. Clear
evidence for the cellular formation of [^{3}H]3-deazaadenosine
5'-triphosphate (c^{3}ATP) and [^{3}H]3-deazaadenosine 5'-di-
phosphate (c^{3}ADP) was obtained. The putative [^{3}H]c^{3}ATP was
eluted from the HPLC column at the same retention time as
UTP and was shifted to the retention time of the putative
[^{3}H]c^{3}ADP after treatment of a portion of the cell extract
with yeast hexokinase plus glucose. The amount of cellular
[^{3}H]c^{3}ATP formed increased with increasing concentrations
of [^{3}H]c^{3}Ado added to the medium. Lymphocytes incubated
for 60 min with 40 μM [^{3}H]c^{3}Ado contained 10 pmol of [^{3}H]-
c^{3}ATP/10^6 cells as compared with their ATP content of
560 pmol/10^6 cells. This relatively small cellular accumulation of c^{3}ATP, together with the co-elution of c^{3}ATP and
UTP, precluded detection of c^{3}ATP present in cell extracts
in previous studies utilizing non-radiolabeled c^{3}Ado
(Zimmerman et al., 1978, 1979). Somewhat surprisingly,
0.1 μM 5-iodotubercidin, a potent inhibitor of adenosine
kinase (Wotring & Townsend, 1979), reduced this cellular
formation of [^{3}H]c^{3}ATP by only 20-30%. However, this
result is consistent with the extremely poor substrate
efficiency of c^{3}Ado found with adenosine kinase purified
from rabbit liver (Miller et al., 1979). Further work is
necessary to identify the enzyme chiefly responsible for
the cellular phosphorylation of c^{3}Ado. In addition, since
microfilaments normally utilize ATP, it will be of interest
to determine whether this metabolically formed c^{3}ATP is
contributing to the disorganization of cellular microfilaments caused by c^{3}Ado.

ACKNOWLEDGEMENTS

    The excellent technical assistance of Mrs. Marvin S.
Winston and Robert L. Veasey is gratefully acknowledged.
We express our appreciation to Dr. Stephen P. Watson for
his guidance in the Quin-2 experiments and to Dr. Thomas A.
Krenitsky for his enthusiastic support of this work.

REFERENCES

Bader, J. P., Brown, N. R., Chiang, P. K. and
    Cantoni, G.L. (1978) Virology 89, 494-505.

Chiang, P. K., Richards, H. H. and Cantoni, G. L. (1977)
    Mol. Pharmacol. 13, 939-947.
Chiang, P. K. (1985) Methods in Pharmacol. 6, 127-145.
Faulstich, H., Trischmann, H. and Mayer, D. (1983) Exp.
    Cell Res. 144, 73-82.
Garcia-Castro, I., Mato, J. M., Vasanthakumar, G.,
    Wiesmann, W. P., Schiffmann, E. and Chiang, P. K.
    (1983) J. Biol. Chem. 258, 4345-4349.
Grunspan-Swirsky, A. and Pick, E. (1978) Immunopharmacol.
    1, 71-82.
Hoffman, J. L. (1979) in Transmethylation (Usdin, E.,
    Borchardt, R. T. and Creveling, C. R., Eds.)
    pp. 181-186, Elsevier/North-Holland, New York.
Ikehara, M. and Fukui, T. (1974) Biochim. Biophys. Acta
    338, 512-519.
Insel, P. A. and Koachman, A. M. (1982) J. Biol. Chem.
    257, 9717-9723.
Kitano, S., Mizuno, Y., Ueyama, M., Tori, K., Kamisaku, M.
    and Ajisaka, K. (1975) Biochem. Biophys. Res. Commun.
    64, 996-1002.
Leonard, E. J., Skeel, A., Chiang, P. K. and Cantoni, G. L.
    (1978) Biochem. Biophys. Res. Commun. 84, 102-109.
May, J. A., Jr. and Townsend, L. B. (1975) J. Chem. Soc.
    Perkin Trans. I, 125-129.
Miller, R. L., Adamczyk, D. L., Miller, W. H.,
    Koszalka, G. W., Rideout, J. L., Beacham, L. M., III,
    Chao, E. Y., Haggerty, J. J., Krenitsky, T. A. and
    Elion, G. B. (1979) J. Biol. Chem. 254, 2346-2352.
Montgomery, J. A., Clayton, S. J., Thomas, H. J.,
    Shannon, W. M., Arnett, G., Bodner, A. J., Kion, I.-K.,
    Cantoni, G. L. and Chiang, P. K. (1982) J. Med. Chem.
    25, 626-629.
Rousseau, R. J., Townsend, L. B. and Robins, R. K. (1966)
    Biochemistry 5, 756-760.
Stopford, C. R., Wolberg, G., Prus, K. L.,
    Reynolds-Vaughn, R. and Zimmerman, T. P. (1985) Proc.
    Natl. Acad. Sci. U.S.A. 82, 4060-4064.
Tsien, R. Y., Pozzan, T. and Rink, T. J. (1982) J. Cell
    Biol. 94, 325-334.
Ueland, P. M. (1982) Pharmacol. Rev. 34. 223-253.
Wessells, N. K., Spooner, B. S., Ash, J. F., Bradley,
    M. O., Luduena, M. A., Taylor, E. L., Wrenn, J. T.
    and Yamada, K. M. (1971) Science 171, 135-143.
Wolberg, G., Hiemstra, K., Burge, J. J. and Singler, R. C.
    (1973) J. Immunol. 111, 1435-1443.

Wolberg, G., Stopford, C. R. and Zimmerman T. P. (1984)
    Proc. Natl. Acad. Sci. U.S.A. 81, 3496-3500.
Wotring, L. L. and Townsend, L. B. (1979) Cancer Res. 39,
    3018-3023.
Zimmerman, T. P., Rideout, J. L., Wolberg, G.,
    Duncan, G. S. and Elion, G. B. (1976) J. Biol. Chem.
    251, 6757-6766.
Zimmerman, T. P., Wolberg, G. and Duncan, G. S. (1978)
    Proc. Natl. Acad. Sci. U.S.A. 75, 6220-6224.
Zimmerman, T. P., Wolberg, G., Stopford, C. R. and
    Duncan, G. S. (1979) in Transmethylation (Usdin, E.,
    Borchardt, R. T. and Creveling, C. R., Eds.)
    pp. 187-196, Elsevier/North-Holland, New York.
Zimmerman, T. P., Schmitges, C. J., Wolberg, G.,
    Deeprose, R. D., Duncan, G. S., Cuatrecasas, P. and
    Elion, G. B. (1980) Proc. Natl. Acad. Sci. U.S.A. 77,
    5639-5643.
Zimmerman, T. P., Iannone, M. and Wolberg, G. (1984) J.
    Biol. Chem. 259, 1122-1126.

MECHANISM-BASED INHIBITORS OF ALKYLTRANSFERASES

James K. Coward
Department of Chemistry
Rensselaer Polytechnic Institute
Troy, NY 12180-3590, U.S.A.

MECHANISTIC STUDIES

Alkyltransferases catalyze the reaction of various cellular nucleophiles with an electrophilic carbon adjacent to electron-deficient trivalent sulfur. In the case of methyltransferases, nucleophilic attack is at the methyl group of S-adenosylmethionine (AdoMet), whereas with the aminopropyltransferases, attack is at the less reactive aminopropyl methylene group of S-adenosyl(3-methylthio)-propylamine (decarboxylated AdoMet, dcAdoMet). Although nucleophilic attack at sp^3 carbon is one of the most extensively studied reactions in organic chemistry, much less is known about the corresponding biochemical reactions catalyzed by the alkyltransferases. Our own mechanistic studies have focused on three areas of investigation: catalysis of non-enzymatic model reactions, kinetics of enzyme-catalyzed reactions, and stereochemistry of enzyme-catalyzed reactions. Since this research is the basis for our inhibitor design and synthesis work, it will be reveiwed briefly here.

The methyltransferase which we have studied most extensively is catechol O-methyltransferase (COMT, E.C.2.1.1.6). This is a small (27K) enzyme, important is the inactivation of catecholamine neurotransmitters and hormones, both in the CNS and periphery (Guldberg & Marsden, 1975). Our steady-state kinetics studies using epinephrine as the catechol substrate indicated that the reaction proceeds by a random sequential kinetic mechanism

427

with strong product inhibition by S-adenosylhomocysteine
(AdoHcy) (Coward et al., 1973) Similar studies using 3,4-
dihydroxybenzoic acid as the catechol substrate suggested
that the reaction proceeds by a non-sequential or "ping-
pong" kinetic mechanism (Borchardt, 1973). This mechanistic
uncertainty was resolved in favor of the sequential,
single-displacement mechanism by using chiral methyl (Floss
& Tsai, 1979) AdoMet and both catechol substrates mentioned above (Woodard et al., 1980). Recent kinetics
studies of the COMT reaction using dopamine as the catechol
substrate have suggested that the sequential binding of
substrates and release of products is ordered (Rivett &
Roth, 1982). The methylation of a catechol requires loss of
a proton during the reaction. We have studied the intramolecular alkylation of a 2-substituted cyclopentanol
(Knipe & Coward, 1979) and an o-substituted phenol (Knipe
et al., 1982), and have observed general base catalysis in
these non-enzymatic model reactions, thus suggesting a
catalytic role for general bases in the COMT active site.

Similar investigations have been carried out with
putrescine aminopropyltransferase (PAPT, E.C.2.5.1.16),
also known as spermidine synthase. Studies with partially
purified PAPT from rat prostate revealed severe substrate
inhibition at high (>40 µM) concentrations of dcAdoMet
(Coward et al., 1977). Product inhibition by 5'-deoxy-5'-
methylthioadenosine (MTA) was not observed in this early
work because of the presence of MTA phosphorylase activity
in the crude enzyme preparation. Subsequent work with
purified PAPT, free of MTA phosphorylase and spermidine
aminopropyltransferase (SAPT, E.C.2.5.1) activities,
demonstrated strong product inhibition by MTA (Hibasami et
al., 1980). A more complete kinetics investigation of the
reaction catalyzed by E. coli. PAPT has been reported
(Zappia et al., 1980) and kinetic evidence for a double-
displacement mechanism was presented. However, product
inhibition studies with MTA were not included in this work
because of the presence of MTA nucleosidase activity in the
partially purified E. coli. enzyme preparation. More recent
studies with purified PAPT from bovine brain have concluded
that the reaction proceeds via a single-displacement
mechanism (Raina et al., 1984). Stereochemical studies
should resolve these mechanistic uncertainties, as in the
case of the COMT reaction discussed above. One such study
employed methionine, chiral at the appropriate methylene
group, as a precursor in a biosynthetic labeling experiment

using intact bacteria (E. coli.) followed by isolation of
spermidine, the product of of interest (Golding &
Nassereddin, 1982). The authors in this work concluded
that the PAPT reaction proceeded via a single-displacement
mechanism, based on ¹H-nmr data. We have chosen to
approach the stereochemical study in a cell-free system
using PAPT, isolated from E. coli., and synthetic
dcAdoMet, chiral at the methylene carbon of interest. The
chiral substrates (R- and S-CHD) were synthesized (Orr et
al., 1984) from R- and S-CHD γ-aminobutyrate (Pontoni et
al., 1983). Preliminary results indicate that the reaction
catalyzed by E. coli. PAPT proceeds via a double-displacement mechanism (G. R. Orr, D. W. Kullberg, and J. K.
Coward, unpublished results). If these results are
confirmed in further experiments, it would be the first
stereochemical demonstration of a double-displacement
reaction mechanism involving an alkyl-transferase.
Similar studies must be undertaken with eukaryotic PAPT
and SAPT, as this result has considerable significance in
the design of new drugs to affect polyamine biosynthesis
(vide infra). As with the methylation of catechols, the
aminopropylation of an amine requires the loss of a proton
during the reaction. We have recently studied the intramolecular alkylation of 2-substituted cyclopentylamines
(R. J. Miller, A. Kuliopulos, and J. K. Coward, unpublished results) and have shown that general base catalysis
also may be operative in these model reactions, provided
that a late transition state (poor leaving group) leads to
the development of considerable positive charge and an
increased transition state acidity of the nucleophilic
amine.

INHIBITOR STUDIES

As mentioned above, methyltransferases and aminopropyltransferases are strongly inhibited by the nucleoside
product of each reaction, AdoHcy and MTA, respectively.
Initially, we focused our synthetic, biochemical, and biological investigations on metabolically stable analogs of
AdoHcy and MTA. These efforts have been reviewed (Coward,
1980; Coward, 1982), and may be summarized as follows.
Tubercidin (7-deaza-adenosine) analogs of AdoHcy (S-tubercidinylhomocysteine, STH) and MTA (methylthiotubercidin,
MTT) are very effective inhibitors of methyltransferases
and aminopropyltransferases, respectively, with Ki values

nearly identical to the natural product inhibitors.   They
are metabolically stable and therefore, any cellular
effects observed are not due to a metabolite of the drug.
As such, these analogs have been useful tools for biochemical and pharmacological research.   Unfortunately,
these analogs are not readily transported in at least one
mammalian cell system, the Novikoff hepatoma (Coward et
al., 1983b), and they are not specific inhibitors of a
particular alkyltransferase of interest but of two entire
groups of enzymes: methyltransferases (STH) and aminopropyltransferases (MTT).

We have approached the latter problem of specificity
by designing and synthesizing a series of potential multi-
substrate adduct inhibitors (Heller et al., 1975) of COMT,
PAPT, and SAPT.   Based on the mechanistic work described
above, we designed 1 as a specific inhibitor of COMT.   The
synthesis of compounds related to 1, e. g., 2 and 3, has

been described (Anderson et al., 1981). As expected,
neither 2, 3, nor the corresponding thioethers were
potent inhibitors of COMT.   This is in contrast to recent
reports using similar methyl sulfonium salts designed to
inhibit indoleamine N-methyltransferase (Benghiat &
Crooks, 1983). The synthesis of molecules such as 1 containing three large sulfur ligands was not accomplished in
our initial studies (Anderson et al., 1981). However,
biochemical data obtained with molecules designed to
inhibit PAPT (vide infra) suggested that 1 is a less

viable synthetic target, and our recent efforts have been
focused on the synthesis of 4. We have utilized the
lactones, α-methylbutyrolactone in the 'a' series and the
the corresponding adenosyl lactone (Lyga & Secrist, 1983)
in the 'b' series, as our entry into this type of molecule.
We have succeeded in synthesizing acetylenic precursors of
4a (X=Y=H) by two independent routes. In addition, several
key intermediates in the 'b' series recently have been
synthesized by an extension of this approach (E. K. Yau and
J. K. Coward, unpublished results).

$$a, \ R = CH_3$$

$$b, \ R =$$

The design of aminopropyltransferase inhibitors has
followed a similar approach as that described above for the
methyltransferase, COMT. As noted above, our recent preliminary stereochemical results indicating that E. coli.
PAPT catalyzes aminopropyl transfer via a double displacement mechanism, will require the assessment of eukaryotic
aminopropyltransferases in order to establish the general-
ity of this mechanism. Nonetheless, our initial synthetic
target as a specific inhibitor of PAPT was 5 and its methyl
sulfonium derivative. The synthesis of these molecules has
been described (Tang et al., 1981). The thioether 5, S-
adenosyl-1,8-diamino-3-thiooctane (AdoDATO), proved to be a
potent and specific inhibitor of rat prostate PAPT, whereas
the methyl sulfonium derivative was much less potent and
specific than 5 (Tang et al., 1980). SAPT, also known as
spermine synthase, was inhibited by several adenosyl methyl
sulfonium compounds, including the simplest $AdoS^+(CH_3)_2$
(Tang et al., 1980; vide infra). AdoDATO has been used to
study the inhibition of spermidine biosynthesis in mammal-

$$\underline{5}$$

ian (Pegg et al., 1982) and bacterial (Pegg et al., 1983)
cells. This new drug is a potent and specific inhibitor
of spermidine biosynthesis in vitro, and should prove to
be useful in future studies on the role of polyamines in
cell growth and differentiation.

The successful synthesis of AdoDATO and its excellent
inhibitory properties, prompted us to undertake the
synthesis of $\underline{6}$ and its methylsulfonium derivatives as

$$\underline{6}$$

potential specific inhibitors of SAPT. Our synthetic
approach has involved the elaboration of ε-substituted
caprolactones to 1,3,12-trisubstituted-9-azadodecanes
(J. K. Coward, A. Y. Black, and K. J. Duff, unpublished
results). These are then coupled to adenosine either via
alkylation with 5'-deoxy-5'-chloroadenosine (Coward et
al., 1983a), or by alkylation of 5'-deoxy-5'-thioadeno-
sine (Anderson et al. (1981). Using these methods, we have
completed the synthesis of a 1,12-desamino derivative of
$\underline{6}$, to be used as a negative control in the enzyme work
with SAPT, similar to the use of the 1,8-desamino derivative of AdoDATO ($\underline{5}$) in previous work with PAPT (Tang
et al., 1980; Tang et al., 1981). Several key intermediates

in the synthesis of $\underline{6}$ have been synthesized by an extension of this approach (J. K. Coward & A. Y. Black, unpublished results).

As noted above, the S-methyl derivative of MTA, $AdoS^+(CH_3)_2$, is a better inhibitor of SAPT than of PAPT (Tang et al., 1980). These data suggested the use of $AdoS^+(CH_3)_2$ as a selective inhibitor of spermine bio-synthesis in mammalian cells if it were transported across the cell membrane. Recent studies in collaboration with Professor A. E. Pegg have shown that this charged sulfonium salt does inhibit spermine biosynthesis in SV40-transformed 3T3 cells (A. E. Pegg & J. K. Coward, unpublished results). Thus, we now have available drugs which will selectively inhibit each step of the polyamine biosynthetic pathway (eq. 1). These may be used in combination for studies on the regulation of this pathway,

$$\text{Ornithine} \longrightarrow \text{Putrescine} \longrightarrow \text{Spermidine} \longrightarrow \text{Spermine} \qquad (1)$$
$$\underset{\text{DFMO}}{\uparrow} \qquad\qquad \underset{\text{AdoDATO}}{\uparrow} \qquad\qquad \underset{AdoS^+(Ch_3)_2}{\uparrow}$$

and the effects of depleting a selected polyamine on cell growth and/or differentiation.

ACKNOWLEDGEMENT

Research in the author's laboratory is supported by the grants from the USPHS, GM30286, CA28097, and CA37606. It is a pleasure to acknowledge the essential contribu-tions of the many students and collaborators whose names are given in the references cited.

REFERENCES

Anderson, G. L., Bussolotti, D. L., and Coward, J. K. (1981) J. Med. Chem. 24, 1271-1277.
Benghiat, E. amd Crooks, P. A. (1983) J. Med. Chem. 26, 1470-1477.
Borchardt, R. T. (1973) J. Med. Chem. 16, 377-382.
Coward, J. K. (1980) in Molecular Action and Targets for Cancer Chemotherapeutic Agents (Sartorelli, A. C., Lazo, J., and Bertino, J. R., Eds.) p. 253-263, Academic Press, New York.

Coward, J. K. (1982) Ann. Rept. Med. Chem. 17, 253-259.

Coward, J. K., Anderson, G. L., and Tang, K.-C. (1983a) Methods Enzymol 94, 286-294.

Coward, J. K., Chaudhari, P. R., Kwiat, M. A. and Hluboky, M. (1983b) Fed. Proc. 42, 1892 (Abstract).

Coward, J. K., Motola, N. C., and Moyer, J. D. (1977) J. Med. Chem. 20, 500-505.

Coward, J. K., Slisz, E. P., and Wu, F. Y H. (1973) Biochemistry 12, 2291-2297.

Floss, H. G. and Tsai, M.-D. (1979) Adv. Enzymol. 50, 243-302.

Golding, B. T. and Nassereddin, I. K. (1982) J. Amer. Chem. Soc. 104, 5815-5817.

Guldberg, H. C. and Marsden, C. A. (1975) Pharmacol. Rev. 27, 135-206.

Heller, J. S., Canellakis, E. S., Bussolotti, D. L., and Coward, J. K. (1975) Biochim. Biophys. Acta 403, 197-207.

Hibasami, H., Borchardt, R. T., Chen, S. Y., Coward, J. K., and Pegg, A. E. (1980) Biochem. J. 187, 419-428.

Knipe, J. O. and Coward, J. K. (1979) J. Amer. Chem. Soc. 101, 4339-4348.

Knipe, J. O., Vasquez, P. J., and Coward, J. K. (1982) J. Amer. Chem. Soc. 104, 3202-3209.

Lyga, J. W. and Secrist, J. A. (1983) J. Org. Chem. 48, 1982-1988.

Orr, G. R., Kullberg, D., and Coward, J. K. (1984) Biochemistry 23, 3350-3351 (Abstract).

Pegg, A. E., Bitonti, A. J., McCann, P. P., and Coward, J. K. (1983) FEBS Lett. 155, 192-196.

Pegg, A. E., Tang, K.-C., and Coward, J. K. (1982) Biochemistry 21, 5082-5089.

Pontoni, G., Coward, J. K., Orr, G., and Gould, S. J. (1983) Tetrahedron Lett. 24, 151-154.

Raina, A., Hyvonen, T., Eloranta, T., Vortilainen, M., Samejima, K., and Yamanoha, B. (1984) Biochem. J. 219, 991-1000.

Rivett, A. J. and Roth, J. A. (1982) Biochemistry 21, 1740-1742.

Tang, K.-C., Mariuzza, R., and Coward, J. K. (1981) J. Med. Chem. 24, 1277-1284.

Tang, K.-C., Pegg, A. E., and Coward, J. K. (1980) Biochem. Biophys. Res. Commun. 96, 1371-1377.

Woodard, R. W., Tsai, M.-D., Floss, H. G., Crooks, P. A., and Coward, J. K. (1980) J. Biol. Chem. 255, 9124-9127.

Zappia, V., Cacciapuoti, G., Pontoni, G., and Oliva, A. (1980) J. Biol. Chem. 255, 7276-7280.

SINEFUNGIN AND DERIVATIVES : SYNTHESIS, BIOSYNTHESIS AND MOLECULAR TARGET STUDIES IN LEISHMANIA

P. Blanchard, N. Dodic, J.L. Fourrey, M. Gèze, F. Lawrence, H. Malina, P. Paolantonacci, M. Vedel, C. Tempête, M. Robert-Géro, and E. Lederer

Institut de Chimie des Substances Naturelles, C.N.R.S., 91190 Gif-sur-Yvette, France

Sinefungin $\underline{1}$ is a natural nucleoside in which an ornithine residue is linked to the 5' end of adenosine by a carbon-carbon bond. Its structure is similar to that of $\underline{S}$-adenosyl-homocysteine (SAH) $\underline{2}$ and that of $\underline{S}$-adenosyl-methionine $\underline{3}$ (Scheme I). It was isolated from cultures of Streptomyces griseolus at Lilly Research Laboratories (Hamill & Hoehn, 1973) and from cultures of S.incarnatus at Rhône-Poulenc Industries in France (Patent 761114 : Rhône Poulenc Industries France, 15th April, 1976)

Sinefungin was shown to inhibit the development of various fungi (Gordee & Butler, 1973) and viruses (Pugh et al., 1978, Vedel et al., 1978, Pugh & Borchardt, 1982) but its major interest resides in its potent antiparasitic activity (Bachrach et al., 1980, Trager et al., 1980, Nadler et al., 1982, Dube et al., 1983, Ferrante et al., 1984,

435

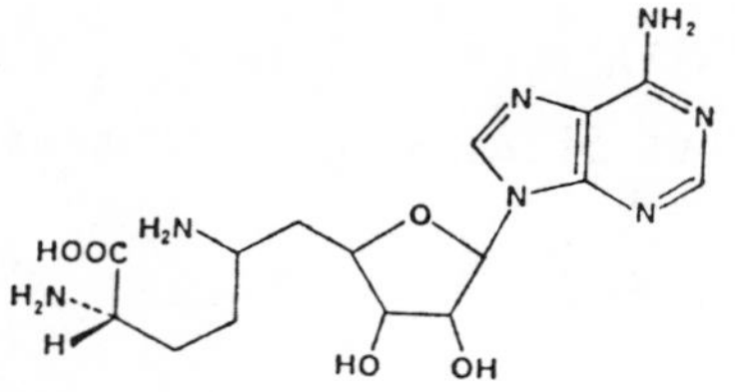

Scheme I

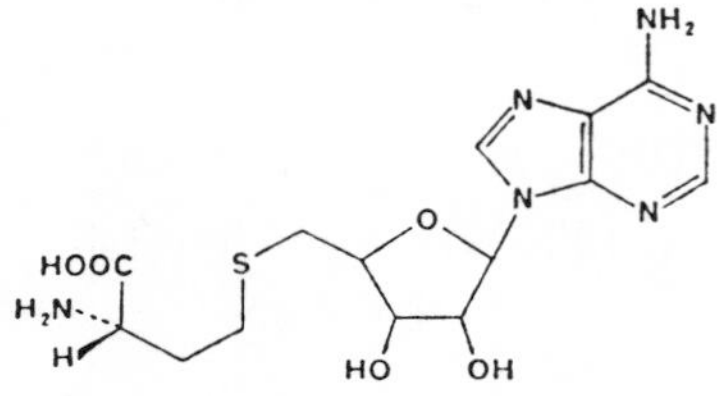

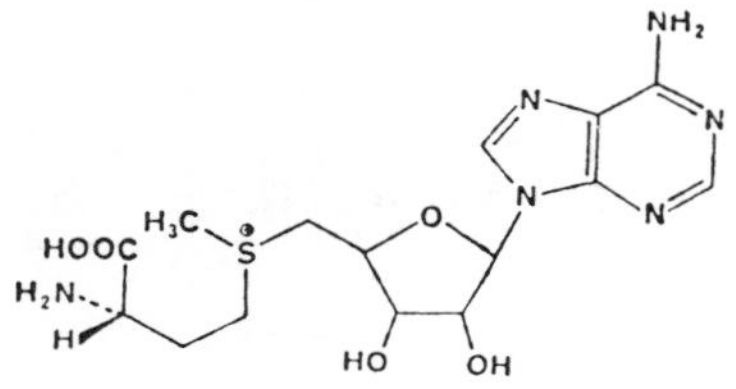

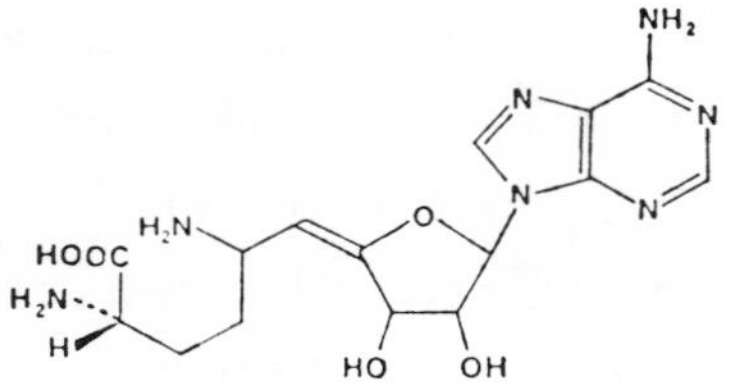

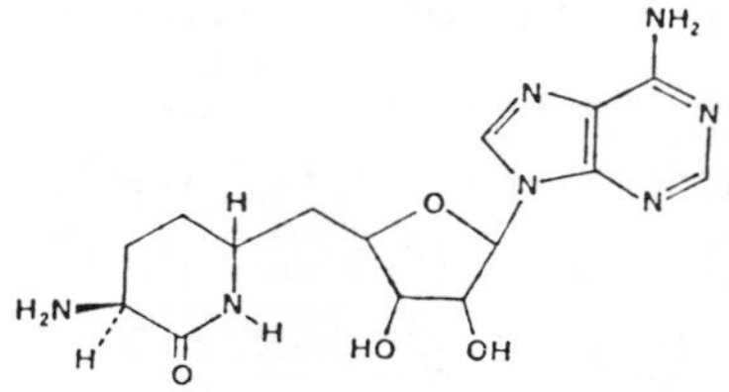

Neal & Croft, 1984, Neal et al., 1985, Paolantonacci et al. , 1985). As this antibiotic is nephrotoxic in vivo several laboratories undertook its chemical synthesis with the aim to prepare structurally related analogues (Mock & Moffatt, 1982, Lugga & Secrist, 1983, Gêze et al., 1983, Moorman, et al., 1983, Mizuno et al., 1984). The total synthesis however, needs many steps, and the overall yield is not satisfactory. Thus, in parallel with our work on chemical synthesis, we started to investigate the biosynthesis of sinefungin with the goal to prepare modified analogues by bioconversion. In this report we also describe our recent results on the inhibition of various Leishmania species by sinefungin and related compounds as well as on their mechanism of action at the molecular level.

Synthesis of Sinefungin and Analogues

Our approach is based on the Horner-Emmons condensation between the cyanomethylphosphonate derivative of adenosine 3 (Scheme II) and a properly chosen aldehyde, (R_2CHO) leading to the α,β unsaturated nitrile 4. Reduction of the latter, followed by partial hydrolysis afforded a mixture of two amides 6. Each amide after HPLC separation underwent a Hoffmann rearrangement in the presence of [bis(trifluoroacetoxy)iodo] benzene providing the expected amine isolated as the amorphous terbutyloxycarbonate 7. This strategy might provide not only the natural sinefungin but also structural analogues. When the aldehyde component was derived from L-allylglycine, the sequence of reaction mentioned above, led to a protected derivative of sinefungin 8. After removal of the protecting groups by treatment with base and acid, a molecule 1 identical in every respect with the naturally occuring sinefungin was obtained. It is impo tant that the two amides 6 could be readily separated by HPLC and that the Hoffmann rearrangement took place with complete retention of the configuration at C-6' providing the corresponding amine.

Using isobutyraldehyde, the same adenosine phosphonate

SCHEME II

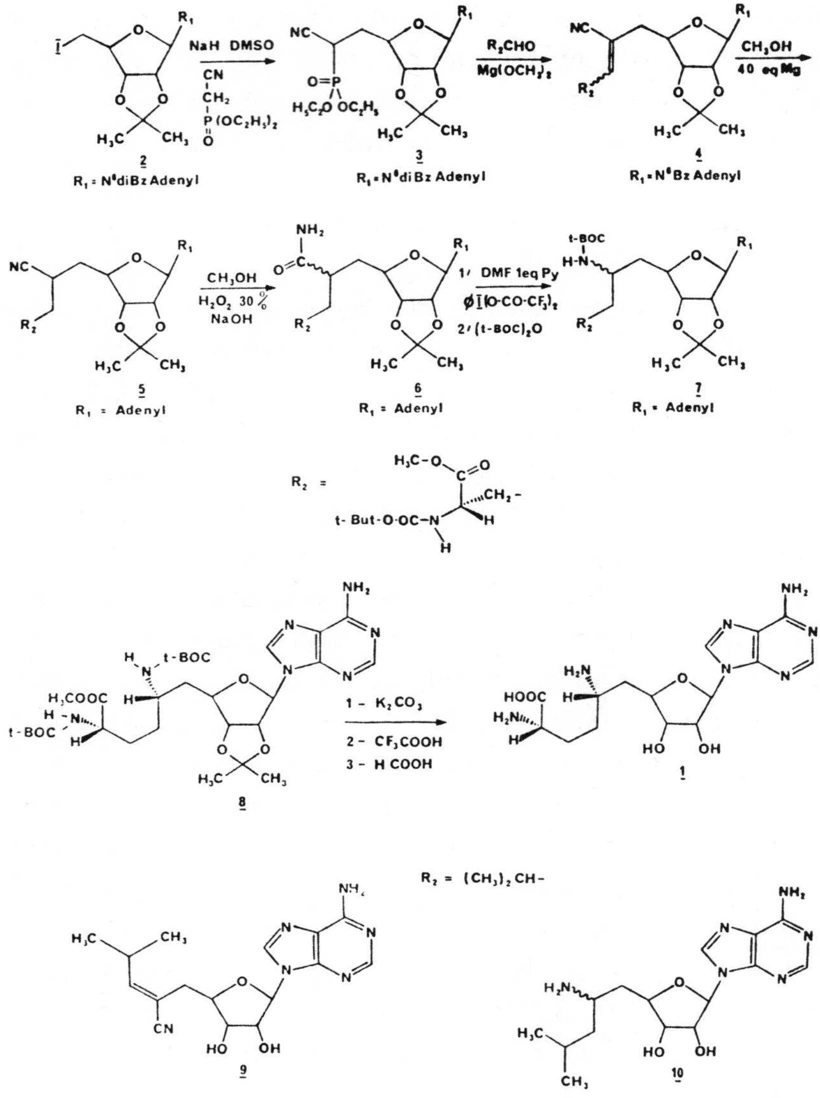
NaH DMSO
CN
CH2
P(OC2H5)2
O
2
R1 = N6diBz Adenyl
3
R1 = N6diBz Adenyl
R2CHO
Mg(OCH3)2
4
R1 = N6Bz Adenyl
CH3OH
40 eq Mg
5
R1 = Adenyl
CH3OH
H2O2 30 %
NaOH
6
R1 = Adenyl
1/ DMF 1eq Py
ØI(O-CO-CF3)2
2/ (t-BOC)2O
7
R1 = Adenyl
R2 =
t- But-O-OC-N
1 - K2CO3
2 - CF3COOH
3 - H COOH
8
1
R2 = (CH3)2CH-
9
10

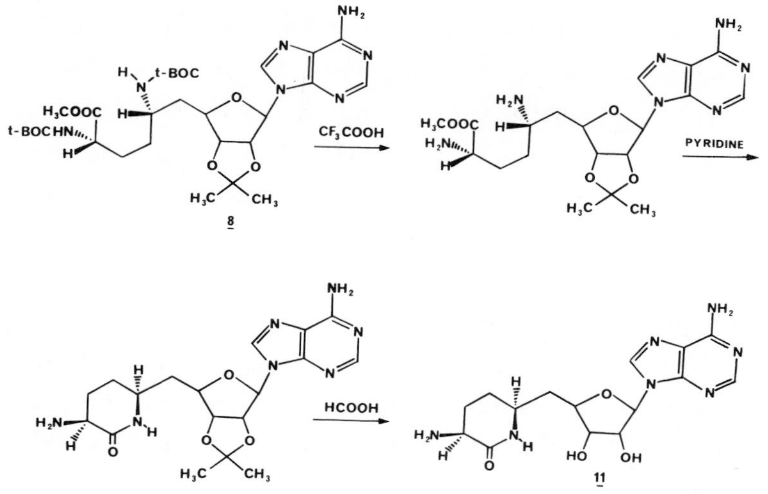

SCHEME III

<u>3</u> and applying the same sequence of reactions, the analogues <u>9</u> and <u>10</u> were obtained (Geze <u>et al</u>, 1983).

The cyclic lactame <u>11</u> was prepared from the fully protected sinefungin <u>8</u> by successive treatment with trifluoroacetic acid and pyridine, followed by the removal of the isopropylidene protecting group (Scheme III).

In order to improve the yield of the synthesis and to obtain a variety of analogues, we are now exploring an alternative approach ; namely the functionalisation of the methyl-2,3-<u>O</u>-isopropylidene-β-D-riboside at the 5' position, followed by acid hydrolysis and acetylation to give the corresponding 1,2,3 tri-<u>O</u>-acetate and finally adenylation.

Studies on Biosynthesis of Sinefungin

One of the strains producing sinefungin is <u>S.</u> <u>incarnatus</u> NRRL 8089, isolated by Rhône Poulenc Industries

in France. As far as we are aware the only work on
sinefungin biosynthesis was performed by Bery and Abott
(1978) with S.griseolus. According to their hypothesis,
based on the incorporation of ^{14}C-labelled compounds into
sinefungin, adenosine and ornithine are condensed by an
unknown mechanism in the terminal step of the biosynthesis.
As the direct condensation between adenosine and ornithine
is hardly conceivable, we decided to reinvestigate this
hypothesis. The understanding of the biosynthetic pathway
and particularly of the last steps, may allow the production
of modified antibiotics by incorporation of structural
analogues of the precursors.

At least three biosynthetic pathways may lead to
ornithine formation:1) hydrolysis of Nα-acetyl ornithine, 2)
transformation of arginine by elimination of the guanido
group, 3) from argininosuccinic acid and citrulline. Thus we
compared the kinetics of incorporation of ^{14}C-U-ornithine
and arginine into the antibiotic. After four hours of
culture 64 percent of the labelled arginine was incorporated
into sinefungin. Surprisingly, ornithine, the presumed
immediate biosynthetic precursor of sinefungin, was
incorporated at a very low extent, (7-8 percent).
Furthermore, most of the ornithine added, remained unchanged
in the culture supernatant. When ^{14}C-U-citrulline was added
to the culture, the incorporation was also very low
indicating that the pathway of sinefungin production does
not proceed via argininocuccinic acid. Incorporation of
uniformly labelled and guanido-group labelled arginine gave
radioactive and unlabelled sinefungin, respectively.
These results indicate that the ornithine moiety of
sinefungin originates from arginine after elimination of the

guanido group. Then we compared the kinetics of ^{14}C-U- ATP and ^{14}C-U-adenosine incorporation into sinefungin. The radioactivity of ATP was incorporated with a high yield : 58 percent after 4 hours of culture. Adenosine incorporation decreased with time, 40 percent after four hours and 28 to 20 percent later during the fermentation process. Free adenosine could be detected all the time the culture lasted.

These results, namely that arginine is incorporated preferentially into sinefungin, suggest that the nitrogen atom of the guanido group may be activated by an enzyme having pyridoxal phosphate as coenzyme. This activation may then produce a very reactive enamine. The latter can then react at the 5' end of adenosine by forming the C-C bond. The elimination of the guanido group would occur at the final step of the biosynthesis. The validity of this hypothesis is now under investigation in our laboratory. Along this line, assays of incorporation of arginine analogues to give sinefungin derivatives have been undertaken (Malina et al., unpublished results).

Antiparasitic Effect of Sinefungin

As shown in Table I sinefungin is very effective against a variety of parasites in vitro.

Among the analogues, A9145C (Scheme I 4) has little effect on Leishmania donovani in comparison to sinefungin, as the minimal leishmanicidal concentrention is > 2.6 µM. The cyclic derivative (Scheme I 5) kills L.donovani promastigotes at 0.26µM and L.tropica promasti gotes at 2.6 µM. The other synthetic analogues (Scheme II 9 and 10) and SAM or SAH were inactive at 10-100 µM.

Table I
Antiparasitic Effect of Sinefungin in vitro

Parasite	Dose [μM]	% inhibition	References
Plasmodium falciparum	0.3-1	78-95	Trager et al (1980)
Trypanosoma cruzi	200-500	62-100	Nadler et al (1982)
Entamoeba histolytica	20-40	100	Ferrante et al (1984)
Leishmania donovani	0.13	100	Paolantonacci et al (1985)
Leishmania tropica	0.26	100	Paolantonacci et al (1985)

In vivo, sinefungin was shown to cure mice, infected with Trypanosoma brucei brucei, T.congolense or T.vivax with a more pronounced effect towards T.congolense. The drug was administered intraperitoneally for a period of 1-3 days. No toxic side effects due to sinefungin treatment were observed in these cases (Dube et al., 1983). The activity of sinefungin was also tested in vivo against Leishmania donovani and L.tropica in mice. In the first case the ED50 value was 320 μg/kg x 5 days. The potency of sinefungin relative to sodium stibogluconate, a known antileishmanial drug, was 73 times superior. No toxicity was observed with the dose schedules used. Sinefungin was also active in vivo against L.major lesions in BALB/C mice. All these experiments are highly promising and designate sinefungin as a potential antiparasitic drug.

Mechanism of Action of Sinefungin in <u>Leishmania</u>

Sinefungin and A9145C (scheme I <u>1</u>, <u>4</u>) are known transmethylase inhibitors in various mammalian and avian cells (Fuller & Nagarajan, 1978, Pugh <u>et al</u>., 1978, Vedel <u>et al</u>., 1978). In an attempt to explain the mechanism of action of the antibiotic, we studied two protein methylases, PMI and PMIII of these parasites. As shown in Table II both activities are present in the two species. SAH and sinefungin are competitive inhibitors of PMI and PMIII with respect to SAM. Sinefungin is a poor inhibitor of PMI compared to SAH but it inhibits very efficiently the PMIII of L.donovani, the ratio Km SAM/Ki sinefungin being 66. Thus, in the case of this parasite, PMIII may be one of the molecular targets of sinefungin (Paolantonacci <u>et al</u>., 1985).

Table II

Apparent kinetic constants[a] of protein methylase I and III
(PMI, PMIII) in <u>L.donovani</u> and <u>L.tropica</u>

		Vm[b]	Km SAM	Ki SAH	Ki sinefungin
PM I[c]	L.donovani	1120	24	3	145
	L.tropica	310	14	19	57
PM III[d]	L.donovani	1560	120	4.8	1.8
	L.tropica	350	37	3	47

a - all kinetic constants are in μM
b - pmole CH_3/mg/h of protein at 27°C
c - PMI = S-adenosylmethionine : protein-arginine
   methyltransferase (EC 2.1.1.23)
d - PMIII = S-adenosylmethionine : protein-lysine
   methyltransferase (EC 2.1.1.25)

As the leishmanistatic effect of sinefungin could not be reversed by addition of high concentrations of methionine in the medium, we studied the effect of this nucleoside on macromolecular biosynthesis. Unexpectedly, sinefungin inhibited very strongly thymidine incorporation into L.donovani and L.tropica promastigotes. The inhibition was concentration dependent, as after 6 hours of contact with 0.026 or 0.26 μM sinefungin, thymidine incorporation into DNA was inhibited by 70 and 91 percent respectively. Thymidine uptake into the cells was not affected. Uridine incorporation was inhibited to a much lesser extent (35 and 61 percent inhibition with respectively 0.026 and 0.26 μM sinefungin) while leucine incorporation was unaffected. In promastigotes of both species there was no inhibition of nucleoside phosphorylation and accumulation of nucleoside triphosphate was observed in treated cells. The DNA, synthesized in the presence and the absence of 0.26 μM sinefungin, was analysed on CsCl gradient. After 6 hours treatment, the synthesys of nuclear DNA and KDNA of L.donovani was 80 and 50 percent inhibited, respectivaly. The DNA polymerase of these promastigotes is not inhibited by sinefungin in vitro. Furthermore sinefungin does not inhibit thymidine incorporation into the host macrophages (Paolantonacci et al., unpublished results).

CONCLUSION

Sinefungin 1, a natural nucleoside, structurally related to S-adenosyl methionine 2 and to S-adenosyl homocysteine 3 inhibits in vitro at submicromolar concentration the development of various parasites.

Its efficiency in vivo against different African Trypanosoma and old world Leishmania has also been demonstrated, and any toxic effect on treated mice could not be observed.

The preparation of sinefungin analogues by chemical synthesis and by biosynthesis with the producer strain Streptomyces incarnatus is now under way.

A clear relationship between the antileishmanial effect of sinefungin and the inhibition of a transmethylase in these parasites could not be established. Sinefungin affects severely by a yet unknown mechanism the DNA synthesis of Leishmania. Host cell (macrophage) DNA synthesis is not inhibited. These results suggest, that sinefungin may be considered as a selective antiparasitic agent of choice.

Acknowledgements : We are grateful to Dr. R.S. Gordee and to Dr. R. Nagarajan (Lilly Research Laboratories Indianapolis, USA) for samples of sinefungin and A9145C. The strain S.incarnatus was provided by Rhône Poulenc Industries France.

This work was supported by the World Health Organisation UNDP/World Bank/WHO Special Programme for Research and Training in Tropical Diseases and from the Fondation de la Recherche Medicale Française.

REFERENCES

- Bachrach, U., Schnur, L.F., El-On, J., Greenblatt, C.L., Pearlman, E., Robert-Géro, M., and Lederer, E., (1980), FEBS Letters, 121, 287-291
- Berry, D.L. and Abbott, B.J., (1978), J. Antibiotics, 31, 185-191
- Dube, D.K., Mpimbaza, G., Allison, A.C., Lederer, E., and Rovis, L., (1983), J. Trop. Med. Hyg., 32, 31-33.

- Ferrante, A., Ljungström, I, Huldt, G., and Lederer, E.,
  (1984), Trans. Ray. Soc. Trop. Med. Hyg., 78, 837-838.
- Fuller, R.W., and Nagarajan, R., (1978), Biochem.
  Pharmacol., 27, 1981-1983
- Gèze, M., Blanchard, P., Fourrey, J.L., and Robert-
  Géro, M., (1983), J. Am. Chem. Soc., 105, 7638-7640.
- Gordee, R.S. and Butler, T.F., (1973), J. Antibiotics, 26
  466-467
- Hamill, R.L., and Hoehn, M.M. (1973), J. Antibiotics, 26,
  463-465
- Lyga, J.W. and Secrist, J.A. III (1983), J. Org. Chem.,
  48, 1982-1983
- Mizuno, Y. Tsuchida, K., and Tampo, H., (1984), Chem.
  Pharm. Bull., 32, 2915-2924
- Mock, G.A., and Moffatt, J.G. (1982), Nucleic Ac. Res.,
  10, 6223-6240
- Moorman, A.R., Martin, T., and Borchardt, R.T., (1983)
  Carbohydr. Res., 113, 233-239
- Nadler, J.P., Lederer, E., Wittner, M., Baum, S.G., and
  Tanowitz, M.B., (1982), Trans. Roy. Soc. Trop. Med.Hyg.,
  76, 285-287
- Neal, R.A., and Croft, S.L., (1984), J. of Antimicrobial
  Chemother., 14, 463-477
- Neal, R.A., Croft, S.L. and Nelson, D.J. (1985), Trans.
  Roy. Soc. Trop. Med. Hyg., 79, 85-122
- Paolantonacci, P., Lawrence, F., and Robert-Géro, M.,
  (1985), Antimicrobial Agents and Chemother., in press.
- Pugh, C.S.G., Borchardt, R.T. and Stone, H.O. (1978), J.
  Biol. Chem., 253, 4075-4077
- Pugh, C.S.G., and Borchardt, R.T., (1982), Biochemistry,
  21, 1535-1541
- Trager, W., Tershakovec, M., Chiang, P.K., and Cantoni,
  G.L., (1980), Exp. Parasitol., 50, 83-89
- Vedel, M., Lawrence, F., Robert-Géro, M., and Lederer, E.,
  (1978), Biochem. Biophys. Res. Comm., 85, 371-376

Subject Index

A

Acetylcholine synthesis in brain,
102
Adenine, 242
formation by adenine phospho-
ribosyltransferase-
deficient cells, 278
formation by methylthio-
adenosine, 276, 278, 289
Adenine analog binding protein,
253
Adenine arabinoside, 265, 267
Adenine
phosphoribosyltransferase-
deficient cells, 278
3-(Adenin-9-yl)-2-hydroxy-
propanoic acids, 402
Adenosine deaminase deficiency,
206
metabolism of neplanocin A,
388
Adenosine-*N*1-oxide, 242
S-Adenosyl-1,8-diamino-3-
thiooctane, 427
S-Adenosylethionine, 62
S-Adenosylhomocysteine, 227,
242, 263, 281, 385, 427,
435
accumulation of, 264, 266,
385, 397
egress from cells, 266

inhibition of catabolism, 264,
265, 385, 409, 417
tissue levels, 151
S-Adenosylhomocysteine analogs
inhibitory profile, 228, 239,
427, 435
naturally occurring, 228, 435
chemically synthesized, 228,
427, 435
S-Adenosylhomocysteine
hydrolase, 227, 239, 253, 263,
385
affinity purification, 397
alternate substrates, 232, 417
amino acid composition, 397
bovine liver, 385
cDNA, 259
competitive inhibitors of, 242,
245, 397, 409
enzyme subunits, 230
gene localization, 253
inactivators of, 244
inactive enzyme, 232
irreversible inactivators of,
245, 385, 397
ligand binding, 253, 256
mouse liver, 397
murine L-929 cells, 385
murine leukemia (L1210) cells,
397

447

neuroblastoma N2a cells, 385
photoaffinity labeling, 254,
    255
quantification with monoclonal
    antibodies, 259
reactivation of, 232, 264, 385
substrates, 248
tightly bound NAD$^+$, 230, 385
S-Adenosylhomocysteine
        hydrolase inhibitors
    antiviral effects, 385, 397,
        409
    aspermatogenic activity, 397
    antibacterial activity, 385
    embryo toxicity, 397
    insect chemosterilant activity,
        397
    teratogenicity, 397
S-Adenosylhomocysteine/S-
        adenosyl-methionine ratio
    in cancer cells, 218
    and differentiation of cells,
        235
    effect of nucleoside analogs,
        229, 266, 385
    and phospholipid
        methyltransferase
    phosphorylation, 94, 97, 98
SAdenosylhomocysteine/methyl-
        thioadenosine nucleo-
        sidase
    bacterial, 289
    inhibitors, 292
    properties, 291
    purification, 290
S-Adenosylhomocysteine-
        Sepharose, 77
S-Adenosylmethionine, 227, 263,
        275, 315, 373, 385, 427,
        435
    and β-adrenergic system, 320
    anti-inflammatory acstion,
        364
    anti-inflammatory effects,
        323
    anti-depressant action, 346
    in brain, 106

as branchpoint metabolite, 229
cardiovascular effects, 342
in cerebrospinal fluid, 318,
    330
in cerebrospinal after
    S-adenosylmethionine
    treatment, 330, 333, 335
consuming pathways, 279, 280
conversion to phosphatidyl-
    choline in vivo in brain,
    106
in depression, 327, 339
and differentiation of HL60
    cells, 72
and dopaminergic system, 320
effects on the central nervous
    system, 319
effects on neurotransmitters,
    336, 339
half-life in brain, 106
and homocysteine metabolism,
    205
in human lymphocytes, 203
infusion in man, 340
metabolism during growth, 279
metabolism vs. multiple drug
    resistance, 283
noradrenergic and cardio-
    vascular effects, 339
in nucleoside-resistant
    cells, 282
oral administration, 317
in osteoarthrosis, 363, 366
pharmacokinetics, 315
physiological hierarchy of
    utilization, 229
in plasma, 329
rate of synthesis in brain, 106
serotoninergic system, 319
side effects, 368
therapeutic effect in
    osteoarthrosis, 367
tissue levels, 151
turnover, 207, 208, 280
urinary excretion, 316
in whole blood, 329

S-Adenosylmethionine decarboxylase, 229, 279, 281, 282, 378,
390
S-Adenosylmethionine
phosphatidylethanolamine
methyltransferase, 62
S-Adenosylmethionine
synthetase, 203
inhibition by products, 211
inhibition of, 210
kinetics, 209
mechanism, 211
multiple forms, 204
purification, 209
Se-Adenosylselenomethionine, 62,
378
Adenovirus, 139
Adenylate cyclase and schizophrenia, 359
β-Adrenergic system and
S-adenosylmethionine, 320
Adriamycin, 223
Aldosterone, stimulation of Na+
transport, 234
5'-Aminoadenosine, 244
2-Aminoethylphosphonic acid, 57
2-Amino-2-methylpropanol, 63
L-2-Amino-4-methoxy-cis-but-3-
enoic acid, 373
Aminopropyltransferases
mechanism-based
inhibitors, 427
Antibacterial drugs, 287
Antifungal drugs, 435
Antiparasitic drugs, 435
Antiviral drugs, 385, 403, 409,
435
9-B-D-Arabinofuranosyl-
adenine, 243
Arginine-N-methyltransferase, 15
from various sources, 18
Aristeromycin, 228, 242, 264
D-Asparagyl residues methylation
of, 3, 6
D-Aspartyl β-methyl esters in
proteins, 3

D-Aspartyl residues
and protein biosynthesis, 7
cellular fates of, 12
formation by racemization, 7
methylation of, 6
2-Azaadenosine, 244
8-Azaadenosine, 242
5-Azacytidine, 113
and differentiation of HL60
cells, 70
2-Aza-3-deazaadenosine, 242
6-Azidoadenosine, 244
8-Azidoadenosine interaction
with S-adenosylhomo-
cysteine hydrolase, 254
8-Azido-cyclicAMP interaction
with S-adenosylhomo-
cysteine hydrolase, 254

B

Bacterial chemotaxis, 43
"memory" system, 44
Bacterial sensory adaptation, 44
Balb/3T12-3 cells, 69
Balb/3T3-A31 cells, 68
Basophilic leukemia cells from
rat, 249
Bone marrow,
effect of methylthioadenosine, 308, 309
Brain phosphatidylcholine, 106
half-life of, 108
pool formed by methylation of
phosphatidylethanol-
amine, 108
Brain S-adenosylmethionine, 106
Butaclamol, 358
5'-n-Butylthioadenosine, 292
Burkitt lymphoma cell line, 127

C

Calcineurin
carboxylmethylation of, 26, 33
immunocytochemical localization in brain, 37

Calmodulin, carboxylmethylation
      of, 358
Calmodulin-stimulated
      phosphatase activity, 34
Cancer, 113, 127, 139, 151
   methionine metabolism and
      transmethylation, 217
Carboxyl-O-methyltransferase
   in erythrocytes, 4
   properties and occurrence of
      two classes, 5
   role in protein repair or
      degradation, 8
Carcinogenesis, 151
Carcinogens, and DNA
      methylation, 221
Carnitine, 55
Catechol-O-methyltransferase
   inhibitors of, 427
Catecholamines, effect of
      S-adenosylmethionine on
      plasma levels, 343
CDP-choline pathway, in
      transformed fibroblasts,
      69
Chemotaxis-negative mutation,
      dominant, 51
2-Chloroadenosine, 264
Chloramphenicol
      acetyltransferase, 139
5'-Chloroformycin, 292
Chlorophenylthio-cyclic AMP, 89
2-Chloro-adeninearabinoside, 244
2-Chloro-adenosine, 244
2-Chloro-3-deazaadenosine, 244
5'-Chloro-5'-deoxy-adenosine,
      244
Choline deficiency and
      carcinogenesis, 215
Clonidine, 347
Clorgyline, 347
Colony forming unit-granulocyte,
      macrophage (CFU-GM)
      assay, 303
Cordycepin, 204
5'-Cyanoadenosine, 244
Cyclic AMP binding protein, 231

Cyclic AMP-adenosine binding
      protein, 253
Cycloleucine, 180, 283, 373
Cytochalasin B, 409
Cytochrome C
   effect of methylation on pI, 21
   methylation of in Euglena
      gracilis, 17
   queuine-related changes, 163
Cytostatic effect of
      methylthioadenosine,
      275

D

3-Deazaadenine, 242
3-Deazaadeninearabinoside, 244,
      265
3-Deazaadenosine, 83, 233, 242,
      264, 265, 283, 409, 417
   and carcinogenesis, 157
   and differentiation of HL60
      cells, 70
7-Deazaadenosine, 409
3-Deazaadenosine 5'-diphosphate,
      424
3-Deazaadenosine 5'-triphos-
      phate, 424
S-3-Deazaadenosylhomocysteine,
      242, 417
1-Deazaaristeromycin, 242
3-Deazaaristeromycin, 233, 242,
      265, 271, 409
   W1-L2 human B cells resistant
      to, 260
7-Deazaaristeromycin, 409
3-Deazaaristeromycin 5'-triphos-
      phate, 424
3-Deazaaristeromycinylhomo-
      cysteine, 242
3-Deazaguanosine, 245
Dementia and S-adenosyl-
      methionine in cerebro-
      spinal fluid, 331
Demethylation products, 11
2'-Deoxyadenosine, 244
2'-Deoxycoformycin, 268

Depression, 352
    and S-adenosylmethionine, 327
Diazepam, 245
Dicytostelium discoideum, 163
2', 3'-Dideoxyadenosine, 244
Differentiation and DNA
        methylation, 127
Difluoromethylornithine, 278, 281
Dihydroalprenolol binding to
        membranes, 323
(s)-9-(2, 3-Dihydroxypropyl)
        adenine, 402
N, N-Dimethyladenosine, 245
Dimethylphosphatidylethanol-
        amine, 58
Dimethyltrypotamine, 352
    and methionine, 354
DNA
    CpG sites, 113
    delayed methylation of, 113
    demethylation, 113, 127
    hememethylated sites, 113,
        127
    HpaII sites, 113, 127, 139
    hypomethylation, 113, 127,
        151
    maintenance methylase, 113,
        127
DNase I hypersensitivity, 113
DNA methylation
    and cancer, 221
    and differentiation, 113, 127
    and neoplastic
        transformation, 121
    and oncogens, 222
    effect of chemical transforma-
        tion agents, 121
    eukaryotic, 113, 127
    gene expression, 113, 127
    gene suppression, 139
    insect virus promoters, 139
    pattern of, 113, 127, 139
    prokaryotic, 139
    tissue specific patterns, 127
    viral, 139
DNA methyltransferases
    and early development, 120

    eukaryotic, 113
    level of, 118
    prokaryotic, 139
Dopamine stimulation of protein
        carboxymethylation, 358
Dopamine release and synthesis,
        effects, of protein carboxy-
        methyltransferase
        inhibition, 38
Dopaminergic system
    and S-adenosylmethionine, 320
    and protein carboxymethyl-
        transferase, 26

E

Eicosanoid system interaction
        with S-adenosyl-
        methionine, 324
Epidermal growth factor, 82
Epstein-Barr virus, 127
D-Eritadenine, 228, 264, 265, 402
Erythro-9-(2-hydroxyl-3-nonyl)
        adenine, 245
Ethionine, 63, 151, 179, 283

F

2-Fluoroadeninearabinoside, 244
Folate
    in cerebrospinal fluid in
        depression, 332
    deficiency in depression, 335
Formycin A, 242
S-Formycinylhomocysteine, 292
S-Formycinylhomocysteine-
        Sepharose, 290

G

Gene expression
    DNA methylation, 139
    regulation of, 113
Gene suppression,
        methylation mediated, 113
Glucagon and phospholipid methyl-
        transferase, 89, 91, 94, 95

Granulocyte–macrophage
    progenitor, cell, 302
Granulopoiesis, 301
    and methylthioadenosine, 306,
        308
Guanidoacetic acid, 63
Guanine, 245

H

Hematopoiesis, 301
Hematopoietic progenitor cells,
    301
Hepatocytes, 266, 267
    and phospholipid methyl-
        transferases, 91, 94, 95
Histamine, release from lung
        mast cells, 234
HL-60 cells, 69, 302, 303, 307
Homocysteine, 263, 264, 266
    and cancer, 151, 217
    and dimethyltryptamine
        production, 354
    distribution of, 266
    free and protein-bound in
        tissues, 266, 267
    in hepatocytes exposed to
        3-deazaaristeromycin,
        268
    and methotrexate, 269
    in plasma and urine during
        methotrexate therapy,
        270
    source of, 233, 267
    turnover in hepatocytes, 267
Homocysteine egress effect of
        methotrexate, 269
    and rate of transmethylation
        reactions, 280
Homovanillic acid in cerebro-
        spinal fluid in
        depression, 332
2-Hydroxyadenosine, 248
N^6-Hydroxyadenosine, 248
5-Hydroxyindole acetic acid in
        cerebrospinal fluid in
        depression, 332

Hypoxanthine phosphoribosyltrans-
        ferase-deficient cells,
        276

I

Immunoblotting of protein
        carboxymethyltransfer-
        ase, 30
Influenza virus methylation
        pattern in mRNA, 193

Inosine, 242
Insulin release from pancreatic
        islets, 234
L-Isoaspartyl a-methyl esters in
        proteins, 3
L-Isoaspartyl residues
        cellular fates of, 12
        formation by deamination, 7
        and protein biosynthesis, 7
S-Isobutylthio-(ethoxymethyl)
        adenine, 245
S-Isobutylthio-3-deazaadenosine,
        244, 292
S-Isobutylthioadenosine, 244,
        292
S-Isobutylthiotubercidin, 245
Iron-dependent methylthiolation,
        166

L

Leishmania, 435
Leukocyte metabolism of
        3-deazaaristeromycin,
        409
Leukocyte cytoskeleton, effect of
        3-deazaaristeromycin,
        409
Leukocyte mocrofilaments effects
        of 3-deazaaristero-
        mycin, 409
Lipoprotein secretion dependence
        on methylation pathway,
        83
Lipoproteins, 59

Lithium and response to physiological challenge, 346
Liver carcinomas, 151
Liver microsomes, phosphatidylethanolamine methyl-
transferase in, 77
Lymphocyte AdoMet
synthetase, 209
Lymphocyte-mediated cytolysis,
inhibition of, 409
Lysine N-methyltransferase, 15
from higher organisms, 19
from lower organisms, 20
Lysolecithin, 59

M

Macrophage chemotaxis inhibition
of, 234
Macrophage phagocytosis,
inhibition of, 409
Mania, 353
Melittin, 70
Membrane viscosity effect of
aging and S-adenosyl-
methionine, 321
Mescaline, 352
Methionine
amount in cancer cells, 219
analogs, 373
in cerebrospinal fluid in
depression, 332
deficiency and carcinogenesis,
151
effect in schizophrenia, 353
metabolism in cancer cells,
215
in plasma during methotrexate
therapy, 271
Methionine adenosyltransferase,
283
in depression, 352
inhibitors, 373
in schizophrenia, 352
Methionine adenosyltransferase
activity and antide-
pressant medication, 356

and neuroleptic therapy, 356
Methionine dependence of cancer
cells, 217, 218
Methotrexate, 269
3-Methoxy-4-hydroxyphenyl-
glycol, 340
in urine during S-adenosylmethionine treatment,
343
Methyl-accepting chemotaxis
proteins in *H. halobium,*
47
Methyl-accepting site
mutations at, 49
result of amidolysis, 46, 51
Methyl-accepting transducer
proteins, 43, 49
N^6-Methyladenosine, 242
determination of, 191
in mRNA, 189
Methylated amino acids, natural
occurrence of, 16
O-Methylbufotenin, 352
Methylcholine, 55
5-Methylcytosine, 113, 151
Methylgloxal-bis-guanylhydra-
zone, 278, 281
7-Methylguanosine
in mRNA, 190
in TRNA, 163
2'-O-Methylnucleosides
in mRNA, 190
5'-Methyltetrahydrofolate, 263
Methyltetrahydrofolate-
homocysteine methyl-
transferase, 233
5'-Methylthio-3-deazaadenosine,
292
Methylthioacyclo adenosine, 245
Methylthioadenosine, 275, 287,
427
and cell proliferation, 301,
302
and granulocyte-macrophage
progenitor cells, 305
cleaving enzymes in
prokaryotes, 288

and differentiation, 301
   of HL-60 cells, 305, 310
effect on bone marow, 306
excretion from cells, 278, 280
excretion of and tumor burden,
   279
fluorometric assay, 279
mechanism of toxicity, 282
metabolic effects of, 281
pathways of formation, 287
in plasma and urine, 279
Methylthioadenosine nucleosidase,
   427
Methylthioadenosine phosphorylase, 302, 303, 427
and arsenate, 293
deficiency in somatic cell
   hybrids, 277
deficient lymphoblasts, 277
distribution of, 293
gene localization, 277
from human placenta, 289
kinetic parameters, 296, 297
purification and properties,
   293, 294
various deficient cells, 275
5'-Methylthioformycin, 292, 297
2-Methylthio-N^6-(isopentenyl)
   adenosine, in t-RNA, 163
5-Methylthioribose-1-phosphate,
   276, 289
5'-Methylthiotubercidin, 292, 427
Methyltransferases
   competitive inhibitors of, 227
   mechanism-based inhibitors,
   427
3-Methoxy-4-hydroxyphenylglycol
   in cerebrospinal fluid in
   depression, 332
Monoamine oxidase inhibitors and
   response to physiological
   challenge, 345
Monoclonal antibodies and
   S-adenosylhomocysteine
   hydrolase, 254, 258
Monomethylphosphatidylethanola
   mine, 58

Murine erythroleukemia cell line,
   127, 163
Myelin basic protein (MBP)-
   methylating enzyme, 17

N

Na^+/H^+-antiport, 72
Neplanocin A, 181, 228, 244, 264,
   265, 385
   analogs, 385
S-Neplanocylhomocysteine, 385
Neuroblastoma N2a cells, 385
Noradrenergic system and
   S-adenosylmethionine,
   346
Norepinephrine and
   S-adenosylmethionine, 339
   effect of S-adenosylmeth-
   ionine on urinary metabo-
   lites, 343
Nuclear polyhedrosis virus, 139
Nucleocidin, 244
S-Nucleosidylcysteine, 249
S-Nucleosidylhomocysteine, 248,
   249

O

Oncogene rasH, 217
One-carbon cycle in neuropsychiatry, 351
Ornithine decarboxylase, 279,
   281, 282
   stimulation of activity, 281
Osteoarthrosis, 364

P

Periodate oxidized adenosine,
   265, 409
Periodate oxidized 3-deaza-
   adenosine, 219
Periodate oxidized
   3-deazaaristeromycin, 409
Phorbol esters, 70, 71

Phosphatase activity of
    calcineurin and
    carboxylmethylation, 34
Phosphatidyl-O-(N-trimethyl)
    homoserine, 57
Phosphatidylcholine, 55, 58, 75
    biosynthesis by transmethyl-
        ation in brain, 102
    molecular species in
        synaptosomes, 104
    newly-synthesized in
        synaptosomes, 103
    pathways of biosynthesis, 102
    pools in brain, 102
    rate constant of synthesis in
        brain, 108
    rate of synthesis in brain, 106
    as source of free choline in
        brain, 101
    synthesis via transmethylation
        in vivo, 105
Phosphatidylethanolamine, 58
    concentration in cells, 79
Phosphatidylethanolamine
    methylation activation by
        cAMP-dependent protein
        kinase, 76
    and biological signal
        transmission, 75, 83
    and calmodulin-dependent
        protein kinase, 81
    effect of cAMP analogs, 80
    inhibition by free fatty acids,
        82
    insulin and ACTH, 85
    and lack of biological
        response, 84
    number of enzymes
        involved, 77
    pH dependency, 78
    in the absence of enzyme
        activity, 83
Phosphatidylethanolamine
    methyltransferase(s), 75
    analysis of, 90
    ^{32}P-labeled tryptic peptides,
        93

purification, 76
    topology of, 78
Phosphatidylmethylcholine, 55
Phosphatidylsulfocholine, 57
Phosphoaminoacids, 92
Phospholipase A2 and cellular
    differentiation, 69
Phospholipid metabolism in
    transformed fibroblasts,
    68
Phospholipid methylation,
    67, 385
    and differentiation, 67
    regulation by phosphorylation,
        89
    and schizophrenia, 356
    and signal transmission, 358
    in transformed fibroblasts, 69
Phospholipid methyltransferase
    effect of S-adenosylmeth-
        ionine on phosphorylation
        of, 93
    in hepatocytes, 91
    phosphorylation of 94, 98
    stimulation by cAMP plus ATP,
        89
Phospholipids, amounts in red
    blood cells in
    schizophrenics, 356
Phosphorylation, 95
    of phospholipid methyltrans-
        ferase, 90, 92, 93, 96
Phosphorylcholine cytidyl-
    transferase, 64
Pineal gland, 322
Polyamines, 302, 379, 390
    inhibitors of synthesis, 278
    kinetics of synthesis, 280
    metabolism during growth, 279
Prolactin mRNA, distribution of
    N^6-methyladenosine, 191
Protein carboxylmethylation, 25,
    43, 358
    and chemotaxis, 43 358
    inhibition, 385
    and neurotransmitter release,
        358

possible function in nervous tissue, 25
Protein methyl esters, demethylation of, 10
Protein methylation, 3, 15
    inhibitors of, 435
Protein methyltransferases specificity of, 17
Protein phosphatase-1 or-2A, 81
Protein-O-carboxylmethyltransferase
    from bovine brain, 29
    characterization of 29
    from human erythrocytes, 29
    lectin chromatography of the bovine enzyme, 32
    immunocytochemical localization in brain, 36
    immunoreactivity, 25
Purine nucleoside phosphorylase, 295
Purine riboside (nebularine), 248
Putrescine, effects of methylthio-adenosine on levels of, 281
Putrescine aminopropyl-transferase, inhibitors of, 427
Pyrazomycin, 242

Q

Queuine, 163
Queuine analogs in chemotherapy, 163
Queuosine-t-RNAs, 163

R

Restriction endonucleases, 113, 127, 139
Retinoic acids, 70, 71
    and differentiation of HL-60 cells, 303
Ribosylthymine in t-RNA, 163
m-RNA capped structures, 189
m-RNA methylation, 189, 385
    inhibition by neplanocin A, 385

inhibition by S-tubercidinyl-homocysteine, 189
    viral, 189, 385
r-RNA methylation, 175
    effects of adenosine, 181
    effects of cycloleucine, 180
    effects of ethionine, 180
    effects of poly(I):poly(C), 180
    relationship to RNA maturation, 175
r-RNA processing
    in E. coli, 175
    in eukaryotic cells, 175
t-RNA hypomethylation, 163
t-RNA methylation, 163
    in cancer cells, 220, 222
    interdependence with formylation of initiator t-RNAs, 166
    tissue specificity, 163
t-RNA-transglycosylase, 167

S

Sangivanmycin, 245
Schizophrenia, 352
    methionine reaction, 353
Selenomethionine, 373
Serine hydroxymethyltransferase
    in plasma of schizophrenic patients, 359
    in schizophrenia, 352
Serotoninergic system and S-adenosylmethionine, 319
Sinefungin, 228, 409, 435
    antifungal activity, 435
    antiparasitic activity, 435
    antiviral activity, 435
    biosynthesis of, 435
    synthetic analogs, 409, 435
Spermidine, 281
Spermidine aminopropyl-transferase, 427
Spermidine synthase, 427
Spermine, 281
    inhibition of synthesis by methylthioadenosine, 276

Spiperone binding, to
        membranes, 323
Succinimide intermediate, 10
Sulfhydryl compounds, 63
Sulfhydryl methyltransferase, 63

T

Transcription-initiation
        factors, 117
Transcriptional inactivation, 139
Transducer mutants, 49
Transducer protein
    methyl-accepting glutamyl
        residues of, 45
    model for disposition in
        membrane, 45
    occurrence in bacteria, 46, 49
    recognition by immunoblotting,
        47
Transducers in *E. coli,* 45
Transmethylation
    in cancer cells, 215
    kinetics of reactions, 280
Transmethylation pathway
    and phosphatidylcholine
        synthesis in vivo in
        brain, 105
    and brain phosphatidyl-
        choline, 108
Trimethylaminoethylphosphonic
        acid, 57
Tubercidin, 228, 243
S-Tubercidinylhomocysteine, 243,
        292, 427
    inhibition of cellular mRNA
        methylation, 190
    inhibition of influenza virus
        protein synthesis, 192
    inhibition of influenza virus
        mRNA methylation, 193

V

Vaccinia virus multiplication
        inhibition by neplanocin A,
        391

Vanillylmandelic acid, 341
    in urine during S-adenosyl-
        methionine treatment,
        343
Vincristin, 223

W

Wybutosine, in t-RNA, 163

X

Xenopus laevis oocytes, 139
Xylosyladenine, 204

Z

Z-type DNA, 113
Zimelidine, 346

DATE DUE

DATE DUE			
OCT 0 1 1990			
JUL 2 1 1999			